Glaucoma

Editor

STEFANO PIZZIRANI

VETERINARY CLINICS
OF NORTH AMERICA:
SMALL ANIMAL PRACTICE

www.vetsmall.theclinics.com

November 2015 • Volume 45 • Number 6

ELSEVIER

1600 John F. Kennedy Boulevard • Suite 1800 • Philadelphia, Pennsylvania, 19103-2899

http://www.vetsmall.theclinics.com

VETERINARY CLINICS OF NORTH AMERICA: SMALL ANIMAL PRACTICE Volume 45, Number 6
November 2015 ISSN 0195-5616, ISBN-13: 978-0-323-41360-2

Editor: Patrick Manley
Developmental Editor: Meredith Clinton

Veterinary Clinics of North America: Small Animal Practice (ISSN 0195-5616) is published bimonthly by Elsevier Inc., 360 Park Avenue South, New York, NY 10010-1710. Months of issue are January, March, May, July, September, and November. Business and Editorial Offices: 1600 John F. Kennedy Blvd., Ste. 1800, Philadelphia, PA 19103-2899. Customer Service Office: 3251 Riverport Lane, Maryland Heights, MO 63043. Periodicals postage paid at New York, NY and additional mailing offices. Subscription prices are $310.00 per year (domestic individuals), $500.00 per year (domestic institutions), $150.00 per year (domestic students/residents), $410.00 per year (Canadian individuals), $621.00 per year (Canadian institutions), $455.00 per year (international individuals), $621.00 per year (international institutions), and $220.00 per year (international and Canadian students/residents). To receive student/resident rate, orders must be accompanied by name of affiliated institution, date of term, and the *signature* of program/residency coordinator on institution letterhead. Orders will be billed at individual rate until proof of status is received. Foreign air speed delivery is included in all *Clinics* subscription prices. All prices are subject to change without notice. **POSTMASTER:** Send address changes to *Veterinary Clinics of North America: Small Animal Practice*, Elsevier Health Sciences Division, Subscription Customer Service, 3251 Riverport Lane, Maryland Heights, MO 63043. Customer Service (orders, claims, online, change of address): Elsevier Periodicals Customer Service, Elsevier Health Sciences Division Subscription **Customer Service 3251 Riverport Lane Maryland Heights, MO 63043. Tel: 1-800-654-2452 (U.S. and Canada); 314-447-8871 (outside U.S. and Canada). Fax: 314-447-8029. E-mail: journalscustomerservice-usa@elsevier.com (for print support); journalsonlinesupport-usa@elsevier.com (for online support).**

Reprints. For copies of 100 or more of articles in this publication, please contact the Commercial Reprints Department, Elsevier Inc., 360 Park Avenue South, New York, NY 10010-1710. Tel.: 212-633-3874; Fax: 212-633-3820; E-mail: reprints@elsevier.com.

Veterinary Clinics of North America: Small Animal Practice is also published in Japanese by Inter Zoo Publishing Co., Ltd., Aoyama Crystal-Bldg 5F, 3-5-12 Kitaaoyama, Minato-ku, Tokyo 107-0061, Japan.

Veterinary Clinics of North America: Small Animal Practice is covered in *Current Contents/Agriculture, Biology and Environmental Sciences, Science Citation Index, ASCA, MEDLINE/PubMed (Index Medicus), Excerpta Medica, and BIOSIS.*

Contributors

EDITOR

STEFANO PIZZIRANI, DVM, PhD
Diplomate, American College of Veterinary Ophthalmologists; Diplomate, European College of Veterinary Surgeons (inactive); Associate Professor, Comparative Ophthalmology, Department of Clinical Sciences, Cummings School of Veterinary Medicine, Tufts University, North Grafton, Massachusetts

AUTHORS

ANTHONY F. ALARIO, DVM
Diplomate, American College of Veterinary Ophthalmologists; Head Ophthalmologist, VCA Capital Area Veterinary Emergency and Specialty, Concord, New Hampshire

GILLIAN BEAMER, VMD, PhD
Diplomate, American College of Veterinary Pathologists; Assistant Professor, Department of Infectious Disease and Global Health, Tufts University, North Grafton, Massachusetts

ELLISON BENTLEY, DVM
Diplomate, American College of Veterinary Ophthalmologists; Clinical Professor of Comparative Ophthalmology, Department of Surgical Sciences, School of Veterinary Medicine, University of Wisconsin-Madison, Madison, Wisconsin

DINELI BRAS, DVM, MS
Diplomate, American College of Veterinary Ophthalmologists; Ophthalmology Department, Centro de Especialistas Veterinarios de Puerto Rico (CEVET), Guaynabo, Puerto Rico; Veterinary Specialists Center of Puerto Rico, San Juan, Puerto Rico

HAIYAN GONG, MD, PhD
Professor, Ophthalmology and Anatomy and Neurobiology, Boston University School of Medicine, Boston, Massachusetts

ANDRÁS M. KOMÁROMY, DrMedVet, PhD
Diplomate, American College of Veterinary Ophthalmologists; Diplomate, European College of Veterinary Ophthalmologists; Associate Professor, Department of Small Animal Clinical Sciences, Veterinary Medical Center, College of Veterinary Medicine, Michigan State University, East Lansing, Michigan

FEDERICA MAGGIO, DVM
Diplomate, American College of Veterinary Ophthalmologists; Ophthalmology Department, Tufts Veterinary Emergency Treatment and Specialties (Tufts VETS), Walpole, Massachusetts

GILLIAN J. McLELLAN, BVMS, PhD, MRCVS
Diplomate, European College of Veterinary Ophthalmologists; Diplomate, American College of Veterinary Ophthalmologists; Diploma in Veterinary Ophthalmology; Assistant Professor, Departments of Ophthalmology and Visual Sciences and Surgical Sciences; McPherson Eye Research Institute, University of Wisconsin-Madison, Madison, Wisconsin

PAUL E. MILLER, DVM
Diplomate, American College of Veterinary Ophthalmologists; Clinical Professor of Comparative Ophthalmology, Department of Surgical Sciences, School of Veterinary Medicine, University of Wisconsin-Madison, Madison, Wisconsin

SIMON M. PETERSEN-JONES, DVetMed, PhD, DVOphthal
Diplomate, European College of Veterinary Ophthalmologists; Professor, Department of Small Animal Clinical Sciences, Veterinary Medical Center, College of Veterinary Medicine, Michigan State University, East Lansing, Michigan

STEFANO PIZZIRANI, DVM, PhD
Diplomate, American College of Veterinary Ophthalmologists; Diplomate, European College of Veterinary Surgeons (inactive); Associate Professor, Comparative Ophthalmology, Department of Clinical Sciences, Cummings School of Veterinary Medicine, Tufts University, North Grafton, Massachusetts

STEPHANIE PUMPHREY, DVM
Diplomate, American College of Veterinary Ophthalmologists; Staff Ophthalmologist, VCA South Shore, South Weymouth, Massachusetts

CHRISTOPHER M. REILLY, DVM, MAS
Diplomate, American College of Veterinary Pathologists; Assistant Professor of Clinical Pathology, Microbiology and Immunology, School of Veterinary Medicine, University of California, Davis, California

TRAVIS D. STRONG, DVM, MS
Ophthalmology Resident and Adjunct Instructor, Lloyd Veterinary Medical Center, Iowa State University College of Veterinary Medicine, Ames, Iowa

LEANDRO B.C. TEIXEIRA, DVM, MS
Diplomate, American College of Veterinary Pathologists; McPherson Eye Research Institute; Assistant Professor, Department of Pathobiological Sciences, University of Wisconsin-Madison, Madison, Wisconsin

Contents

In order to understand the pathophysiology, select optimal therapeutic options for patients and provide clients with honest expectations for cases of canine glaucoma, clinicians should be familiar with a rational understanding of the functional anatomy of the ocular structures involved in this group of diseases. The topographical extension and the structural and humoral complexity of the regions involved with the production and the outflow of aqueous humor undergo numerous changes with aging and disease. Therefore, the anatomy relative to the fluid dynamics of aqueous has become a pivotal yet flexible concept to interpret the different phenotypes of glaucoma.

Glaucoma is a common ocular condition in humans and dogs leading to optic nerve degeneration and irreversible blindness. Primary glaucoma is a group of spontaneous heterogeneous diseases. Multiple factors are involved in its pathogenesis and these factors vary across human ethnic groups and canine breeds, so the clinical phenotypes are numerous and their classification can be challenging and remain superficial. Aging and oxidative stress are major triggers for the manifestation of disease. Multiple, intertwined inflammatory and biochemical cascades eventually alter cellular and extracellular physiology in the optic nerve and trabecular meshwork and lead to vision loss.

Primary glaucomas are a leading cause of incurable vision loss in dogs. Based on their specific breed predilection, a genetic cause is suspected to be responsible, and affected dogs should be excluded from breeding. Despite the high prevalence of primary glaucomas in dogs, their genetics have been studied in only a small number of breeds. The identification of canine glaucoma disease genes, and the development of genetic tests, will help to avoid the breeding of affected dogs in the future and will allow for earlier diagnosis and potentially more effective therapy.

The diagnosis of glaucoma is highly dependent on a working understanding of the clinical signs and available diagnostic procedures. Clinical signs may be attributable to increased intraocular pressure and/or complex alterations in the physiology or molecular biology of the anterior segment, retinal ganglion cells, and optic nerve. Many diagnostic procedures seek to more fully characterize these alterations and to identify which clinical features increase the risk of overt primary angle closure glaucoma (PACG) occurring. Considerable progress has been made in identifying the anatomic features that predispose an eye to PACG, and in elucidating the role of reverse pupillary block.

Although the clinical classification of primary glaucoma in dogs is quite simple, the phenotypes of glaucoma in most of the species are indeed multiple. Ophthalmologists can often evaluate the dynamic changes of clinical signs at different times in the course of the disease, whereas pathologists are often presented with globes that have undergone abundant therapies and are at the end stage. Therefore, an open collaboration between clinicians and pathologists can produce the most accurate interpretation in the pathology report and improve patient outcomes. This article focuses on the histomorphologic elements that characterize, and are important to, canine primary glaucomas.

Glaucoma is a painful and often blinding group of ocular diseases for which there is no cure. Although the definition of glaucoma is rapidly evolving, elevated intraocular pressure (IOP) remains the most consistent risk factor of glaucoma in the canine patient. Therapy should be aimed at neuroprotection. The mainstay of therapy focuses on reducing IOP and maintaining a visual and comfortable eye. This article discusses the most current ocular hypotensive agents, focusing on their basic pharmacology, efficacy at lowering IOP, and recommended use in the treatment of idiopathic canine glaucoma.

Canine glaucoma is a common cause of vision loss associated with raised intraocular pressure, and leads to damage of the retina and optic nerve head. In most cases, medical treatment alone cannot provide long-term management of intraocular pressure control and preservation of vision. Surgical intervention is usually recommended to either decrease aqueous humor production, or increase its outflow. Among the current available procedures, filtering techniques are aimed at increasing aqueous humor outflow. Proper surgical timing and a combination of cyclodestructive and filtering procedures have been recently suggested to improve the long-term success of surgical treatment in dogs. Bleb fibrosis and surgical failure are still common occurrences in filtration surgery with relapse of glaucoma and vision loss. End stage procedures, such as enucleation, evisceration with intrascleral prosthesis, and chemical ablation of the ciliary bodies are then recommended to address chronic discomfort in buphthalmic and blind eyes.

 Videos on endoscopic cyclophotocoagulation for the surgical treatment of canine glaucoma accompany this article

Medical and surgical management of canine glaucoma can be challenging. The goal of surgical treatment is to manipulate the inflow and/or outflow of aqueous humor. This article describes the inflow-reducing, cyclodestructive techniques. Diode cyclophotocoagulation is the most common cyclodestructive procedure performed in humans and animals. Diode laser energy can be applied via a transscleral (transscleral cyclophotocoagulation [TSCP]) or an endoscopic (endoscopic cyclophotocoagulation [ECP]) approach. ECP provides direct visualization of the targeted ciliary body, allowing safer and more titratable treatment than TSCP techniques, offering a better long-term prognosis for vision and intraocular pressure control. Advancements in diode laser therapy seem promising.

Feline glaucoma is often insidious in onset and slowly progressive with very subtle clinical signs. As a consequence, it is likely that the disease in cats is underdiagnosed. As cats typically present late in the course of disease, prognosis for long-term maintenance of vision is poor. Patient and owner compliance with frequent application of topical medications can be a limiting factor, and represents a serious clinical challenge. This review outlines the clinical features, classification, and pathophysiology of the feline glaucomas and provides current evidence on which to base the selection of appropriate treatment strategies for cats with glaucoma.

Secondary glaucomas are common in dogs, and occur due to obstruction of aqueous humor flow at the pupil, iridocorneal angle, or trabecular meshwork by numerous mechanisms. Secondary glaucoma is suspected based on examination findings, or presence of elevated IOP in an animal with a signalment inconsistent with primary glaucoma. Animals with secondary glaucoma require more diagnostic testing than animals with primary glaucoma. Management is challenging, and treatments used for primary glaucoma may be ineffective or even detrimental. Prognosis for vision and/or globe retention may be better than for primary glaucoma, particularly if underlying causes can be found and addressed promptly.

VETERINARY CLINICS OF NORTH AMERICA: SMALL ANIMAL PRACTICE

Preface

Glaucoma

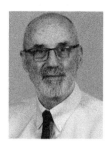

Stefano Pizzirani, DVM, PhD
Editor

I know that I know nothing.
                    —Socrates

With time, I have learned to be humbled by my ignorance and by the infinite, additional speculative thoughts that arise every time I presume I understand something, and I have the illusion that I have reached an endpoint. Opening a single door in the building of knowledge brings the investigator into a room with a multitude of new, mysterious doors. What appeared to be an answer turns out to be only fertile ground for new questions, and new horizons keep expanding exponentially and confusingly.

The same feeling of vast ignorance strikes me when I attempt to define and understand glaucoma. The word "glaucoma" comes from the Greek word "glaucos," which means gray or bluish. The semantics of the word itself seems to prefigure the foggy state of our current knowledge surrounding this group of diseases.

As human beings, we like to classify things in boxes. That's how our minds work best. However, when we try to delve into the finer aspects of the mechanisms and molecular cascades involved in glaucoma, simple categories fail us as we face the confusing, often overlapping but sometimes contradictory nature of a disease that bears a common name but may take very different forms across different species, breeds, and individuals. Things are blurry; multiple shades of gray make the transition between different phenotypes hazy, and we, or at least I, seem to be lost in a state of "quantum confusion."

When asked to coordinate this issue of *Veterinary Clinics of North America: Small Animal Practice*, I was excited and concerned at the same time. My goal in this issue has been to try to illuminate that which is currently known and that which is currently unknown about this group of diseases that we classify under the single term "glaucoma." My challenge has been to provide both practical, useful information and stimulus for further speculation. As veterinarians, we need clear clinical guidance to help our current patients and clients, but we also need to honestly acknowledge the lack

Vet Clin Small Anim 45 (2015) ix–x
http://dx.doi.org/10.1016/j.cvsm.2015.08.004
0195-5616/15/$ – see front matter © 2015 Published by Elsevier Inc.

of specific, in-depth information regarding different forms of glaucoma, particularly in veterinary patients.

It's an ongoing journey. We have made some inroads and changed directions a few times over the years. Our working assumptions about glaucoma are sometimes preliminary and often based on anecdotal evidence. Our numbers are small, and our results are based mostly on retrospective studies, which are truly useful but also constrained by obvious limitations. Each species (and, within each species, each breed and each different stage of disease) likely warrants its own classification scheme and set of treatment recommendations, but the paucity of currently available data makes our job difficult.

I hope this issue will provide rational, useful information to general clinicians while stimulating more questioning and increased collaboration among specialists to further the collection of useful data.

Several people and resources have helped me in the preparation of this issue. I am thankful to the publisher for offering me this opportunity, and I can't value enough the great contributions provided by the authors of this issue.

To all of them goes my sincere gratitude.

Stefano Pizzirani, DVM, PhD
Comparative Ophthalmology
Cummings School of Veterinary Medicine
Tufts University
200 Westboro Road
Grafton, MA 01536, USA

E-mail address:
stefano.pizzirani@tufts.edu

Functional Anatomy of the Outflow Facilities

Stefano Pizzirani, DVM, PhD[a],*, Haiyan Gong, MD, PhD[b]

KEYWORDS

- Aqueous • Formation • Outflow • Trabecular meshwork • Anatomy • Canine

KEY POINTS

- Understanding the composition and function of the outflow system helps to interpret clinical signs, choose therapies, and formulate the prognosis for patients affected with glaucoma.
- Normal intraocular pressure is maintained because there is a balance between aqueous formation and outflow.
- The outflow pathways in dogs have clear morphologic and topographic differences from the corresponding structures in primates.
- The functional anatomy is a dynamic concept and there are physiologic changes that occur with age and tissue remodeling.
- More advanced and extensive changes that are similar to those occurring with aging may occur in glaucoma.

The aqueous humor (AH) is the fluid that fills the anterior and posterior chambers of the eye. Its main roles are to provide nourishment and metabolic waste removal to active metabolic ocular structures that are avascular and to contribute maintaining a normal intraocular pressure (IOP) without altering the refractive status of the eye. Its composition and the fluid dynamics associated with its flow are voluble and undergo changes associated with age and disease. Of particular importance is that the resistance to the outflow of AH from the anterior chamber is influenced by morphologic, physiologic, and biochemical dynamic factors.[1] Beside aqueous nutritional importance, its solutes also participate in establishing the anterior chamber associate immune deviation, and carry and distribute the different proteins and molecules that promote and direct tissue remodeling and changes in the anterior segment that are associated with both age and disease.

The authors have nothing to disclose.
[a] Ophthalmology, Department of Clinical Sciences, Cummings School of Veterinary Medicine, Tufts University, 200 Westboro Road, North Grafton, MA 01536, USA; [b] Ophthalmology and Anatomy and Neurobiology, Boston University School of Medicine, 72 East Concord Street, L905, Boston, MA 02118, USA
* Corresponding author. Department of Clinical Science, Cummings School of Veterinary Medicine, Tufts University, 200 Westboro Road, North Grafton, MA 01536.
E-mail address: stefano.pizzirani@tufts.edu

Vet Clin Small Anim 45 (2015) 1101–1126
http://dx.doi.org/10.1016/j.cvsm.2015.06.005
0195-5616/15/$ – see front matter © 2015 Elsevier Inc. All rights reserved.

Three major distinct aspects of the aqueous need to be considered:

1. Aqueous production
2. Aqueous composition
3. Aqueous outflow

In this review, the authors focus on aqueous outflow and introduce concepts of aqueous production, mentioning some of the dynamic variations in aqueous composition that may influence the physiologic and pathologic changes seen with aging and glaucoma.

The physiologic range of IOP is maintained through the constant balance between aqueous production and aqueous outflow. The pressure gradient within the eye is comprised within specific values that may vary individually in different daily patterns and with aging. A rule of the thumb indicates normal IOP in dogs to be between 12 and 25 mm Hg; however, most dogs tend to have a normal pressure below the 20s.[2–6] IOP values may also vary depending on the time and technique of measurement. The IOP fluctuates during the day with circadian phases that peak and drop at different times of the day, depending on the species. In dogs, like in humans, the highest normal IOP values are measured in the morning, and IOPs are lower in the evening.[3,5] In dogs, a decrease in baseline IOP is associated with increased age[2]; a range of diverse findings has been reported in different human studies.[7] There are differences in ethnic groups, and both positive and negative relationships between increased age and IOP have been described.[8,9] Although the outflow seems to decrease with age, the production of AH may also decrease.[10]

AQUEOUS PRODUCTION

Two mechanisms—passive and active—are responsible for aqueous production and contribute to its composition.[11] Passive diffusion and ultrafiltration of plasma occur in the vascularized ciliary body stroma. The passive mechanisms do not contribute significantly to the formation of AH. Because the ciliary blood vessel endothelia are fenestrated, diffusion of solutes travels according to a concentration gradient, trying to maintain a balance between different tissues/compartments. Substances with high lipid solubility coefficients can easily move across cellular membranes.

Ultrafiltration allows molecules to cross a cell membrane following a hydrostatic force or an osmotic gradient, and it results from differences between the pressure of the ciliary body capillaries and the IOP and solute differences. The hydrostatic pressure of ciliary body capillaries has been estimated to be between 25 and 33 mm Hg,[12,13] whereas the oncotic pressure of vascular proteins is about 14 mm Hg.[14] Hydrostatic and oncotic forces would both actually favor resorption of AH.[15] If we consider the IOP around the value of 15 mm Hg, we can understand how a much higher hydrostatic pressure would be needed to achieve relevant amount of aqueous formation through this passive mechanism.

Passive mechanisms are, however, able to generate a reservoir fluid within the ciliary body.[16] Furthermore, because of the lack of a true epithelium on the anterior surface of the iris, leakage and diffusion of diluted plasma occurs from the ciliary vessels into the anterior chamber.[17]

Basically, AH is secreted across the ciliary epithelium by transferring solutes, mainly NaCl, from the stroma to the posterior chamber of the eye, with a subsequent passive movement of water in the same direction.[18] At least 80% to 90% of AH formation occurs with active mechanisms.[19] Active secretion requires energy that is provided by the hydrolysis of adenine triphosphate and relies mainly on 2 enzymes: an adenosine triphosphatase Na/K pump and carbonic anhydrase. The structural site for active secretion resides in the inner (facing the posterior chamber), nonpigmented ciliary epithelium of the ciliary processes where these 2 enzymes are highly concentrated. Active formation through an adenosine triphosphatase Na/K pump is responsible for more than 70% of the aqueous production.[13,20] Besides the increased concentration of NA^+ ions in the posterior chamber, secondary active transport mechanisms increase the concentration of other solutes, including Cl^-. Active formation is also catalyzed by the enzyme carbonic anhydrase that is particularly present in the nonpigmented epithelium of the ciliary body.[21] The latter accounts for about 40% to 50% of the aqueous production.[22] Carbonic anhydrase catalyzes the reaction $H_2O + CO_2 \leftrightarrow HCO_3^- + H^+$. Bicarbonate moves then in the posterior chamber influencing fluid transport by also affecting Na^+, possibly by regulating the pH for optimal active ion transport.[15] The 2 active mechanisms share some of the pathways, explaining the mathematics of the rate of production. When active release of sodium (Na^+) or bicarbonate ($HCO3^-$) ions into the posterior chamber is mediated by these enzymes, an osmotic gradient is created and the plasma ultrafiltrate can move from the stroma of the ciliary body into the posterior chamber (**Fig. 1**). This mechanism is sensitive to the level of IOP and decreases with increased IOP. However, this effect is insufficient to serve as a protective mechanism against the development of glaucoma.

Posterior Chamber (Aqueous)

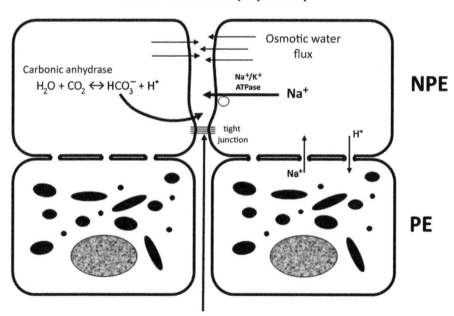

Ultrafiltration

Fig. 1. Mechanism for aqueous secretion. An active movement of Na^+ and HCO_3^- increases the solute concentrations in the posterior chamber in proximity of the ciliary processes and creates a positive osmotic gradient that recalls fluids collected in the ciliary tissues because of diffusion and ultrafiltration. ATPase, adenosine triphosphatase; NPE, nonpigmented epithelium; PE, pigmented epithelium.

The amount of AH production is indirectly calculated by measuring the amount of outflow.[23] Outflow facility (c) indirectly indicates the amount of aqueous production and it can be expressed as μL/min or μL/min/mm Hg. In normal humans, c is about 2.75 $\pm$ 0.63 μL/min (range, 1.8–4.3) or about 0.3 μL/min/mm Hg.[24] In dogs, the total value has been manually calculated with a mean $\pm$ SD equal to 5.22 $\pm$ 1.87 μL/min, whereas when calculated by an automatic software the flow rate was 4.54 $\pm$ 2.57 μL/min.[25] These values grossly mirror the values of 0.24 to 0.30 μL/m/mm Hg reported by Gum and colleagues.[26]

Individual variations are following circadian rhythms and are also influenced by age.[24,27] In humans, AH formation and outflow both decrease with aging.[10,28]

Although the site and the mechanisms of aqueous formation seem to be well-established and described, the mechanisms for outflow are still a large field for research, especially when related to the pathophysiology of the different phenotypes of glaucoma.

PATHWAYS OF AQUEOUS OUTFLOW

The outflow facilities are a complex hydraulic system that allows the AH to exit the eye consistently, yet maintaining a physiologic IOP balanced with aqueous secretion. When the regulation of the outflow is impaired, an increase in IOP occurs. No active transport mechanisms is involved in the outflow. AH passes through the trabecular meshwork (TM) as bulk flow driven by the pressure gradient, which is higher in the eye when compared with the distal outflow vessels.[29,30] The posterior, uveoscleral outflow (USO) is passive and largely independent from the IOP; it is mostly regulated by osmotic gradients.[31]

The pathways of canine aqueous outflow include several different anatomic structures whose nomenclature has been variously and differently described, used, and classified.[32–38] The understanding of the normal morphology and composition of these structures, and the array of dynamic physiologic changes that occur in different breeds and aging are important considerations when pathologic changes are then analyzed and therapeutic agents selected.

Besides an irrelevant corneal and uveal permeability, 2 main, different outflow pathways are usually considered the most essential to IOP balance:

- The anterior/trabecular or conventional outflow
- The posterior or unconventional, or the USO

TRABECULAR OUTFLOW

The anatomic terminology related to the trabecular outflow system (**Figs. 2–4**) includes the following:

- Iridocorneal angle (ICA)
- Ciliary cleft (CC)
- Pectinate ligament (PL)
- The TM system, which includes
  ○ Uveal TM (UTM)
  ○ Corneoscleral TM (CSTM) and uveoscleral TM (USTM)
  ○ Juxtacanalicular tissue (JCT)
- Angular aqueous plexus (AAP)
  ○ Inner wall (IW)
  ○ Inner collector channels
- Radial collector channels
- Episcleral veins and intrascleral venous plexus (ISVP) or circle of Hovius

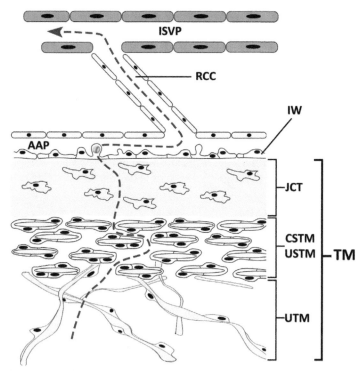

Fig. 2. Aqueous (*red dotted line*) trabecular meshwork (TM) outflow pathway from the ciliary cleft through the trabecular beams of the uveal TM (UTM), the lamellar corneoscleral or uveoscleral trabecula meshwork (CSTM/USTM) and the extracellular matrix of the juxta-canalicular connective tissue (JCT). The fluid moves through the inner wall (IW) endothelial cells by formation of intracellular giant vacuoles that open into the lumen of angular aqueous plexus (AAP). The AAP is connected to larger radial collector channels (RCC) leading to the intrascleral venous plexus (ISVP). (*Adapted from* Swaminathan SS, Oh DJ, Kang MH, et al. Aqueous outflow: segmental and distal flow. J Cataract Refract Surg 2014;40(8):1264; with permission.)

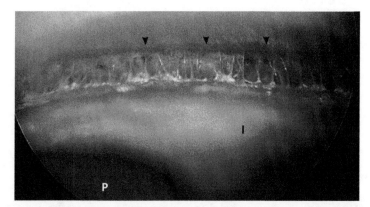

Fig. 3. Normal iridocorneal angle in a dog at gonioscopy. Lightly pigmented iris tissue strands can be observed spanning the peripheral angular space and introducing to the posterior space of the ciliary cleft. The corneoscleral pigmented line (Schwalbe's *line*) is indicated by the arrowheads. I, anterior surface of the iris; P, pupil.

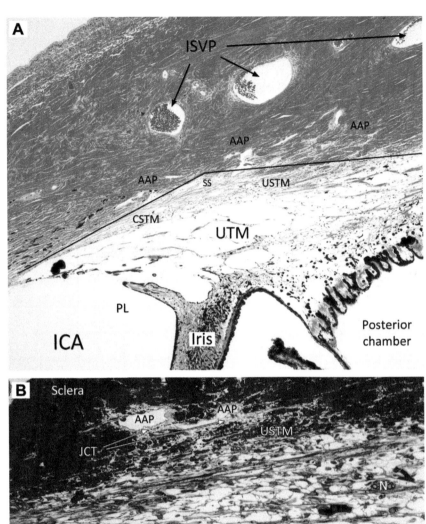

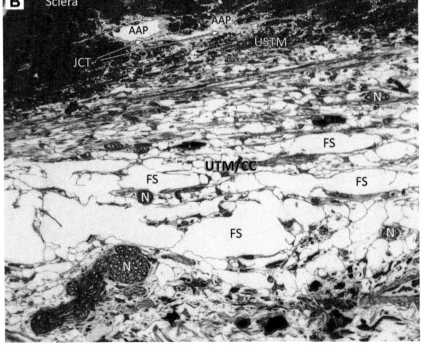

Iridocorneal Angle

The ICA represents the peripheral, circumferential portion of the anterior chamber, where the cornea, sclera, and base of the iris converge. It can be examined clinically with a gonioscopic lens and the gross appearance of the ICA is characterized by the presence of slender strands of uveal tissue, PLs that connect the peripheral base of the iris to the peripheral cornea, just posterior to the deep scleral pigmented line, which approximately corresponds with where the Descemet membrane ends. The junction between the cornea and PL is labeled Schwalbe's line (see **Fig. 3**).

Pectinate Ligaments

The iconic PL is formed by a slender, branching palisade of discrete beams of iris tissue that span the ICA. The number, pattern, length, and thickness of the PLs vary among breeds and individuals.[33,36,39,40] The width of the ICA can also vary depending on breed and age.[41–44] The PLs are composed of a core of collagen and lined by iridal melanocytes and fibroblasts.[33,36] They are usually pigmented unless the dog is sub-albinotic. However, with aging, dispersed pigment from microdamage to the posterior epithelium of the iris may accumulate in the ICA even in dogs with a blue iris. The most anterior ligaments are thicker than the beams that form the UTM more posteriorly. PLs branch and anastomose between themselves and with the beams of the UTM. The morphologic transition between the tougher PLs and the thinner trabecular beams can be gradual or abrupt.

Ciliary Cleft

The CC names the peripheral circumferential space posterior to the ICA. This almost virtual space extends posteriorly to the PLs into the posterior ciliary body with a triangular shape with anterior base. Its anatomic boundaries are represented by the PLs anteriorly, the iris root and the anterior pars plicata of the ciliary body internally, the ciliary body matrix and muscle posteriorly, and the sclera externally. Although it is a separate entity with its own boundaries, some authors include the CC in the posterior part of the ICA. The width and depth of the CC varies in different individuals, breeds and with aging.[33] The CC is the container for the UTM.

The Trabecular Meshwork

The TM system is a useful nomenclature to group the whole proximal (converging) trabecular outflow system. The TM in dogs consists of 3 main different sections listed from internal to external: (1) The cobweblike UTM, (2) the lamellated CSTM and USTM,

◄ ────────────────────────────

Fig. 4. Microphotographs of sagittal sections of canine trabecular outflow tissues. (*A*) Hematoxylin and eosin staining. A partial section of a pectinate ligament (PL) can be recognized anteriorly and separates the iridocorneal angle (ICA) from the ciliary cleft that is filled with irregularly distributed beams of the uveal trabecular meshwork (UTM). It contains the Fontana spaces. The corneoscleral trabecular meshwork (CSTM) and the uveoscleral TM (USTM) are a transition zone between the sclera and the UTM and lie in the scleral sulcus (SS and *continuous line*). Note the wide spreading of the angular aqueous plexus (AAP) in the inner sclera. Three large venous vessels can be seen in the midsclera. They constitute the intrascleral venous plexus (ISVP; *arrows*). (*B*) Toluidine blue staining at higher magnification. The progressive reduction of the Fontana spaces (FS) can be appreciated. Large spaces converge into smaller intertrabecular spaces in the USTM. With this coloration, the translucency of the juxtacanalicular connective tissue (JCT) are appreciated around the angular aqueous plexus. Several nerve bundles (N) are noted within the UTM.

and (3) the nonlamellated cribriform region or JCT. The latter is intimately connected to the IW of channels that form the AAP (see **Fig. 4**).

The Uveal Trabecular Meshwork

The CC contains the UTM, which is a spongiform, cobweblike tissue defined by irregularly anastomosing trabecular beams. The empty spaces between the beams are named Fontana's spaces. Outwards and posteriorly, these spaces reduce progressively because of the increasing interlacing between the beams. The core of the beams are made by connective tissue with collagen and elastin fibers and other extracellular matrix (ECM) proteins.[33] The beams are lined by endothelial cells and their basal membrane; these cells are considered to be an extension of the corneal endothelium and play a substantial role in regulating outflow and IOP.[35] TM cells respond to mechanical strain increasing ECM turnover, altered gene expression, and release of several cytokines.[45] TM cells have phagocytic properties,[46,47] and with age they tend to engulf melanin granules released by the posterior surface of the iris (**Fig. 5**).[48,49] If the TM cells become extremely engulfed, they may slough off from the beam, exposing the underlying ECM. Marked trabecular cell loss has been associated to collapse and fusion of the lamellae and loss of intertrabecular spaces.[50,51] In primates with primary open-angle glaucoma, there is a marked loss of TM cells when compared with normal age-matched eyes.[52,53]

Anterior tendons of the ciliary muscle insert on the elastic fibers of the UTM and JCT,[54] and seemingly the inner scleral tissue, mostly at the outer portion in the posterior half of the CC. The effect of these tendons and their relative muscle on the outflow in dogs has not been well-determined yet, but, considering their anatomic distribution, are likely to help in opening the spaces of the AAP (**Fig. 6**). Myofibroblast-like cells have been reported in different species to be present in the TM, including the outermost region transitioning into the collector channels/Schlemm's canal.[33,54] All this

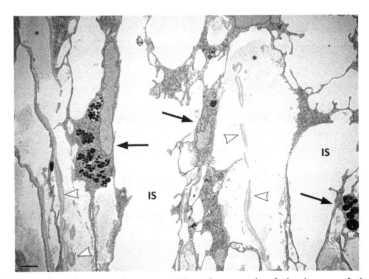

Fig. 5. Transmission electron microscopy. Microphotograph of the beams of the canine uveoscleral trabecular meshwork. The beams are interposed to the intertrabecular spaces (IS). The beams are showing collagen (*asterisks*) and elastin (*arrowheads*) fibers in their core. Black arrows point to trabecular meshwork endothelial cells that line the outside of the beams and have phagocyted melanin granules.

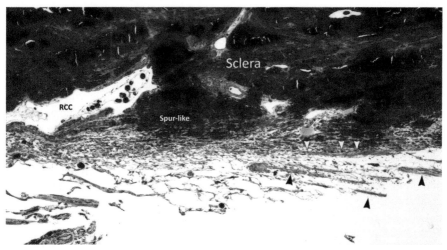

Fig. 6. Semithin section of the posterior trabecular meshwork of a canine eye. Toluidine blue staining. Longitudinal ciliary body muscle fibers are indicated by the arrowheads. They direct to the inner sclera, in an area that reminds scleral spur in primates and that is just posterior to a large radial collector channel (RCC).

region has high content of the elastic fiber system, which is composed of a core of elastin and surrounding microfibrils (fibrillin-1 and microfibrillar-associated protein-1 and -2). The system provides support, resilience, and allows recoiling to regions under biomechanical stress.[55] Elastin deposition and its microfibrillar envelopment, because the thickness of the basal membrane of the endothelial monolayer of the CC increase with age.[35] The thickening of the elastin system with aging is in part owing an increased fibers cross-linking.[56] These changes are associated with an increased stiffness of the tissues of the TM.

The capability of this region to undergo constant modifications associated with muscular activity matches with the diffuse presence of nerve endings (see **Fig. 4**). Both parasympathetic (from the ciliary ganglion) and sympathetic (from the cranial cervical ganglion) systems innervate the ciliary body.[26] Sensorial nerves are also provided by branches of the V cranial nerve.

Parasympathetic fibers can be assumed to be the most influential on the longitudinal ciliary muscle in dogs. Other neurotransmitters may play a role in the outflow. Nitrovasodilators in bovine induce relaxation of the myofibroblast-like cells in the TM, increasing the outflow.[57,58] Nitrous oxide has also shown interesting effects in reducing the IOP in normotensive and dogs with primary open-angle glaucoma.[59]

Collagen V and VI are also present. The nonfibrillar collagen type IV is associated with the endothelial basal membranes, together with laminin, fibronectin and perlecan.[54,60] Fibronectin and laminin are also found interspersed within the ECM in the beams of TM and in the JCT.[61] The beams of the UTM thicken with age and glaucoma in dogs.[1,35] Fibronectin is among the major protein components of the ECM of the TM and, although few controversial opinions, increased deposit of fibronectin in trabecular tissues with aging and glaucoma is consistently reported.[56,61–63]

UTM cells also undergo modulating production of several non-structural proteins that regulate ECM turnover and remodeling, including, but not limited to, transforming growth factor beta-2 (TGFβ2), stromelysin, secreted protein acidic and rich in cysteine (SPARC), trombospondin-1 and -2, bone morphogenic protein-7, tenascin-C, matrix metalloproteinases and their inhibitors.[64-68] In addition, TM cells can express several receptors that can be activated by cytokines present in the aqueous (aquecrine/paracrine response) or by growth factors produced by the TM cells themselves (autocrine response).[69] These highly convoluted and variably dynamic mechanisms of cellular and matrix communication, which only represent a partial portion, constitute part of the complex mechanisms that regulate tissue homeostasis, remodeling, and changes that occur physiologically and pathologically in the outflow pathways. The boundaries between homeostasis and disease, innate or/and adaptive immune reactions, parainflammation and inflammation are not sharp and often overlapping.[70,71] These interactions are not well defined or at least not well understood as a whole yet. In adjunct, polymorphic alleles in coding genes or/and promoters and enhancers and linkage disequilibrium with major histocompatibility complex haplotypes can have an influence on individual diversity in the dynamic cascades involving these factors or can explain breed predisposition to specific multifactorial diseases.

Corneoscleral and Uveoscleral Trabecular Meshwork

The CSTM and the USTM are essentially the same tissue that assumes different names depending on its location and the relationship with surrounding tissues (**Fig. 7**). The CSTM and the UTMS place in the innermost part of the sclera, occupying the scleral sulcus, a circular, shallow, and wide triangular groove with its outer apex approximately corresponding with the base of the iris (see **Fig. 4**). Their inclusion within the CC is questionable. In primates, the scleral sulcus is the site that harbors the TM and an equivalent

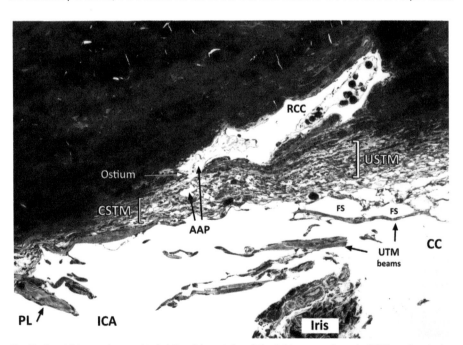

Fig. 7. Semithin section and toluidine blue stain of the iridocorneal angle (ICA) and anterior ciliary cleft (CC). The corneoscleral and uveoscleral trabecula meshwork (CSTM and USTM) are the same, lamellar, more compact tissue than the uveal trabecular meshwork (UTM). The name changes depending on anterior (more corneal) or posterior (uveal) position. An ostium between inner collector channels (ICC) and a radial collector channel (RCC) is indicated with the arrow. FS, Fontana spaces; PL, pectinate ligament.

scleral modification can be observed in canine eyes that have been sectioned after fixation with agents that tend to better preserve the ocular anatomy (see **Fig. 4**). The scleral sulcus extends from the peripheral edge of Descemet's membrane to the posterior boundaries of the CC. The morphologic cobweblike network pattern of the UTM differs from the more organized and compact arrangement of the connective lamellae in the CSTM and USTM. The lamellae are disposed in tangentially oriented parallel layers band with evidently and progressively reduced intertrabecular spaces while approaching the AAP. These spaces are still lined by endothelial cells. As mentioned, the CSTM and the USTM share similar anatomy and organization and their division is purely made for anatomic nomenclature dictated by their location.

The CSTM is cranial and fades into the cornea approximately around the inner limbal area. The USTM is more posterior and represents the outer boundary of the posterior CC. The CSTM and the USTM represent the transition tissue between the UTM and the JCT (**Fig. 8**).

The Cribriform Region or Juxtacanalicular Tissue and the Inner Wall of Inner Collector Channels

The whole anterior outflow system can be imagined as an hourglass with sand replaced by the aqueous. The proximal, converging spaces are inner to the eye and can be identified with the anterior chamber, the cleft with the UTM, the CSTM and the USTM, whereas the distal, progressively diverging spaces are represented by the lumen of the AAP, radial collector channels, the larger outer collector channels, the episcleral veins, and the ISVP. The scientific consensus is that the site of higher

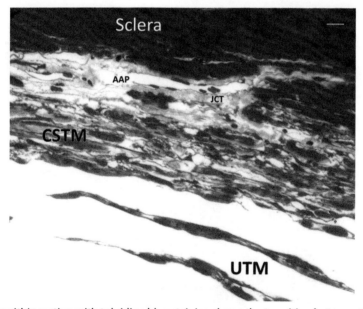

Fig. 8. Semithin section with toluidine blue staining shows the transition between the uveal trabecular meshwork (UTM) represented by irregularly distributed beams of connective tissue lined by endothelial cells into a more lamellar and organized tissue represented by the corneoscleral trabecular meshwork (CSTM). Small, interlamellar spaces can be seen. The justacanalicular connective tissue (JCT) is a thin layer rich in extracellular matrix that surround the inner wall of the endothelial cells of angular aqueous plexus (AAP). Bar = 10 μ.

A

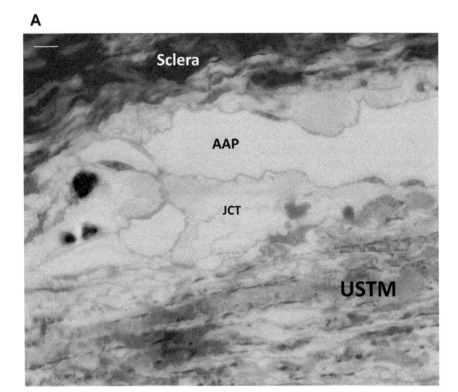

B

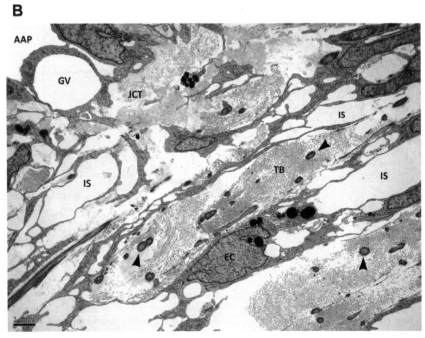

resistance is represented by both the thin layer of JCT around the AAP and their endothelium that represents the IW.[54,72–75] This critical area, its structural and functional characteristics, and the changes that occur with aging and disease are the primary region of interest in the normal regulation and dysregulation of IOP. In dogs, in which closed angle glaucoma is the most common phenotype of the disease, other anatomic regions may be of interest as well.

The JCT (also called the endothelial meshwork or the cribriform region) is the outermost region of the TM and lies underneath the IW of the AAP. Despite some morphologic differences between primate and nonprimate mammals, the JCT has been identified in dogs and bovines.[35,36,76,77] The tissue is extremely thin and likely variable in thickness and composition at different sites.[78] Its thickness is reported to vary between 5 to 10, 7 to 14, and 2 to 20 μ.[74,78–80] The JCT represents a nonlamellar, loose, and not well organized tissue. Fibroblastlike cells are embedded into an almost fluid fibrillary ECM abundant in proteoglycans and glycosaminoglycans (GAGs), and rich in unarranged elastin and collagen fibers.[74,75] The cells are kept in mutual contact with each other as well as the IW endothelial cells by extensions of their cytoplasmic membranes.

In dogs, the JCT is not as compact as in humans (**Fig. 9**).[33] Electron-lucent or "empty" spaces have been described in the JCT. These spaces may actually be filled with GAGs[35] and seem to be empty owing to sample processing (see **Fig. 9**). On histologic and transmission electron microscopy sections, the JCT is dogs is more discernible in proximity of the IW of the AAP (see **Figs. 8** and **9**).

The spaces of Fontana and the intertrabecular spaces of the CSTM and USTM are large enough not to offer resistance to the aqueous flow. The ECM of the JCT is then considered to assume a pivotal role in the regulation of IOP in both normal and open angle glaucomatous eyes.[81] The elastic fibers allow plasticity of the tissue in response to fluctuations in IOP.[79] However, collagen cross-linking occurs with age and it is increased in glaucoma, making the ECM stiffer.[82,83] GAGs and their associated proteoglycans, particularly dermatan sulfate, chondroitin sulfate, hyaluronic acid[84] and versican[79] separate the cells from the fibrillar collagen and have a primary role in modulating resistance.[79] Numerous other structural and functional proteins are present, like fibronectin, laminin, collagen types I, III, IV, V, and VI (but not type II), and some of them actively participate in ECM remodeling like myocilin, trombospondin-1, and SPARC.[74,79,85,86] Trombospondin-1 is one of the activators of latent transforming growth factor beta-2 abundantly present within the anterior segment,[87,88] whereas SPARC is a matricellular protein known to regulate ECM in many tissues and is highly expressed in the TM. SPARC-null mice demonstrated a lower IOP, which is associated with a more uniform outflow pattern and decreased collagen fibril diameter.[85]

Fig. 9. (A) Semithin section with toluidine blue staining of the angular aqueous plexus (AAP) region in a canine eye. The lamellar organization of the uveoscleral trabecular meshwork (USTM) can be recognized at the bottom. Some interlamellar spaces can be seen. The transition region between the USTM and the AAP is represented by a loose translucent tissue, the juxtacanalicular connective tissue (JCT). Bar = 5 μ. (B) Transmission electron microscopy. A microphotograph of a same corresponding area shows the trabecular beams (TB) of the USTM. The beams are constituted by collagen fibers and larger elastin fibers (*arrowheads*). Endothelial trabecular meshwork cells line the beams and engulf melanin granules (EC). Intertrabecular spaces (IS) are reducing toward the JCT. A giant vacuole (GV) can be seen within the cytoplasm of an endothelial cell of the inner wall of the angular aqueous plexus (AAP).

With age, the components of the ECM of this region tend to accumulate plaques of amorphous material supposedly derived from the sheaths of the elastic fibers and collagen VI,[72,89] and the outflow resistance increases proportionally.[74]

The JCT is separated from the lumen of the AAP by a monolayer of endothelial cells. The endothelium of the IW has 2 opposite functions. Although it allows aqueous percolation from the underlying JCT through the formation of giant vacuoles and pores, at the same time it prevents blood products from entering the eye if elevated episcleral venous pressure exceeds IOP because of the presence of tight junctions. For the latter reason, the endothelium should be considered part of the blood–aqueous barrier along with the ciliary epithelium, the iris vascular endothelium, and the posterior iris epithelium.[90] The basement membrane of endothelial cells of Schlemm canal in humans and the basement membrane of the AAP in dogs are not continuous.[36,80] This feature, associated with the presence of intercellular continuous tight junctions, categorizes the AAP in between lymphatic channels and venules.[91] The discontinuity of the basal lamina creates a direct connection between the ECM of the JCT and the IW. The transit of the aqueous from the JCT to the AAP lumen occurs through the formation of endothelial giant vacuoles and intracellular pores or directly through the intercellular pores formed between 2 neighbor cells.[80,92]

AH filters through the TM as bulk flow that is influenced by, and positively correlates with the pressure gradient; no active transport is involved.[74] Several studies have demonstrated a pivotal role of GAGs and their protein complexes, proteoglycans, in regulating the flow through the TM, in particular in the JCT and IW.[93–96] All of the normal GAGs have been identified, with hyaluronic acid or hyaluronan and chondroitin sulfate being the most preponderant.[81] The hydrophilic properties of their moieties are able to absorb fluids easily. Although initial publications assigned to GAGs a contributing role in flow resistance,[1,96–98] more recent works have shown that primary open-angle glaucoma is actually associated with a loss of hyaluronic acid from the TM and that treatment with chondroitinases and hyaluronidase intracamerally in monkey eyes does not change the outflow facility or IOP.[99,100]

The composition of the JCT and the IW of the Schlemm's canal in primates and of the AAP in dogs has been thoroughly described both ultrastructurally and functionally.[33,35,36,54,79] It would be a mistake though to think about this area as a stable, uniform tissue. The JCT must be considered a dynamic tissue undergoing continuous remodeling.[79,101] Dynamic changes both structurally and in the ECM occur with age and different conditions.[35,74] Nonstructural proteins and molecules are produced and released during tissue remodeling and under the influence of cytokines and growth factors present in the aqueous at different times.[70,79] The influence of different cytokines and growth factors (ie, tumor necrosis factor-α, transforming growth factor beta-2) and matricellular proteins on ECM permeability have been extensively studied to understand and differentiate dynamic changes seen in aging and glaucoma.[89,101]

The most common phenotypes of glaucoma in dogs are those classified as angle closure glaucoma. In these cases, the consistent pathologic finding is the collapse/closure of the CC. Whether these changes are the consequence of a primary obstruction starting in the JCT/AAP or a primary event into the CC itself or if both sites can simultaneously be affected is unknown. Glaucoma is an age-related disease in most of the instances and the histologic changes that occur with aging in normal canine eyes are described mostly with pigment dispersion, increased number of melanin-laden macrophages within the CB, CC, and AAP, and visible collagen deposition in the CB.[102] In humans and dogs, an increased permeability of the blood–aqueous barrier with aging has been described,[103–106] supporting the idea that its protein content and quality vary and may influence and explain the dynamic remodeling of the outflow tissues.

The intertrabecular spaces, the loose matrix of JCT and the giant vacuoles in the IW endothelium are the expression of how the aqueous permeates through the outer CSTM/USTM and JCT into the AAP. The fine mechanisms by which the fluid passes through the tissue into the lumen are still, however, under investigation. The bulk flow of the aqueous is a passive mechanism that follows pressure gradients. IOP is higher than pressure within the outer draining venous system. Episcleral pressure both in humans and dogs has been measured between 8 and 12 mm Hg.[107,108] However, in dogs, an unknown role is also played by the ISVP and vortex veins,[36,97] whereas in primates the distal outflow is regulated only through the episcleral and anterior ciliary veins.[109] The morphologic presence of giant vacuoles within the endothelial cells of Schlemm's canal (better seen under flow condition or perfusion-fixed eyes) with or without basal opening and micron-sized (0.5–1.5 μ) pores on the luminal surface of the endothelial cells have been documented in primates, dogs, rabbits, and bovine.[35,36,92,110] Pores of the IW cells can be observed with both transmission electron microscopy and scanning electron microscopy.[35,92] The endothelial surface of the AAP is also covered by a thin layer of glycocalix that may play a role in regulating aqueous outflow resistance.[111]

Endothelial pores are nonuniformly distributed[112] and their density proportionally reflects the segmental pattern of higher AH outflow through the TM/JCT.[113] IW pore density proportionally increases with increased perfusion in normal eyes.[114] However, the density of the pores decreases on the endothelial surface of Schlemm's canal in human glaucomatous eyes.[114]

Besides the formation of giant vacuoles, pynocytic, intracytoplasmic microvesicles have been observed; however, their role and relevance in aqueous outflow is unknown.[35] The giant vacuoles are seen most commonly within the endothelial cells that line the inner side of the AAP, facing the JCT.[92] Studies using eyes perfused with a tracer have shown that tracer accumulation corresponds to the location of collector channel ostia[109] and with regions of JCT containing less versican.[115]

The anterior outflow is not uniformly distributed over the circumference of the meshwork, but has a segmental pattern in adult humans,[116] bovine,[117,118] porcine,[115] nonhuman primates, and mice.[85] The areas of preferential flow correspond to areas of lower resistance and are located in the proximity of the radial collector channels and vary with their distribution.[119] Sectorial flow may occur because some collector channels reside near larger episcleral venules, the final destination of aqueous.[109] Although the nasal[116] and inferior[120] quadrants have been suggested to be more active,[109] no consistency in the pattern of segmental outflow is yet accepted.[116] The segmental portions of active outflow decrease in glaucomatous patients or with increasing IOP.[117,121]

ANGULAR AQUEOUS PLEXUS

Tripathi[37] was the first to use the nomenclature of "angular aqueous plexus (AAP)" to name the complex pattern of the inner-scleral venous aqueous outflow in nonprimate mammals and to recognize, despite morphologic differences, the anatomic and functional similarity of these canalicular structures with Schlemm's canal in primates.[36,37]

The AAP in dogs is a complex, tangled vascular network that expands from the Schwalbe's line anteriorly to the end of the CC posteriorly, spanning for hundreds of microns. The plexus occupies the inner sclera at the transition zone between the cornea and the outer uvea. The area seems to be similar to a triangular scleral sulcus, with the outer vertex corresponding more or less with the transition area between the ICA and the CC (see **Fig. 4**; **Fig. 10B**).

The plexus is made by several channels that have different diameters and directions and lie in different layers at different depths in the inner sclera (see **Fig. 10**). They represent the first, distal dilation after the JCT and IW. Thin, inner channels are close to the CSTM and USTM and form an intricate network with incomplete circumferential, oblique and meridional tangential directions. These channels are lined by endothelial cells that are

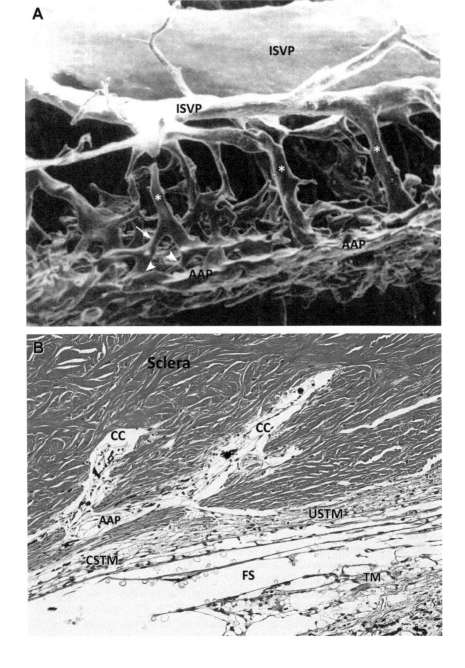

the true functional equivalent of the IW of Schlemm's canal in primates and represent the AAP in dogs.[36,37] The plasma membranes of the endothelial cells adhere with tight junctions and for this reason are considered part of the blood–aqueous barrier.[75]

The multiple tangential channels forming the AAP merge then into perpendicular, radial collector channels through openings called "ostia." Because the tangential channels may be displaced in different planes, short radial collector channels may be present together with longer and larger outer radial channels. As many as 30 to 35 external collector channels have been reported in the human eye.[84] Radial channels have different, anterior (corneoscleral) and posterior (uveoscleral) distributions (see **Fig. 10**). High variability, however, exists and complex patterns of anastomoses can be seen at light microscopy depending not only on the species of animal, but also on the different sections of an individual eye.[36,37] The complex patterns of anastomoses can also be clearly observed in luminal casts.[38] The histologic sectorial changes in radial channels may reflect the sectorial distribution of the collector channels described in primates, mice and bovines. Preferential outflows may occur in different sectors, which is confirmed by pigment deposition in the near JCT, as described for other species.[74,109] Unevenly distributed radial collector channels are present in primates, more being on the nasal than on the temporal side of the eye.[84]

Larger radial collector channels direct to the outer sclera and anastomose with the anterior ciliary veins or the ISVP (or the venous circle of Hovius); both drain into the orbit via the ophthalmic vein (the former) and via the vortex veins (the latter).[38] There are 2 to 4 large venous vessels that compose the ISVP, which is located in the outer third of the sclera. The anterior venules are usually smaller and the caliber of the vessels increases posteriorly (**Fig. 11**).

POSTERIOR, UVEOSCLERAL, OR UNCONVENTIONAL OUTFLOW

The uveoscleral or unconventional outflow represents the amount of aqueous that once has entered the TM escapes the trabecular outflow and directs posteriorly where it can filter through the porosity of the loose connective tissue and its ECM in the ciliary body. The connective tissue between the longitudinal bundles of the ciliary muscle is loose and permeable. After percolating through the ECM of the ciliary body, the aqueous collects into the uveoscleral space, a virtual space between the posterior ciliary body/anterior choroid and the sclera; from here, the AH can reach the posterior

◀―――

Fig. 10. (*A*) Luminal cast of the canine trabecular outflow pathway. The vessels of the outflow at the level of the angular aqueous plexus (AAP) display a complex and tangled network made by smaller channels oriented tangentially in different planes and directions. Larger radial collector channels (*asterisks*) connect the network to larger venous vessels in the outer sclera, the intrascleral venous plexus (ISVP). Radial channels are displaced at different anterior and posterior sites. Irregular patterns of anastomoses are present among all the channels and shorter radial channels are seen (*arrow*). The connections between almost perpendicular inner and radial channels are called ostia (*arrowheads* and **Fig. 7**). (*B*) Microphotograph of a histologic sagittal section of the inner scleral region at the level of the scleral sulcus in a normal canine eye showing the complex anastomotic pattern of the drainage system in dogs. Hematoxylin and eosin staining. Two large, radial collector channels (CC) are visible anteriorly and posteriorly. These collector channels convey the aqueous filtered through the complex system represented by trabecular meshwork (TM), CSTM, uveoscleral TM (USTM), and angular aqueous plexus (AAP). Fontana spaces (FS) are present between the beams of the TM. (*Adapted from* Van Buskirk EM. The canine eye: the vessels of aqueous drainage. Invest Ophthalmol Vis Sci 1979;18:226; with permission.)

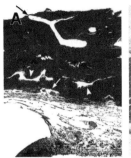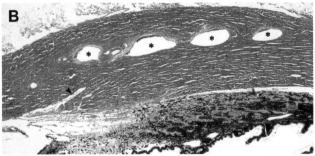

Fig. 11. The scleral outflow systems. (*A*) The complex angular aqueous plexus (AAP) and collector channels are displaced in different layers with different directions and different sizes in the inner sclera. The arrowheads indicate collector channels. The white arrow points to an ostium between AAP and a short radial collector channel. In the outer sclera an aqueous vein can be seen directed to the limbus and to the anterior ciliary veins (*black arrow*) (toluidine blue). (*B*) Longitudinal section of the sclera corresponding to the ciliary body area. Four large scleral veins representing the intrascleral venous plexus (ISVP) are indicated with asterisks. The arrowhead points to a large, radial collector channel directing to the ISVP area (Hematoxylin and eosin).

suprachoroidal space. This flow is passive and mostly independent from IOP. It is driven by a positive osmotic gradient between the colloids in the choroidal and scleral blood vessels and the uveal tissue of the posterior ciliary body. Furthermore, the hydraulic conductivity of the scleral tissue is able to absorb and remove 4.3 µL/min in humans.[122]

In normal dogs, the USO allows full permeability to 1 µ spheres that can easily reach the suprachoroidal space and the connected vascular outflow. In glaucomatous dogs, this ability is reduced significantly.[123] The unconventional outflow represents 15% of the total outflow in normal Beagles, whereas it is reduced to 3% in glaucomatous Beagles.[124] It is only 3% in normal cats.[125] The normal rate of outflow through the unconventional pathway varies in different species and decreases with age.[31,56] In nonhuman primates, 40% to 60% of the aqueous leaves the globe through this pathway, whereas in people several rates have been reported, ranging between 12% and 54%.[31] The lower values are associated with advanced age.[31] In particular the reduction in outflow in normal people has been quantified in about 7% to 10% per decade.[31]

In younger primates, the connective tissue between the muscular bundles in the ciliary body is sparse. In aging dogs, the loose connective tissue between the muscular bundles of the longitudinal ciliary muscle accumulates large melanin-laden macrophages that progressively obstruct and likely activate or contribute to remodeling the region (see **Fig. 12**).[102]

The most recent calculations of the amount of flow through the USO in humans have provided higher values than early studies, increasing the actual relevance of the unconventional outflow. High variability is determined by age. Healthy humans between 20 and 30 years of age showed rates of USO between 36% and 54%, whereas people of 60 years or older had rates between 12% and 42%.[10] This is likely to happen in dogs as well. Unfortunately, the USO has been limitedly investigated only Beagles in the 1980s.[123]

Along with the decreased outflow that occurs with age, there is also a decrease in aqueous production and the clinical influence of the decreased facility in normal patients is limited by this factor.[10]

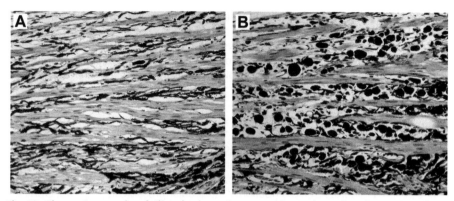

Fig. 12. Photomicrographs of ciliary body sections posterior to the trabecular meshwork in 2 normal eyes from different dogs. (*A*) Ten month old male Labrador. The longitudinal bundles of the ciliary muscle alternate with connective tissue mostly filled with fusiform dendritic melanocytes representing the normal pigmented component of uveal ocular tissue. (*B*) Fifteen year old spayed female Labrador. The intermuscular spaces present a large number of plump large pigmented cells representing infiltrating macrophages melanin-laden (melanophages).

The point of greatest resistance is considered the ECM of the posterior ciliary body. The connective spaces between the longitudinal muscular bundles decrease with age and become less permeable.[10] The composition, tightness, and permeability of the ECM of the ciliary body can also differ and change depending on several physiologic, pharmacologic, and inflammatory factors. The contraction or relaxation of the longitudinal ciliary muscle has some influence on the rate of the outflow. Atropine increases the permeability of the ciliary muscle in nonhuman primates, whereas pilocarpine decreases it.[126] However, the overall clinical effect of pilocarpine on IOP may be different because of the contraction of the tendons of the ciliary muscles also opens the Fontana spaces, hypothetically shifting the outflow to the anterior pathways. Tendons of the longitudinal ciliary muscle, the only ciliary muscle present in dogs, are directed to the posterior half of the scleral sulcus. According to this morphologic interpretation, ciliary muscle contraction might open the radial collector channels (see **Fig. 6**).

The USO is the target for powerful medications used to treat glaucomas in dogs. Because the anterior outflow is usually collapsed in advanced glaucoma, decreasing AH production and increasing the posterior outflow are the most rationale pharmacologic goals. Synthetic prostaglandins increase the USO by increasing the permeability of the ECM in the ciliary body. The effect is mediated by the increased expression of matrix metalloproteinases that remodel the ECM of the ciliary body.[127]

SUMMARY

Knowledge of the anatomic and physiologic background of aqueous dynamics is important for the clinician. Glaucoma is a heterogeneous group of diseases with multiple phenotypes. Accurate evaluation of the clinical conditions is pivotal to understanding the possible therapeutic options and prognosis for an affected patient. It is also important to shift the consideration of anatomy from a steady perspective to a dynamic process in which age is a clear influencing factor and is affecting the structure and the function of ocular outflow.

Moreover, a remarkable benefit of knowing the pathophysiology and relative functional anatomy of the region resides in the possible establishment of predictive models in cases of early disease. The attention to details at the beginning of the disease may allow the clinician to reach the longest control over a pathologic condition that unfortunately is associated with a high occurrence of blindness and patient discomfort.

REFERENCES

1. Gum GG, Samuelson DO, Gelatt KN. Effect of hyaluronidase on aqueous outflow resistance in normotensive and glaucomatous eyes of dogs. Am J Vet Res 1992;53(5):767–70.
2. Gelatt KN, MacKay EO. Distribution of intraocular pressure in dogs. Vet Ophthalmol 1998;1(2–3):109–14.
3. Giannetto C, Piccione G, Giudice E. Daytime profile of the intraocular pressure and tear production in normal dog. Vet Ophthalmol 2009;12(5):302–5.
4. Leiva M, Naranjo C, Pena MT. Comparison of the rebound tonometer (ICare) to the applanation tonometer (Tonopen XL) in normotensive dogs. Vet Ophthalmol 2006;9(1):17–21.
5. Martin-Suarez E, Molleda C, Tardon R, et al. Diurnal variations of central corneal thickness and intraocular pressure in dogs from 8:00 am to 8:00 pm. Can Vet J 2014;55(4):361–5.
6. Andrade SF, Palozzi RJ, Giuffrida R, et al. Comparison of intraocular pressure measurements between the Tono-Pen XL(R) and Perkins(R) applanation tonometers in dogs and cats. Vet Ophthalmol 2012;15(Suppl 1):14–20.
7. David R, Zangwill L, Stone D, et al. Epidemiology of intraocular pressure in a population screened for glaucoma. Br J Ophthalmol 1987;71(10):766–71.
8. Baek SU, Kee C, Suh W. Longitudinal analysis of age-related changes in intraocular pressure in South Korea. Eye (Lond) 2015;29(5):625–9.
9. Wong TT, Wong TY, Foster PJ, et al. The relationship of intraocular pressure with age, systolic blood pressure, and central corneal thickness in an Asian population. Invest Ophthalmol Vis Sci 2009;50(9):4097–102.
10. Toris CB, Yablonski ME, Wang YL, et al. Aqueous humor dynamics in the aging human eye. Am J Ophthalmol 1999;127(4):407–12.
11. Millar C, Kaufman PL. Aqueous humor: secretion and dynamics. In: Tasman W, Jaeger EA, editors. Duane's foundations of clinical ophthalmology, vol. 2. Philadelphia: Lippincott-Raven; 1995. p. 1–51.
12. Bill A. Blood circulation and fluid dynamics in the eye. Physiol Rev 1975;55(3): 383–417.
13. Cole DF. Secretion of the aqueous humour. Exp Eye Res 1977;25(Suppl): 161–76.
14. Caprioli J. The ciliary epithelia and aqueous humor. In: Hart WM, editor. Adler's physiology of the eye. Clinical application. 9th edition. St Louis (MO): Mosby; 1993. p. 228–47.
15. Goel M, Picciani RG, Lee RK, et al. Aqueous humor dynamics: a review. Open Ophthalmol J 2010;4:52–9.
16. Gabelt BT, Kaufman PL. Aqueous humor hydrodynamics. In: Kaufman PL, Albert A, editors. Adler's physiology of the eye. Clinical application. 10th edition. St Louis (MO): Mosby; 2003. p. 237–89.
17. Freddo TF. A contemporary concept of the blood-aqueous barrier. Prog Retin Eye Res 2013;32:181–95.

18. Civan MM, Macknight AD. The ins and outs of aqueous humour secretion. Exp Eye Res 2004;78(3):625–31.
19. Green K, Pederson JE. Contribution of secretion and filtration to aqueous humor formation. Am J Physiol 1972;222(5):1218–26.
20. Bonting SL, Becker B. Studies on sodium-potassium activated adenosine triphosphatase. Xiv. Inhibition of enzyme activity and aqueous humor flow in the rabbit eye after intravitreal injection of ouabain. Invest Ophthalmol 1964;3:523–33.
21. Bhattacherjee P. Distribution of carbonic anhydrase in the rabbit eye as demonstrated histochemically. Exp Eye Res 1971;12(3):356–9.
22. Lutjen-Drecoll E, Lonnerholm G, Eichhorn M. Carbonic anhydrase distribution in the human and monkey eye by light and electron microscopy. Graefes Arch Clin Exp Ophthalmol 1983;220(6):285–91.
23. McLaren JW. Measurement of aqueous humor flow. Exp Eye Res 2009;88(4): 641–7.
24. Schneider TL, Brubaker RF. Effect of chronic epinephrine on aqueous humor flow during the day and during sleep in normal healthy subjects. Invest Ophthalmol Vis Sci 1991;32(9):2507–10.
25. Ward DA, Cawrse MA, Hendrix DV. Fluorophotometric determination of aqueous humor flow rate in clinically normal dogs. Am J Vet Res 2001;62(6):853–8.
26. Gum GG, Gelatt KN, Esson DW. Physiology of the eye. In: Gelatt KN, editor. Veterinary ophthalmology, vol. 1, 4th edition. Ames (IA): Wiley-Blackwell; 2007. p. 149–82.
27. Naushad M, Alothman ZA, Khan MR. Removal of malathion from aqueous solution using De-Acidite FF-IP resin and determination by UPLC-MS/MS: equilibrium, kinetics and thermodynamics studies. Talanta 2013;115:15–23.
28. Gaasterland D, Kupfer C, Milton R, et al. Studies of aqueous humour dynamics in man. VI. Effect of age upon parameters of intraocular pressure in normal human eyes. Exp Eye Res 1978;26(6):651–6.
29. Van Buskirk EM, Brett J. The canine eye: in vitro studies of the intraocular pressure and facility of aqueous outflow. Invest Ophthalmol Vis Sci 1978;17(4):373–7.
30. VanBuskirk EM, Grant WM. Influence of temperature and the question of involvement of cellular metabolism in aqueous outflow. Am J Ophthalmol 1974;77(4): 565–72.
31. Alm A, Nilsson SF. Uveoscleral outflow–a review. Exp Eye Res 2009;88(4):760–8.
32. Samuelson DA. A reevaluation of the comparative anatomy of the eutherian iridocorneal angle and associated ciliary body musculature. Vet Comp Ophthalmol 1996;6(3):153–72.
33. Samuelson DA. Ophthalmic anatomy. In: Gelatt KN, Gilger BC, Kern TJ, editors. Veterinary ophthalmology, vol. 1, 5th edition. Ames (IA): Wiley-Blackwell; 2013. p. 39–170.
34. Samuelson DA, Gelatt KN. Aqueous outflow in the beagle. I. Postnatal morphologic development of the iridocorneal angle: pectinate ligament and uveal trabecular meshwork. Curr Eye Res 1984;3(6):783–94.
35. Samuelson DA, Gelatt KN. Aqueous outflow in the Beagle. II. Postnatal morphologic development of the iridocorneal angle: corneoscleral trabecular mesh work and angular aqueous plexus. Curr Eye Res 1984;3(6):795–807.
36. Bedford PG, Grierson I. Aqueous drainage in the dog. Res Vet Sci 1986;41(2): 172–86.
37. Tripathi RC. Ultrastructure of the exit pathway of the aqueous in lower mammals. (A preliminary report on the "angular aqueous plexus"). Exp Eye Res 1971; 12(3):311–4.

38. Van Buskirk EM. The canine eye: the vessels of aqueous drainage. Invest Ophthalmol Vis Sci 1979;18(3):223–30.
39. Read RA, Wood JL, Lakhani KH. Pectinate ligament dysplasia (PLD) and glaucoma in Flat Coated Retrievers. I. Objectives, technique and results of a PLD survey. Vet Ophthalmol 1998;1(2–3):85–90.
40. Bedford PG. Gonioscopy in the dog. J Small Anim Pract 1977;18(10):615–29.
41. Pearl R, Gould D, Spiess B. Progression of pectinate ligament dysplasia over time in two populations of Flat-Coated Retrievers. Vet Ophthalmol 2015;18(1): 6–12.
42. Bjerkas E, Ekesten B, Farstad W. Pectinate ligament dysplasia and narrowing of the iridocorneal angle associated with glaucoma in the English Springer Spaniel. Vet Ophthalmol 2002;5(1):49–54.
43. Ekesten B, Narfstrom K. Correlation of morphologic features of the iridocorneal angle to intraocular pressure in Samoyeds. Am J Vet Res 1991;52(11): 1875–8.
44. Crumley W, Gionfriddo JR, Radecki SV. Relationship of the iridocorneal angle, as measured using ultrasound biomicroscopy, with post-operative increases in intraocular pressure post-phacoemulsification in dogs. Vet Ophthalmol 2009;12(1):22–7.
45. WuDunn D. Mechanobiology of trabecular meshwork cells. Exp Eye Res 2009; 88(4):718–23.
46. Samuelson DA, Gelatt KN, Gum GG. Kinetics of phagocytosis in the normal canine iridocorneal angle. Am J Vet Res 1984;45(11):2359–66.
47. Gasiorowski JZ, Russell P. Biological properties of trabecular meshwork cells. Exp Eye Res 2009;88(4):671–5.
48. Pizzirani S, Desai SJ, Pirie CG, et al. Age related changes in the anterior segment of the eye in normal dogs. Vet Ophthalmol 2010;13(6):421.
49. Cracknell KP, Grierson I, Hogg P, et al. Melanin in the trabecular meshwork is associated with age, POAG but not Latanoprost treatment. A masked morphometric study. Exp Eye Res 2006;82(6):986–93.
50. Gottanka J, Johnson DH, Grehn F, et al. Histologic findings in pigment dispersion syndrome and pigmentary glaucoma. J Glaucoma 2006;15(2):142–51.
51. Rohen JW, van der Zypen E. The phagocytic activity of the trabecular meshwork endothelium. An electron-microscopic study of the vervet (Cercopithecus aethiops). Albrecht Von Graefes Arch Klin Exp Ophthalmol 1968;175(2): 143–60.
52. Alvarado J, Murphy C, Juster R. Trabecular meshwork cellularity in primary open-angle glaucoma and nonglaucomatous normals. Ophthalmology 1984; 91(6):564–79.
53. Grierson I, Howes RC. Age-related depletion of the cell population in the human trabecular meshwork. Eye 1987;1(Pt 2):204–10.
54. Lutjen-Drecoll E. Functional morphology of the trabecular meshwork in primate eyes. Prog Retin Eye Res 1998;18(1):91–119.
55. Hann CR, Fautsch MP. The elastin fiber system between and adjacent to collector channels in the human juxtacanalicular tissue. Invest Ophthalmol Vis Sci 2011;52(1):45–50.
56. Gabelt BT, Kaufman PL. Changes in aqueous humor dynamics with age and glaucoma. Prog Retin Eye Res 2005;24(5):612–37.
57. Wiederholt M, Sturm A, Lepple-Wienhues A. Relaxation of trabecular meshwork and ciliary muscle by release of nitric oxide. Invest Ophthalmol Vis Sci 1994; 35(5):2515–20.

58. Stumpff F, Strauss O, Boxberger M, et al. Characterization of maxi-K-channels in bovine trabecular meshwork and their activation by cyclic guanosine monophosphate. Invest Ophthalmol Vis Sci 1997;38(9):1883–92.
59. Impagnatiello F, Borghi V, Gale DC, et al. A dual acting compound with latanoprost amide and nitric oxide releasing properties, shows ocular hypotensive effects in rabbits and dogs. Exp Eye Res 2011;93(3):243–9.
60. Marshall GE, Konstas AG, Lee WR. Immunogold ultrastructural localization of collagens in the aged human outflow system. Ophthalmology 1991;98(5): 692–700.
61. Hann CR, Springett MJ, Wang X, et al. Ultrastructural localization of collagen IV, fibronectin, and laminin in the trabecular meshwork of normal and glaucomatous eyes. Ophthalmic Res 2001;33(6):314–24.
62. Babizhayev MA, Brodskaya MW. Fibronectin detection in drainage outflow system of human eyes in ageing and progression of open-angle glaucoma. Mech Ageing Dev 1989;47(2):145–57.
63. Faralli JA, Schwinn MK, Gonzalez JM Jr, et al. Functional properties of fibronectin in the trabecular meshwork. Exp Eye Res 2009;88(4):689–93.
64. Tripathi RC, Chan WFA, Li J, et al. Trabecular cells express the TGF-beta2 gene and secrete the cytokine. Exp Eye Res 1994;58(5):523–8.
65. Fuchshofer R, Yu AH, Welge-Lussen U, et al. Bone Morphogenetic Protein-7 Is an Antagonist of Transforming Growth Factor beta 2 in Human Trabecular Meshwork Cells. Invest Ophthalmol Vis Sci 2007;48(2):715–26.
66. Alexander JP, Samples JR, Van Buskirk EM, et al. Expression of Matrix Metalloproteinases and Inhibitor by Human Trabecular Meshwork. Invest Ophthalmol Vis Sci 1991;32(1):172–80.
67. Rhee DJ, Haddadin RI, Kang MH, et al. Matricellular proteins in the trabecular meshwork. Exp Eye Res 2009;88(4):694–703.
68. Flugel-Koch C, Ohlmann A, Fuchshofer R, et al. Thrombospondin-1 in the trabecular meshwork: localization in normal and glaucomatous eyes, and induction by TGF-beta1 and dexamethasone in vitro. Exp Eye Res 2004;79(5):649–63.
69. Wordinger RJ, Clark AF, Agarwal R, et al. Cultured human trabecular meshwork cells express functional growth factor receptors. Invest Ophthalmol Vis Sci 1998;39(9):1575–89.
70. Xu H, Chen M, Forrester JV. Para-inflammation in the aging retina. Prog Retin Eye Res 2009;28(5):348–68.
71. Medzhitov R. Origin and physiological roles of inflammation. Nature 2008; 454(7203):428–35.
72. Overby DR, Stamer WD, Johnson M. The changing paradigm of outflow resistance generation: towards synergistic models of the JCT and inner wall endothelium. Exp Eye Res 2009;88(4):656–70.
73. Gong H, Freddo TF. The washout phenomenon in aqueous outflow – Why does it matter? Exp Eye Res 2009;88(4):729–37.
74. Tamm ER. The trabecular meshwork outflow pathways: structural and functional aspects. Exp Eye Res 2009;88(4):648–55.
75. Johnson M. 'What controls aqueous humour outflow resistance?' Exp Eye Res 2006;82(4):545–57.
76. Gong H, Yang CY. Morphological and hydrodynamic correlations with increasing outflow facility by rho-kinase inhibitor Y-27632. J Ocul Pharmacol Ther 2014;30(2–3):143–53.
77. Scott PA, Overby DR, Freddo TF, et al. Comparative studies between species that do and do not exhibit the washout effect. Exp Eye Res 2007;84(3):435–43.

78. Ten Hulzen RD, Johnson DH. Effect of fixation pressure on juxtacanalicular tissue and Schlemm's canal. Invest Ophthalmol Vis Sci 1996;37(1):114–24.

79. Keller KE, Acott TS. The juxtacanalicular region of ocular trabecular meshwork: a tissue with a unique extracellular matrix and specialized function. J Ocul Biol 2013;1(1):3.

80. Gong H, Ruberti J, Overby D, et al. A new view of the human trabecular meshwork using quick-freeze, deep-etch electron microscopy. Exp Eye Res 2002; 75(3):347–58.

81. Acott TS, Kelley MJ. Extracellular matrix in the trabecular meshwork. Exp Eye Res 2008;86(4):543–61.

82. Sethi A, Mao W, Wordinger RJ, et al. Transforming growth factor-beta induces extracellular matrix protein cross-linking lysyl oxidase (LOX) genes in human trabecular meshwork cells. Invest Ophthalmol Vis Sci 2011;52(8): 5240–50.

83. Last JA, Pan T, Ding Y, et al. Elastic modulus determination of normal and glaucomatous human trabecular meshwork. Invest Ophthalmol Vis Sci 2011;52(5): 2147–52.

84. Gong H, Tripathi RC, Tripathi BJ. Morphology of the aqueous outflow pathway. Microsc Res Tech 1996;33(4):336–67.

85. Swaminathan SS, Oh DJ, Kang MH, et al. Secreted protein acidic and rich in cysteine (SPARC)-null mice exhibit more uniform outflow. Invest Ophthalmol Vis Sci 2013;54(3):2035–47.

86. Ueda J, Wentz-Hunter K, Yue BY. Distribution of myocilin and extracellular matrix components in the juxtacanalicular tissue of human eyes. Invest Ophthalmol Vis Sci 2002;43(4):1068–76.

87. Daniel C, Wiede J, Krutzsch HC, et al. Thrombospondin-1 is a major activator of TGF-beta in fibrotic renal disease in the rat in vivo. Kidney Int 2004;65(2): 459–68.

88. Kuchtey J, Kuchtey RW. The microfibril hypothesis of glaucoma: implications for treatment of elevated intraocular pressure. J Ocul Pharmacol Ther 2014; 30(2–3):170–80.

89. Rohen JW, Futa R, Lutjen-Drecoll E. The fine structure of the cribriform meshwork in normal and glaucomatous eyes as seen in tangential sections. Invest Ophthalmol Vis Sci 1981;21(4):574–85.

90. Johnstone MA, Grant WG. Pressure-dependent changes in structures of the aqueous outflow system of human and monkey eyes. Am J Ophthalmol 1973; 75(3):365–83.

91. Kizhatil K, Ryan M, Marchant JK, et al. Schlemm's canal is a unique vessel with a combination of blood vascular and lymphatic phenotypes that forms by a novel developmental process. PLoS Biol 2014;12(7):e1001912.

92. Tripathi RC, Tripathi BJ. The mechanism of aqueous outflow in lower mammals. Exp Eye Res 1972;14(1):73–9.

93. Grierson I, Lee WR. Acid mucopolysaccharides in the outflow apparatus. Exp Eye Res 1975;21(5):417–31.

94. Lerner LE, Polansky JR, Howes EL, et al. Hyaluronan in the human trabecular meshwork. Invest Ophthalmol Vis Sci 1997;38(6):1222–8.

95. Usui T, Nakajima F, Ideta R, et al. Hyaluronan synthase in trabecular meshwork cells. Br J Ophthalmol 2003;87(3):357–60.

96. Knepper PA, Goossens W, Palmberg PF. Glycosaminoglycan stratification of the juxtacanalicular tissue in normal and primary open-angle glaucoma. Invest Ophthalmol Vis Sci 1996;37(12):2414–25.

97. Van Buskirk EM, Brett J. The canine eye: in vitro dissolution of the barriers to aqueous outflow. Invest Ophthalmol Vis Sci 1978;17(3):258–71.
98. Barany EH. The action of different kinds of hyaluronidase on the resistance to flow through the angle of the anterior chamber. Acta Ophthalmol 1956;34(5): 397–403.
99. Hubbard WC, Johnson M, Gong H, et al. Intraocular pressure and outflow facility are unchanged following acute and chronic intracameral chondroitinase ABC and hyaluronidase in monkeys. Exp Eye Res 1997;65(2):177–90.
100. Gong H, Freddo TF. Hyaluronic-Acid in the Normal and Glaucomatous Human Outflow Pathway. Invest Ophthalmol Vis Sci 1994;35(4):2083.
101. Fuchshofer R, Tamm ER. Modulation of extracellular matrix turnover in the trabecular meshwork. Exp Eye Res 2009;88(4):683–8.
102. Pizzirani S, Desai SJ, Pirie CG, et al. Age related changes in the anterior segment of the eye in normal dogs. Paper presented at: 41st Annual Meeting of the American College of Veterinary Ophthalmologists. San Diego, CA, October 6–9, 2010.
103. Oshika T, Kato S, Sawa M, et al. Aqueous flare intensity and age. Jpn J Ophthalmol 1989;33(2):237–42.
104. Onodera T, Gimbel HV, DeBroff BM. Aqueous flare and cell number in healthy eyes of Caucasians. Jpn J Ophthalmol 1993;37(4):445–51.
105. Satoh K, Takaku Y, Ohtsuki K, et al. Effects of aging on fluorescein leakage in the iris and angle in normal subjects. Jpn J Ophthalmol 1999;43(3):166–70.
106. Pizzirani S, Rankin AJ, Meekins JM, et al. Anterior chamber fluorophotometry in normal dogs of different ages. Paper presented at: 45th Annual Meeting of the American College of Veterinary Ophthalmologists. Fort Worth, October 8–11, 2014.
107. Talusan ED, Schwartz B. Episcleral venous pressure. Differences between normal, ocular hypertensive, and primary open angle glaucomas. Arch Ophthalmol 1981;99(5):824–8.
108. Gelatt KN, Gum GG, Merideth RE, et al. Episcleral venous pressure in normotensive and glaucomatous beagles. Invest Ophthalmol Vis Sci 1982;23(1): 131–5.
109. Hann CR, Fautsch MP. Preferential fluid flow in the human trabecular meshwork near collector channels. Invest Ophthalmol Vis Sci 2009;50(4):1692–7.
110. Inomata H, Bill A, Smelser GK. Aqueous humor pathways through the trabecular meshwork and into Schlemm's canal in the cynomolgus monkey (Macaca irus). An electron microscopic study. Am J Ophthalmol 1972;73(5):760–89.
111. Yang CY, Huynh T, Johnson M, et al. Endothelial glycocalyx layer in the aqueous outflow pathway of bovine and human eyes. Exp Eye Res 2014;128:27–33.
112. Allingham RR, de Kater AW, Ethier CR, et al. The relationship between pore density and outflow facility in human eyes. Invest Ophthalmol Vis Sci 1992;33(5): 1661–9.
113. Braakman ST, Read AT, Chan DW, et al. Colocalization of outflow segmentation and pores along the inner wall of Schlemm's canal. Exp Eye Res 2015;130: 87–96.
114. Johnson M, Chan D, Read AT, et al. The pore density in the inner wall endothelium of Schlemm's canal of glaucomatous eyes. Invest Ophthalmol Vis Sci 2002; 43(9):2950–5.
115. Keller KE, Bradley JM, Vranka JA, et al. Segmental versican expression in the trabecular meshwork and involvement in outflow facility. Invest Ophthalmol Vis Sci 2011;52(8):5049–57.

116. Chang JY, Folz SJ, Laryea SN, et al. Multi-scale analysis of segmental outflow patterns in human trabecular meshwork with changing intraocular pressure. J Ocul Pharmacol Ther 2014;30(2–3):213–23.

117. Battista SA, Lu Z, Hofmann S, et al. Reduction of the available area for aqueous humor outflow and increase in meshwork herniations into collector channels following acute IOP elevation in bovine eyes. Invest Ophthalmol Vis Sci 2008; 49(12):5346–52.

118. Zhu JY, Ye W, Gong HY. Development of a novel two color tracer perfusion technique for the hydrodynamic study of aqueous outflow in bovine eyes. Chin Med J 2010;123(5):599–605.

119. Parc CE, Johnson DH, Brilakis HS. Giant vacuoles are found preferentially near collector channels. Invest Ophthalmol Vis Sci 2000;41(10):2984–90.

120. Dvorak-Theobald G. Further studies on the canal of Schlemm; its anastomoses and anatomic relations. Am J Ophthalmol 1955;39(4 Pt 2):65–89.

121. Cha E, Jin R, Gong H. The relationship between morphological changes and reduction of active areas of aqueous outflow in eyes with primary open angle glaucoma. Paper presented at: ARVO 2013 Annual Meeting. Seattle, WA, May 5–9, 2013.

122. Jackson TL, Hussain A, Hodgetts A, et al. Human scleral hydraulic conductivity: age-related changes, topographical variation, and potential scleral outflow facility. Invest Ophthalmol Vis Sci 2006;47(11):4942–6.

123. Barrie KP, Gum GG, Samuelson DA, et al. Morphologic studies of uveoscleral outflow in normotensive and glaucomatous beagles with fluorescein-labeled dextran. Am J Vet Res 1985;46(1):89–97.

124. Barrie KP, Gum GG, Samuelson DA, et al. Quantitation of uveoscleral outflow in normotensive and glaucomatous Beagles by 3H-labeled dextran. Am J Vet Res 1985;46(1):84–8.

125. Bill A. Formation and drainage of aqueous humour in cats. Exp Eye Res 1966;5: 185–90.

126. Bill A. Effects of atropine and pilocarpine on aqueous humour dynamics in cynomolgus monkeys (Macaca irus). Exp Eye Res 1967;6(2):120–5.

127. Lim KS, Nau CB, O'Byrne MM, et al. Mechanism of action of bimatoprost, latanoprost, and travoprost in healthy subjects. A crossover study. Ophthalmology 2008;115(5):790–5.e4.

Definition, Classification, and Pathophysiology of Canine Glaucoma

 CrossMark

Stefano Pizzirani, DVM, PhD

KEYWORDS

- Canine • Glaucoma • Primary glaucoma • Secondary glaucoma • Open angle
- Closed angle • Goniodysgenesis

KEY POINTS

- Glaucoma is a group of diseases with optic nerve degeneration and blindness as a final outcome.
- In primary glaucoma the main risk factors are age, breed, gender, and goniodysgenesis.
- Classification is based on clinical evaluation and assessment of the iridocorneal angle and ciliary cleft with gonioscopy and ultrasound biomicroscopy.
- Cellular and extracellular progressive changes occur at the level of the lamina cribrosa and in the trabecular meshwork and are responsible for retinal ganglion cell degeneration and decreased outflow.
- Mechanical and vascular theories are predominant to explain the pathogenesis of the disease, leading to oxidative stress and molecular inflammation, which in turn contribute to disease progression.

DEFINITION

Glaucoma is a heterogeneous group of progressive disorders characterized by retinal ganglion cell (RGC) apoptosis and a specific optic neuropathy (glaucomatous optic neuropathy [GON]) associated with cupping of the optic disc. In human patients, peripheral visual field loss and tunnel vision are common initial clinical signs, which may eventually progress to irreversible blindness.[1,2] Primary glaucoma is considered a bilateral disease, although both eyes may not be affected simultaneously.

This definition is widely accepted in medical ophthalmology. Compared with the common definition used in veterinary medicine, several interesting points emerge.

Disclosure: The author has nothing to disclose.
Ophthalmology, Department of Clinical Science, Cummings School of Veterinary Medicine, Tufts University, 200 Westboro Road, North Grafton, MA 01536, USA
E-mail address: stefano.pizzirani@tufts.edu

Vet Clin Small Anim 45 (2015) 1127–1157
http://dx.doi.org/10.1016/j.cvsm.2015.06.002
0195-5616/15/$ – see front matter © 2015 Elsevier Inc. All rights reserved.

First, glaucoma is a group of diseases with many different phenotypes. This variation expands the possible causes and means that its classification is not straightforward.

Second, increased intraocular pressure (IOP), which has historically been a common definition for the disease in small animals, is not mentioned in the accepted definition used by physician ophthalmologists. Increased IOP is considered an important, but not necessary, major risk factor.[3–5] IOP values in humans are not considered sensitive or specific to make a diagnosis or suggest prognosis,[6] because IOP can be normal in patients affected with normotensive glaucoma (NTG).[7]

Unlike in people, increased IOP has historically been a requirement for the diagnosis of clinical glaucoma in dogs,[8] despite pattern-electroretinography (pERG) changes and posterior-segment blood flow abnormalities having been reported before the onset of clinical signs of primary open-angle glaucoma (POAG) in dogs,[9–11] suggesting that pathologic changes in the retina can occur before any increase in IOP. Furthermore, glaucoma is a progressive disease in humans and in dogs even with a controlled normalized IOP, suggesting that additional pathophysiologic mechanisms must be involved.[12]

Recently, an updated version of the definition of glaucoma in animals included increased IOP as a constant risk factor.[8] The differences between the definitions commonly used in physician-based and veterinary ophthalmology may in part relate to the anatomic and functional differences between the 2 species (ie, differences in angle morphology; presence or absence of a central retinal artery), but likely follow largely from small animals with glaucoma typically being initially assessed at an advanced stage of disease. A few factors are responsible for this:

- The inability of nonhuman patients to communicate verbally
- The reliance of the veterinarian on information provided by the pet owner
- The different levels of attentiveness displayed by pet owners regarding changes to their pet's eyes or vision
- The better tolerance dogs are likely to have for initial, prodromic signs not associated with acute pain
- The possibility for dogs to display apparently normal visual behavior until the point at which significant, usually bilateral, vision loss has occurred

Although people undergo regular and periodic assessments when they age, and can report and be tested for peripheral visual field deficits, dogs continue to behave normally even with substantial loss of retinal function.

Besides increased IOP, several other risk factors are considered of major importance and correlate with an increased likelihood of disease occurrence. These factors include:

- Age
- Familial history
- Breed and presence of goniodysgenesis
- Gender
- Systemic blood hypotension

Age

The incidence of primary glaucoma is strongly correlated with aging in several species. Data in **Fig. 1** compare the exponential relationship between age and the incidence of primary glaucoma in humans and the more commonly affected canine

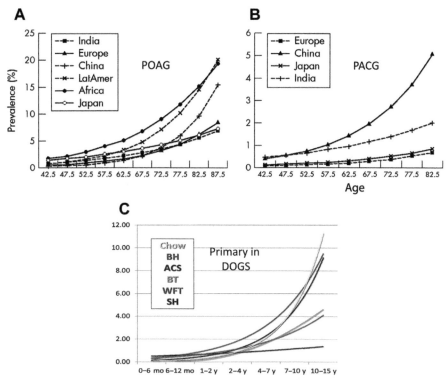

Fig. 1. The prevalence model data showing age-specific incidence of (*A*) POAG and (*B*) primary angle-closure glaucoma (PACG) for the major human ethnic groups in which qualifying studies have been performed. (*C*) An equivalent prevalence model correlated with age in 6 breeds of dogs commonly affected with primary glaucoma. ACS, American Cocker Spaniel; BH, Basset Hound; BT, Boston Terrier; SH, Siberian Husky; WFT, Wire-haired Fox Terrier. (*From* Quigley HA, Broman TA. The number of people with glaucoma worldwide in 2010 and 2020. Br J Ophthalmol 2006;90(3):263; with permission.)

breeds. The variation of the slopes in different breeds of dogs with primary glaucoma clearly reflects the variations seen in different human ethnic groups.[13]

Preexisting age-related changes of the trabecular meshwork (TM) may play a role in the development of increased outflow resistance and increased IOP in various types of glaucoma when other concomitant conditions are present.[14,15] Changes that normally occur with age in the anterior segment of dogs are[15]:

- Progressive exfoliation of the pigmented neuroepithelium (PNE) of the iris at the pupillary edge and vacuolization/hypertrophy of the middle iris PNE. With increasing age, pupillary atrophy and/or pigmented fibrosis can be observed.
- Pigment dispersion in the ciliary cleft and pigment phagocytosis by trabecular endothelial cells.
- Pigment uptake by the nonpigmented ciliary epithelium of the ciliary processes closer to the iris.
- Progressive increase in deposition of collagen at the base of the ciliary processes.
- Increased accumulation of melanin-laden macrophages in the TM, base of the iris, and uveoscleral outflow pathways.

The ultrastructural changes in the TMs of glaucomatous human patients are similar to, albeit more pronounced than, those observed in the normal TM in nonglaucomatous elderly humans.[16–19] These changes include thickening of basal membranes and trabecular beams, their enlargement or collapse, partial loss of endothelial cells and the accumulation of materials such as pigment granules, and an increase in electrodense plaques and collagen.[20] Furthermore, it has been shown that outflow resistance increases normally with age.[21]

In the author's opinion, the increased incidence of the disease with age indicates that associated tissue remodeling may differentially affect tissue homeostasis if it occurs in the presence of other predisposing factors (structural changes such as goniodysgenesis, genetic polymorphisms, metabolic variations, and so forth). We have shown that aging is associated with increased friction between the posterior epithelium of the iris and the increasing size and hardness of the lens.[15,22] The lens may play an essential role in the pathogenesis of primary angle-closure glaucoma (PACG). Clinical studies in human patients suggest that lensectomy and intraocular lens implantation may offer successful IOP control. Lensectomy may eliminate pupillary block and widen the angle.[23] Whether or not removal of the lens decreases physical contact between posterior iris and lenticular tissue in dogs has not been established; it likely does not, considering that following extracapsular lens extraction the friction between the capsulorrhexis edge and the posterior iris epithelium still exists and can often be clinically noted after surgery as pigmentation of the capsulorrhexis edge or anterior chamber pigment dispersion.

The incidence of primary glaucoma in people increases after 40 years of age, which corresponds with increases in both volume and stiffness of the lens.[13] This finding parallels the increased incidence of the disease with age in canine breeds predisposed to PACG, in which the lens is supposed to reach its adult size around 2 years of age[15,22] (discussed later).

Gender

Men are more predisposed to POAG than women, at a ratio 1.37:1.[24] In contrast, PACG more commonly affects women of specific ethnic groups, and is thought to be correlated with a shallower anterior chamber in women.[25] In dogs, in which PACG is the most common form of glaucoma, the overall female/male ratio of the incidence of primary glaucoma is about 2:1.[26–28]

A recent study using high-resolution ultrasonography has shown the angle opening distance (AOD) to be smaller in female than in male dogs. The study used normal beagles, a breed predisposed to POAG,[27] so the correlations between gender differences in the anterior chamber depth and PACG in dogs are so far speculative.

The involvement of immune-mediated and autoimmune mechanisms in glaucoma is discussed later. However, gender association with autoimmune diseases is well documented in people, with women more predisposed to this set of diseases. For example, 60% to 75% of patients affected with rheumatoid arthritis, multiple sclerosis, and myasthenia gravis are women.[29]

Familial History

Genetics have always been considered an important risk factor for development of glaucoma, both in humans and dogs.[30–32] Since the advent of genome-wide association studies (GWAS), the ability to identify causative genes in complex diseases has powerfully increased. Glaucoma is a multifactorial disease, and genetics are not the sole determining factor for the presence of the disease. Nevertheless, it is incontrovertible that a familial history of glaucoma increases an individual's risk of developing the disease. The genetic aspects of glaucoma are discussed by Komár-omy and Petersen-Jones.[33]

Breed and Goniodysgenesis

These 2 factors are associated, and in several predisposed breeds a correlation be-tween glaucoma and developmental defects of the angle has been suggested.[34–36] Goniodysgenesis, a defect in the development of the angle associated with decreased angle width and/or malformation of the pectinate ligament, has genetic causes in humans and likely in dogs, considering its high incidence in specific breeds.[37,38] Wyman and Ketring[39] reported an incidence of 63% in normotensive basset hounds, whereas in normotensive flat-coated retriever and Bouviers the inci-dences of different grades of goniodysgenesis were 35% and 75% respectively.[35,40] The rate of goniodysgenesis in a control group of arbitrarily chosen breeds was 6%.[35]

However, the highest overall incidence of glaucoma in the predisposed breeds does not exceed 6%,[26] whereas the reported incidence of goniodysgenesis can be up to 10 times higher.[39,40] Rates of glaucoma in colonies of predisposed breeds descending from the same ancestor and in which strict genetic connections can be assumed reach 10%.[41] This phenomenon is well recognized in people as well, leading one physician glaucoma specialist to ask the question: "Why are there 10 persons with gonioscopically narrow angles for every 1 who develops ACG?"[42] Clearly, goniodys-genesis alone is insufficient and other factors need to be present or induced to trigger the disease.

Goniodysgenesis varies in severity, morphology, and circumferential involvement. Involvement of 75% or more of the circumference of the angle is associated with an extremely high risk of glaucoma, whereas involvement of less than 25% is usually considered a variation of normal.[35]

A few studies have also reported the grade of goniodysgenesis to be dynamic and to progress with age in certain normotensive dogs.[36,43]

CLASSIFICATION OF GLAUCOMAS

A clear, comprehensive classification of the canine glaucomas is impossible. Glau-coma is considered a multifactorial disease in which numerous genes with varying numbers of alleles and related protein products are involved. Epigenetics may also cause the same genes and proteins to undergo differential regulation and expression. Just as an example, if 100 genes are estimated to be involved in a process and each of them have 5 alleles, then 7,888,609,052,210,118,054,117,285,652,827,862,296, 732,064,351,090,230,047,702,789,306,640,625 genotypes are possible. The relation-ship between genotype, phenotype, and environmental or acquired factors is even more complex. The boundaries between different forms of glaucoma, and even those between normal and affected individuals, become hazy in this context.

The efforts to persevere in the attempt to create a schematic classification of dis-ease are motivated by the following goals[6]:

- To be able to distinguish between healthy, affected, and at-risk patients
- To establish standardized inclusion criteria for each group to define the severity of glaucoma
- To optimize therapy based on an individual's disease phenotype
- To describe progression of visual deficits in a simple format
- To predict and monitor the progression of the disease
- To provide a common language for both clinical and research purposes

The following simplistic categories have historically been adopted to simplify and organize the multiple phenotypes seen clinically and should be considered as large containers, in which multiple, different disease entities may be present.

Canine glaucomas can be classified according to a possible cause as:

- Congenital
- Primary
- Secondary

All glaucomas can also be classified based on the gonioscopic morphology of the iridocorneal angle (ICA) as:

- Open-angle glaucoma
- Narrow-angle glaucoma
- Closed angle[8]

In addition, a pragmatic method of classification takes into account the stage of the disease (discussed by Miller and Bentley[44]).

- Early noncongestive
- Acute or congestive
- Chronic/end stage

These classifications can be used in combination to offer a better, more inclusive description of the clinical condition of an individual patient. Classification has important ramifications for treatment and prognosis. For example, primary glaucoma is considered a bilateral condition and although the fate of the affected eye is often poor, clinicians should focus on preventing or delaying the onset of the disease in the fellow eye by starting prophylactic treatment and suggesting periodic monitoring.[45,46]

Congenital Glaucoma

Congenital glaucoma is a severe form of glaucoma that develops immediately after birth or within the first few months of life. The term congenital may suggest the condition is present at birth; however, although the angle abnormalities may be present at birth, the IOP increase may occur later. Increased IOP is caused by obstruction of aqueous outflow by a severe dysgenesis of the neural crest tissue involved in the formation of the anterior segment, including the TM (**Fig. 2**).[47–49] Several different genes (PAX6, PITX2/RIEG1, LTPB2, FOXC1, CYP1B1)[32,38,50–52] regulate differentiation of tissues involved in TM and ICA formation. Their pleomorphisms or mutations may cause defects in the development of outflow pathways.[50,53–56]

Anterior segment dysgenesis-related glaucoma of this type may be considered as a severe variant of PACG, in which congenital tissue malformations assume a fundamental, primary mechanical role in the development of disease. Congenital glaucomas in dogs and cats are often accompanied by associated anterior segment anomalies, similar to severe Peters and Axenfeld anomalies in humans. Corneal changes are common along with severe buphthalmia caused by the increased elasticity of the scleral tissue in younger individuals. Although congenital glaucomas are developmental in nature and likely involve genetic causes, they can be unilateral. More that 50% of people with some forms of anterior chamber dysgenesis develop glaucoma at some point during their lives, complicating the view of what constitutes a congenital glaucoma.[32,57]

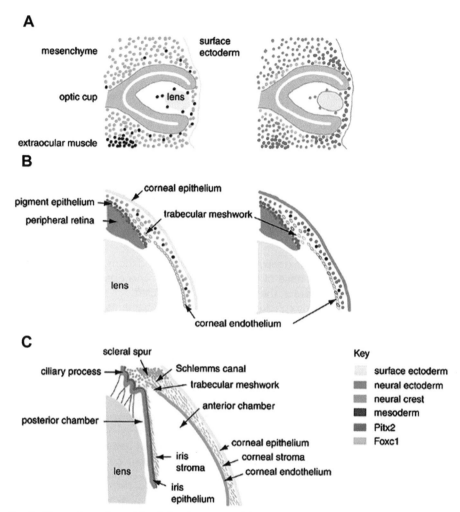

Fig. 2. The embryonic and fetal development of the anterior segment of the eye. (*A*) Optic cup stage. (*B*) Formation of anterior chamber. (*C*) Mature anterior segment depicting the lens, iris, iridocorneal angle, and the cornea. Key shows the color coding used to represent the embryonic origin of the anterior segment tissues in the right-hand plates, and the pattern of expression of the Foxc1 and Pitx2 genes in the left-hand plates, based on published expression data. (*From* Sowden JC. Molecular and developmental mechanisms of anterior segment dysgenesis. Eye (Lond) 2007;21(10):1311; with permission.)

Primary Glaucoma

The term primary (or idiopathic) glaucoma in dogs is used to refer to glaucomas that seem to occur spontaneously for unknown and intrinsic reasons and are thought to be caused by inherent defects in the multiple and complex mechanisms of IOP regulation.[37] No other grossly recognizable ocular disease should be present, like trauma, neoplasia, severe inflammation, lens luxation, or hemorrhage.

Secondary glaucomas occur after other ocular diseases that lead to alterations of the fluid dynamics within the eye. Canine secondary glaucomas will be discussed by Pumphrey.[58]

Primary glaucomas are divided into 2 subcategories, according to the appearance of the ICA.

Primary angle-closure glaucoma

PACG is by far the most common form of primary glaucoma in dogs. It probably has a genetic predisposition[59] and is more common in certain breeds, with American cocker spaniels and basset hounds significantly overrepresented.[26] Because most diagnoses are made in clinically advanced cases, inclusion criteria for PACG include the presence of characteristic clinical signs in the affected eye, absence of signs of other ocular diseases, and gonioscopic abnormalities of the ICA and pectinate ligaments in the fellow, unaffected eye. Angle morphology in the unaffected eye has been found to serve as an accurate indicator of underlying angle morphology in the affected eye, which may be distorted by buphthalmia or secondary angle closure, or may be impossible to visualize because of corneal edema.[22,35,40] Gonioscopic evaluation of the ICA should take into consideration 3 aspects:

- The distance between the deep pigmented scleral band (corresponding with the Schwalbe line) and the base of the peripheral iris.[60] This observation also provides an indirect estimate of the width of the ciliary cleft.
- The conformation and morphology of the pectinate ligaments (PLs).
- The percentage of the circumference of the ICA affected by any noted abnormalities.

These aspects need to be evaluated and considered independently, although their implications are similar.

ICA width is assessed subjectively. Accuracy and reproducibility depend on the clinical experience of the investigator. The span of the PLs over a normal angle in English and American cocker spaniels and basset hounds has been gonioscopically estimated to be 1.5 to 2 mm.[37] The measurements taken on histologic sections show the ICA width to be about 1 mm or less in normal adult beagles. However, variations exist between individuals and breeds. It should also be remembered that these values may change with aging and that scoring should be repeated periodically, especially in patients initially examined at a young age.[36,45,61]

The gonioscopic scoring system for the ICA opening follows the classification suggested by Shaffer[62] (**Table 1**). Ekesten and Narfstrom[34] adapted a similar scoring system for dogs (**Fig. 3**).

Table 1 Gonioscopic scoring system for ICA	
Score	**Number of ICA Degrees Visible**
Grade 4	35–45
Grade 3	20–35
Grade 2	20
Grade 1	≤10
Grade 0	0

Data from Shaffer RN. Primary glaucomas. Gonioscopy, ophthalmoscopy and perimetry. Trans Am Acad Ophthalmol Otolaryngol 1960;64:112–27; and Ekesten B, Narfstrom K. Correlation of morphologic features of the iridocorneal angle to intraocular pressure in Samoyeds. Am J Vet Res 1991;52(11):1875–8.

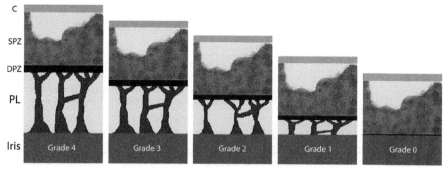

Fig. 3. The different grades of ICA scores at gonioscopy according to the Shaffer scale modified by Ekesten. The width of the ICA decreases from grade 4 (wide open) to 0 (closed) and PLs shorten. Deep pigmented zone (DPL) and superficial pigmented zone (SPZ) are visible. C, conjunctiva. (*Adapted from* Ekesten B. Gonioscopy: some basic principles. J Br Assoc Vet Ophthalmol 1997;2:8–14. *Courtesy of* B. Ekesten, Uppsala, Sweden.)

Normal PLs are usually thin, regular, single strands of iridal tissue spanning the ICA. PL morphology varies considerably between different dogs and even between portions of the ICA within the same animal. When PL dysplasia (PLD) is present, it may take a variety of forms. Less severe forms show larger interligament wide connections, often at the iridal base. More severe PLD is represented by solid sheets of tissue spanning between varying numbers of ligaments. Small holes may be seen between larger sheets, and thin sheets of tissue can be seen covering a normal wide cleft (**Fig. 4**).

Van der Linde-Sipman[40] described 4 degrees of PLD in Bouviers (**Table 2**). Note that only in advanced grades are thicker and shorter, stout, wide sheets of dysplastic ligaments associated with a narrowing of the ICA.[40,63]

Another PLD nomenclature system has been adopted by the European College of Veterinary Ophthalmologists and is accessible online (http://www.ecvo.org/inherited-eye-diseases/ecvo-manual). This classification blends the angle width

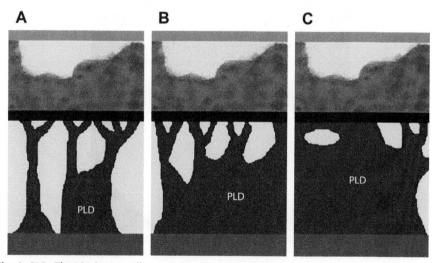

Fig. 4. PLD. The ICA is normally open; however, wider of irislike tissue are occluding the ICA (*A–C*). (*Adapted from* Ekesten B. Gonioscopy: some basic principles. J Br Assoc Vet Ophthalmol 1997;2:8–14. *Courtesy of* B. Ekesten, Uppsala, Sweden.)

Table 2 Degrees of PLD	
Grade	**Description**
1 (Normal)	Single pectinate strands: single insertion on the corneal side Two to 4 strands may originate from a common base at the iris Some connections between adjacent strands may be present Thickness of the strands may vary slightly between dogs
2	Four to 10 PL strands coalesced with broad strands
3	Ten or more PL strands coalesced forming small sheets of tissue Narrowed iridocorneal angle in about 30% of normal eyes
4	Broad solid sheets of iridal tissue with or without flow holes Narrowed iridocorneal angle in about 45% of normal eyes
5	Broad sheets with very short strands on the corneal side No normal pectinate present Narrowed iridocorneal angle in about 46% of normal eyes

and PLD together in a classification using fibrae latae, lamina, and occlusio as categories.

This classification assumes that the PLD is always associated with a narrowing of the ICA, which is not the experience of the author (**Fig. 5**). Although the definitions and scoring criteria seem to be precise and straightforward, consensus about PLD scoring does not exist yet and there are significant limitations created by the extensive variability between dogs and by the subjective interpretations required of the examiner.

Predisposition to disease can be estimated using the overall scores. Once the width and the morphology of the PLs have been evaluated, it is important to determine the degree of ICA circumference involved if changes are found. An important correlation between disease occurrence and the circumferential extension of the defects has

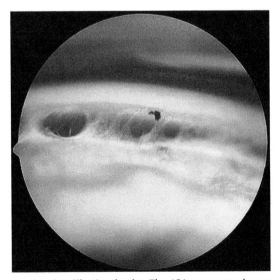

Fig. 5. PLD in a normotensive Siberian husky. The ICA presents abnormal sheets of tissue alternating with large holes. Despite the subalbinotic breed, pigment dispersion is present in the ICA, indicating its origin from the posterior pigmented epithelium of the iris. The ICA width is normal.

been reported.[40,63] Less than 25% of circumference involved is considered a normal variation, whereas more than 75% is highly associated with the occurrence of glaucoma.[34,63]

Ultrasonography biomicroscopy (UBM) using probes of 35 to 50 MHz, although less commonly available, is a useful means for assessment of angle opening and ciliary cleft width and provides valuable supplementary information to gonioscopy.

Primary open-angle glaucoma

This is the most common form of glaucoma in humans and the least common in dogs. The considerable amount of literature regarding POAG in dogs is the result of specific colonies of beagles having provided a spontaneous model of disease for the study of human POAG. Affected animals are gonioscopically normal at early stages of the disease in glaucomatous eyes (or are gonioscopically normal in the fellow eye when gonioscopy is not reliable or possible in the glaucomatous eye). The ICA progressively closes because of the effects of increased IOP in the moderate to late stages of POAG. Clinical signs may be observed as early as 6 to 18 months of age in beagles.[64]

About 30% of humans with POAG may have an IOP within normal ranges and are classified as having NTG.[65] In this case diagnosis is made on retinal and optic nerve findings. Whether an equivalent normotensive form exists in dogs is still a matter of debate. Pattern-ERG findings in predisposed beagles with early stage disease (absence of clinical signs with mean IOP of 27.7 mm Hg) already show signs of RGC damage.[9,10] POAG is uncommonly encountered in veterinary clinical practice. Because its signs are insidious and develop slowly over the course of several months, diagnosis on client-owned pets is usually made only in clinically advanced cases.

PATHOGENESIS AND PATHOPHYSIOLOGY OF PRIMARY GLAUCOMA

A current view of the pathogenesis of glaucoma must account for multiple factors (**Fig. 6**). Numerous genetic/epigenetic, age-related, immunologic, and vascular factors interact to activate a series of cascades with optic nerve degeneration as a common final outcome.

Ocular damage in the course of glaucoma, primarily GON, follows from mechanisms that lead to outflow obstruction (and subsequent increased IOP) and RGC apoptosis.

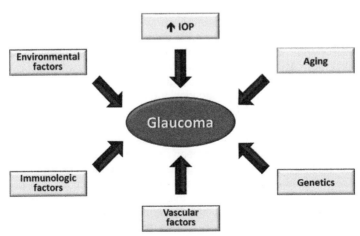

Fig. 6. Glaucoma is a multifactorial disease. Several of the main contributing factors are indicated.

Although not mutually exclusive, the two factors are not necessarily linked, because in humans RGC apoptosis may occur without increased IOP.

In dogs, however, increased IOP seems to be a prerequisite. The only possible reason for an increase in IOP is a decrease in aqueous outflow. In normal canine eyes, the primary site for flow resistance in the TM has been identified in the extracellular matrix (ECM) of the juxtacanalicular connective tissue (JCT) and in the inner wall of the angular aqueous plexus, which in dogs is analogous to the Schlemm canal in primates.[66] Because the 2 main types of primary glaucoma in dogs (PACG and POAG) refer to disruptions in different portions of the ICA and cleft, the obstruction of the outflow in the two forms may have different causes.

Primary Angle-closure Glaucoma

The pathogenesis and the pathophysiology of PACG are still unknown. A recent GWAS compared genotypes of affected and nonaffected basset hounds. Two allelic variants, positioned on chromosomes 14 and 20 respectively, were found with higher frequency in affected dogs. The stronger candidate gene was COL1A2, suggesting a likely contribution of collagen mutations to the pathogenesis of PACG in dogs. The obvious histologic finding in PACG is the collapse of the ciliary cleft. Whether this specific finding occurs secondary to an already increased IOP generated elsewhere in the outer outflow pathways (ie, JCT) or whether it is primarily generated by slow progressive intrinsic mechanisms in the cleft itself is unknown. Both mechanisms could be present at the same time. However, it is interesting to note that a progressive, age-related decrease in the ciliary cleft width has been documented in dogs with normal ICA, in dogs with different grades of goniodysgenesis, and in early glaucomatous dogs.[36,43,61]

Because of clear anatomic differences, the theories applied to PACG in human patients cannot automatically be applied to veterinary medicine. PACG in people is considered a disorder of ocular anatomy.[23,67] In ethnic groups predisposed to PACG the anterior chamber is shallower, the lens larger, and the filtration angle width is decreased.[68] The apposition of the peripheral iris with the peripheral cornea or formation of peripheral anterior synechiae can cause the obstruction of the TM, which in primates is located anterior to the iris base.[23] Miller and colleagues[69] hypothesized that similar mechanisms involving the position of the iris might be responsible for some forms of PACG in dogs. A reverse pupillary block with flattening and attachment of the iris tip to the lens and subsequent anterior bowing of the base of the iris secondary to increased aqueous humor pressure in the posterior chamber has been suggested. Ekesten and Torrang[22] also proposed that age-related increased lens thickness may cause pupillary block and be a contributor to PACG in Samoyeds with goniodysgenesis.

In the opinion of this author, age-related pigment dispersion, tissue remodeling, and modest but constant inflammatory reactions and fibrosis are responsible for the progressive, irreversible closure of the ciliary cleft and also produce qualitative and quantitative ECM modifications of the outflow pathways (**Fig. 7**).[70] The presence of pigment dispersion and mononuclear inflammatory infiltrates in the anterior segment of canine eyes enucleated because of PACG has been also reported by other investigators.[71] A pivotal role in pathogenesis may be assigned to macrophages (discussed later) and TM cells. TM cell levels decrease with age in normal individuals, and do so more rapidly in glaucomatous patients, in whom they show clear pathologic changes.[17,72,73] TM cells are extremely susceptible to mitochondrial dysfunction and oxidative stress, both of which increase with age and can be major contributors to cell loss.[74,75] In addition, TM cells are able to release/produce humoral factors and express cytokine receptors whose upregulation or downregulation may further contribute to

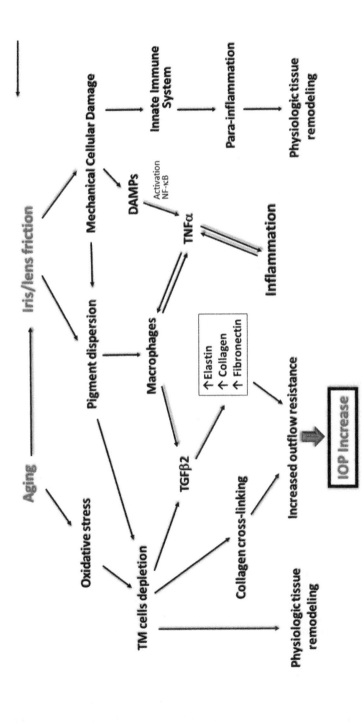

Fig. 7. IOP increases when the resistance to aqueous outflow increases. The obstruction of the outflow facilities occurs because of a progressive deposition of ECM in the TM. Several mechanisms and factors may interact to contribute to ECM deposition and collapse of the ciliary cleft. DAMPs, damage-associated molecular patterns; NF-κB, nuclear factor kappa B; TGFβ2, transforming growth factor beta-2; TNFα, tumor necrosis factor alpha.

the changes seen in glaucoma and explain increased outflow resistance.[76–78] In particular, increased expression and activation of transforming growth factor beta-2 (TGFβ2) or downregulation of metalloproteinases may be associated with fibrosis and decreased outflow.[79,80]

Primary Open-angle Glaucoma

Although the pathogenesis of POAG in dogs is still obscure and the pathophysiologic mechanisms not completely described, the obstruction seems to affect the outer corneoscleral and the uveoscleral TM, with increased deposition of membranelike materials, collagen type VI, and elastin material, causing thickening and increased stiffness of the ECM of the JCT.[81]

POAG in beagles has recently been linked to a mutation in a region of the metalloproteinase gene ADAMTS10. This mutation found in beagles affected with POAG would support an altered processing of ECM and/or defects in microfibril structure that would eventually contribute to a decreased outflow and subsequently to an increased intraocular pressure.[31,82]

THEORIES AND MECHANISMS

The main end point in all forms of glaucoma is GON, the characteristic features of which are interlinked: RGC death, activation of glial cells, tissue remodeling, and changes in blood flow (**Fig. 8**).[83]

The cascades that cause RGC apoptosis are extremely complex. The RGCs are the innermost neurons of the retina and their axons form the optic nerve. All the photic information collected by photoreceptors is eventually carried to the brain by the RGC axons, which travel in the nerve fiber layer of the retina and converge to form the optic nerve at the optic disc. Axons are not myelinated while traveling inside the eye, but become myelinated (and are then visible as the whitish head of the optic nerve) at the level of the lamina cribrosa, a specialized portion of the sclera in the posterior pole of the globe. The lamina cribrosa is a round structure of about 1 to 2 mm diameter where the lamellae of connective tissues that form the scleral wall assume a specific configuration. The lamina cribrosa, which contains numerous cell bodies (mainly those of astrocytes), is considered a highly specialized form of ECM, different from the scleral tissue. The lamellae of the lamina cribrosa have pores that are aligned to allow passage of RGC axons while maintaining normal IOP and normal axonal function. The axons carry visual information to the lateral geniculate body in the midbrain, where they have their first synapses with cerebral neurons. The axons contain the axoplasm, the equivalent of cytoplasm in nonneuronal cells. However, its composition differs from the cytoplasm of cells in other tissues. The characteristic features of the axoplasm are the presence of bidirectional flow of molecules and neurotransmitters, and a large mitochondrial population, necessary for providing energy to a cell with high metabolic needs.

Axoplasmic flow is a physiologic phenomenon, energy dependent, and is responsible for transit of metabolic products along the axon. There are 2 flow directions, 1 away from the cell body (orthograde) and 1 toward the cell body (retrograde). Although RGCs deliver visual neurotransmission to the lateral geniculate body neurons orthogradely with membrane-related mechanisms, at the same time they receive vital neurotrophic factors via retrograde flow. When axoplasmic flow is obstructed, major disruptions in cell physiology occur and RGCs die via apoptosis. Apoptosis causes cytoplasmic and nuclear condensation and fragmentation of DNA.[84] Degenerated debris of apoptotic cells are removed by rapid phagocytosis by the surrounding cells, and apoptotic cellular death was previously not considered to cause inflammation.[85]

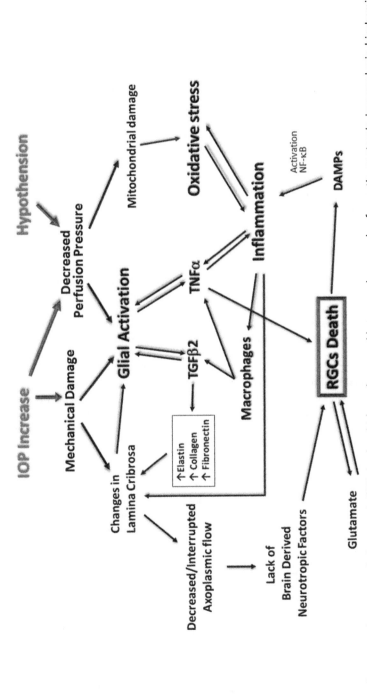

Fig. 8. The eventual outcome of glaucoma is RGC death, which can be caused by a complex cascade of genetic, anatomic, immunologic, biochemical, mechanical, and vascular events.

The concept of apoptosis as a noninflammatory process has recently been called into question and molecular inflammation has now been associated with apoptosis.[86,87] The release of molecules from dying cells is able to trigger a series of receptors that activate and upregulate further release of growth factors and inflammatory cytokines.

In glaucoma, obstruction of the axoplasmic flow in the axons of the RGCs occurs at the level of the lamina cribrosa and this event is considered pivotal in the pathophysiology of GON.[88] An IOP of 30 to 35 mm Hg compromises 87% of axoplasmic flow in beagles with POAG.[89] One of the most detrimental consequences of the interruption of axoplasmic flow is the impeded delivery of neurotrophic factors to the cell body, which in turn promotes apoptosis. Brain-derived neurotrophic factor is the most essential peptide for RGC survival.[90–92] Axonal loss after RGC death and modifications in the ECM of the lamina cribrosa cause optic nerve cupping that is visible on fundic examination.

Overall, 2 major pathogenic theories have been suggested to account for RGC loss: mechanical and vascular. These events may be independent primary events, may occur in association with one another, or may have a sequential or causative relationship.[93]

Increased IOP is considered the main causative factor for the changes observed at the level of the optic cup; however, mechanical stress cannot explain the phenotypes that in people are associated with normal IOP. Vascular hypotension and its associated consequences are considered responsible for inducing laminar changes, optic nerve cupping, and RGC apoptosis. Vascular damage in the retina has been associated with glutamate redistribution in dogs with glaucoma.[94] Furthermore, vascular dysregulation leads to ischemia and reperfusion injury, thereby inducing oxidative damage. Oxidative damage has been shown to affect both TM cells and RGCs.[95–97]

Mechanical Theory

Increased, unsustainable IOP can induce stretching of the scleral lamina cribrosa and secondary damage to RGC axons.[98] As mentioned earlier, the lamina cribrosa has a unique anatomy. The lamellae display pores that are aligned to allow the passage of the RGC axons. In glaucoma, the lamellae that form the lamina cribrosa rotate and collapse. Axon paths are distorted and squeezed and the axoplasmic flow is severely and irreparably compromised.[99] The lamina cribrosa is also considered a specialized form of ECM, in which modifications and remodeling occur under mechanical and hypotensive vascular stress. Astrocytes are the major glial cell component of the optic nerve head. Astrocytes express mechanoreceptors that are sensitive to pressure changes that activate them from the quiescent form. Activated astrocytes can significantly contribute to collagen deposition and gliosis (scarring). These intrinsic modifications of the laminar ECM may also contribute to permanently decreased levels of axoplasmic flow.[89]

At the same time, increased IOP also affects ocular blood vessels and decreased tissue perfusion. There is consensus regarding reduction of ocular blood flow in glaucoma.[100] Ocular perfusion pressure corresponds with the mean systemic blood pressure minus IOP, and it is important in regulating the ocular blood flow. Either systemic hypotension or increased IOP can cause a dysregulation of the ocular perfusion.

Vascular Theory

The vascular hypothesis presumes primary tissue ischemia. Both primary and secondary vasospasm syndromes can cause decreased ocular perfusion.[101] The occurrence of primary or secondary hypoxia is well established in glaucomatous eyes and hypoxia of 6 hours' duration is sufficient to induce permanent damage in RGCs.[102] Moreover, low blood pressure in humans is considered a major risk factor and the association between systemic hypotension and glaucomatous damage is well documented.[103]

Ischemic tissue damage and reperfusion injury lead to tissue remodeling, and cellular and ECM changes may then be responsible for an increased resistance to outflow in the TM and in the posterior ciliary body, and axon compression at the level of the lamina cribrosa.[104] This theory provides a pathogenetic mechanism for NTG in people and could explain retinal changes discovered with pERG before the onset of clinical signs in beagles.[9,10] Color Doppler imaging in glaucomatous beagles has shown decreased blood velocities and increased pulsatility and resistive indexes in orbital and ocular arteries compared with normal beagles. Retinal artery blood flow velocities were not different in the two groups.[105] Affected beagles investigated with the same modality during a 4-year longitudinal study showed the blood flow abnormalities to be progressive and to occur ahead of increases in IOP.[11] Whether the changes observed in dogs can be translated to humans is uncertain. Vascular anatomy differs significantly between primates and dogs. Primates have a central retinal artery that supplies the arterial venules and choroidal vascular regulation is separate from retinal vascular regulation. However, the optic nerve is supplied by short posterior ciliary arteries in both species.[83,106,107] Similarities in the vascular pathogenesis of GON could be possible in different species.

Pathophysiologic Mechanisms

The mechanical and vascular theories of RGC damage involve common mechanisms that include:

- Mitochondrial dysfunction
- Oxidative stress
- Activation of glial cells
- Tissue remodeling
- Deprivation of neurotrophic factors
- Glutamate excitotoxicity
- Immune-mediated mechanisms

All these mechanisms are linked and some can trigger or influence each other. This list represents only those mechanisms that have received the most research attention. Likely other molecular and biochemical phenomena are involved, of which clinicians may not yet be fully aware. The sheer number of potential mechanisms also highlights the limitations of some of the therapeutic approaches that target specific single mediators of disease.

Metabolomic and proteomic studies may provide a wider understanding of the dynamic changes that occur in the eye as a whole.[108]

Mitochondrial dysfunction

Mitochondria are plentiful in RGC axons and are essential for neuronal function. Mitochondria are more numerous in RGC axons than in the somata, providing the high level of energy that is necessary for nerve conduction.[109] They are very sensitive to dysregulation of axoplasmic flow,[89,110] and undergo degenerative damage when axoplasmic flow is compromised in glaucoma.[111] Reactive oxygen species (ROS) are normal end products of the energy-producing mitochondrial aerobic respiration (or oxidative phosphorylation) and are potentially harmful for cells when they accumulate; however, in normal conditions, a mitochondrial reducing enzymatic system neutralizes ROS, which are used as a signaling system. Mitochondria are the major producers of ROS in mammalian cells.[112]

There is evidence that mitochondrial function decreases with age and this is correlated with a decreased efficacy of the ROS scavenging system, which alters the redox balance. Mitochondrial dysfunction corresponds with a decreased production in ATP, which provides energy for cellular functions.[113] Neurons are more susceptible than other cells to cellular damage secondary to decreases in mitochondrial function because their high metabolic rate necessitates high levels of ATP for regulating transmembrane ion transport.[114] Primary or secondary ischemic damage to RGC axons and/or ECM modifications causing compression to axons and altered flow are both events that occur during glaucoma and, when combined with the effects of age, cause even further mitochondrial dysfunction with subsequent higher rate of neuronal loss. Mitochondrial dysfunction also contributes to increased RGC susceptibility to inflammatory cytokines and toxic substances released by glial cells in the extracellular space.[109] Furthermore, increased amounts of ROS are released into the surrounding milieu, activating other important pathologic cascades in nearby cells and tissues. The most dramatic consequence of ROS accumulation is oxidative stress. Oxidative damage leads to accumulation of damaged/misfolded proteins; increased mutagenesis rate; and last, but not least, to inflammation.[115]

Oxidative stress

Oxidative stress is tightly linked to mitochondrial function.[96,116] Oxidative stress is involved in aging changes and in the pathogenesis of a large number of age-related diseases, especially neurodegenerative disorders.[117,118] Each cell is normally provided with enough antioxidant capacity to buffer the damage caused by excessive accumulation of ROS and reactive nitrogen species (RNS). When ROS and RNS production exceeds the normal tolerance of cells, oxidative stress perpetuates severe damage to mitochondrial and cellular proteins, lipids, and nucleic acids, and may activate molecular patterns of inflammation.[96,119]

Both increased IOP and hypoxia are able to induce oxidative stress and reperfusion injury in the retina.[102] Nitric oxide (NO) is an important RNS. At physiologic levels NO is an important vasodilator and neurotransmitter generated at low levels by 2 constitutive isoforms of the enzyme NO synthase (NOS). The 2 isoforms are secreted by nervous tissue (nNOS or NOS-1) and by endothelial cells (eNOS or NOS-3). In pathologic conditions like infections, inflammation, or ischemic injury, macrophages produce high levels of a third, inducible isoform (iNOS or NOS-2). NOS-2 produces high levels of NO that cause oxidative stress, leading to cell and tissue damage.[120] Endothelin-1 is a protein expressed by glial cells after reperfusion injury. Endothelin-1 induces vasospasm and contributes to increased hypoxia.[83] Levels of endothelin-1 and NO are both significantly increased in the aqueous and in the vitreous of American cocker spaniels with PACG.[12] Other markers for oxidative stress are also increased in the early stages of PACG in dogs.[121]

In addition, and perhaps most significantly, oxidative stress is also able to stimulate an immune reaction, activating glial cells or macrophages, upregulating the expression of tumor necrosis factor alpha (TNFα), and increasing the antigen-presenting abilities of resident cells.[118]

Activation of glial cells

In the normal optic nerve, quiescent astrocytes are vital for RGCs health. They are the most widespread glial cell type and support optic nerve fibers at the lamina cribrosa in most mammals.[1] Astrocytes are intimately connected with each other and communicate through gap junctions, forming a syncytium. They create the structural interface between RGC axons, connective tissue, and vasculature.[122] Astrocytes normally produce collagen and elastin and maintain the homeostasis of the ECM in the lamina cribrosa. They also provide neurotrophic factors to axons and contribute to removal of glutamate from the extracellular space.[1,123,124]

Normal quiescent astrocytes become activated by mechanical and hypotensive stresses and then assume a predominant role in the development of GON. Activated astrocytes produce increased amounts of collagen and elastin and release cytokines,[125] among which TNFα is the most important. This activation is responsible for elastosis of the lamina (disorganized deposition of ECM material) and the formation of a glial scar that eventually compresses optic nerve axons and contributes to RGC death.[122,126] Astrocytes express type 1 and type 2 receptors for TGFβ2, which is the fibrosis-inducing cytokine eventually responsible for laminar elastosis. TGFβ2 also increases the expression of fibronectin and type I, IV, and VI collagen in optic nerve astrocytes.[20,127]

At the same time, activated glial cells represent a source themselves for TGFβ2 production.[128]

Microglia are the other glial cell type populating the optic nerve tissue, retina and central nervous system. Although astrocytes are structurally supportive, microglia are the equivalent of tissue-resident macrophages and have defensive, immunologic roles. Like astrocytes, they are quiescent cells in their normal state.[1] Mechanical, vascular, and also biochemical stimuli (TNFα) can activate microglia and disrupt homeostasis.[129] Activated microglia become migratory, antigen-presenting cells that trigger immune responses and upregulate cell receptors. Activated microglia induce upregulation of proinflammatory mediators (TNFα, interleukin [IL]-1β, IL-6, cyclooxygenase-2, and NOS-2) and TGFβ2, and subsequent release of neurotoxic substances (NO, endothelin-1) contributing to GON.[90,130,131]

Glutamate

Glutamate is an essential amino acid and the most common and diffuse excitatory neurotransmitter in the nervous system, including the retina.[132] Glutamate acts through 2 main classes of receptors but it is its binding to the N-methyl-D-aspartate (NMDA) subtype that seems to be responsible for RGC toxicity. The degenerative effects of an excess of glutamate on the inner retina and optic nerve were first reported many years ago.[133] In glaucoma, an excess release of extracellular glutamate has been reported from damaged retinal cells along with increased activation and channeling of NMDA receptors.[134,135] Intracellular glutamate levels were lower in glaucomatous dogs compared with normal dogs, leading to the speculation that, in patients with glaucoma, more of the amino acid is present extracellularly.[136] The activation of NMDA receptors corresponds with an increased influx of Ca^{++} ions within the cells, leading to extrinsic activation of caspases and eventual cellular apoptosis.[132] This phenomenon, called glutamate excitotoxicity, received much attention in several species, dogs included, in the late 1990s and early 2000s[89,134–137] and seemed to suggest new neuroprotective therapeutic strategies.[138,139] Although glutamate release from photoreceptors and its accumulation in Mueller cells was later reported in dogs with primary glaucoma, its role in excitotoxicity is still not clear.[140]

More recently there has been a lack of reproducibility in the initial data and conflicting findings have been reported.[12,141–143] However, a well-documented case of scientific fraud has undermined the value of this information and more work needs to be done to determine the true role of glutamate in GON.[143–145]

Immune-mediated and autoimmune mechanisms

It is becoming obvious that immune-mediated and autoimmune mechanisms connect and regulate the numerous events that induce the functional and structural pathologic changes noted in glaucoma, both in the anterior chamber and at the level of the optic nerve.[146–149] An increasing, substantial body of evidence supports a strong relationship between aging, age-related diseases and neurodegeneration, and oxidative stress and low-grade, chronic, subclinical molecular inflammation.[119,150]

Normal tissue homeostasis requires tissue remodeling to adjust to even normal stress stimuli. Parainflammation is an innate response of damaged tissues to induce tissue remodeling and maintain intraocular homeostasis.[151] The ECM in the TM normally responds by increasing or decreasing its permeability to adjust to physiologic IOP fluctuations, and proteins like metalloproteinases are involved in this recoiling process.[152] These responses may lead to pathologically important changes when the pressure stress is high, with age, or with genetic variations in the translation of proteins involved with ECM modifications.[153–157]

In glaucomatous human patients the blood-aqueous barrier is often disrupted and the quality of the proteins and cytokines present varies from that expressed in normal aqueous.[158] In the author's opinion, immunologic mechanisms are also involved in the outflow obstruction in dogs, and the role of mononuclear cells, particularly macrophages, is crucial. Pigment dispersion and mononuclear inflammatory infiltrates have been associated with PACG in dogs.[70,71] Mild flare and faint signs of uveitis are common findings in acutely presented glaucomatous dogs and pigment dispersion and floating cells in the anterior chamber have been noted by the author in patients that subsequently developed increased intraocular pressures.

Aging in dogs is greatly associated with pigment dispersion and phagocytosis.[159] Lens stiffness and volume increase with age, thereby increasing friction between the lens and the posterior iris surface. This friction leads to a low-grade but progressive damage of the posterior epithelium of the iris and anterior capsule with release of pigment granules from the posterior iris pigmented epithelium. This pigment can easily be found in the TM, phagocytized by the trabecular endothelial cells, dispersed free between the beams and lamellae of the TM, engulfing macrophages at the collector channel ostia, at the base of the ciliary processes and iris, and also accumulating between the longitudinal bundles of the ciliary muscle in the posterior ciliary body. These changes are the expression of microdamage to the tissues of the anterior segment.

Alarmins are endogenous damage-associated molecular patterns released by damaged cells. They can activate the production of several proinflammatory cytokines (TNFα, IL-1β, and IL-6) and trigger both innate and adaptive immune systems.[160] The balance and the interaction between the two defensive systems are labile and they may easily overlap. Complex genetic and epigenetic factors drive the responses in different directions. In particular, alarmins can link to receptors for advanced glycation end-products (RAGE) on mononuclear or glial cells and activate an important nuclear transcription factor (nuclear factor kappa B [NF-κB]) that is mostly responsible for inducing production of proinflammatory cytokines. Alarmins are also able to activate antigen-presenting cells (APCs),[160] which may activate adaptive autoimmune responses.

Macrophages are quickly recruited to phagocytize materials present in the outflow pathways.[161] An increased number of melanin-laden macrophages accumulate in the TM and free melanin is phagocytized by trabecular cells. With time, largely engulfed TM cells slough off the trabecular beams exposing the underlying collagen and elastin. Age-related oxidative stress is also considered one of the possible causes for cellular depletion in the TM.[95] Endothelial trabecular cells decrease consistently with age, more in dogs than in humans.[162] Age and TM cell depletion are associated with cross-linking, fusion, thickening, and increased stiffness of the collagen beams.[73,163]

Humans with POAG show greater than average, excessive cell loss of TM cells.[164] All this may affect the outflow facilities (both trabecular and uveoscleral), with a substantial decrease in the permeability of the tissues. It has long been considered that accumulation and stiffness of the ECM components in the TM is the major reason for a decreased filtering ability of the JCT. Several possible mechanisms have been proposed and TGFβ2, a cytokine that stimulates fibrosis and collagen deposition, has been the focus of extensive research. TGFβ2 is abundantly present in a latent form in the anterior segment. Macrophages are a major source for production and activation of TGFβ2.[165]

Few normal ocular tissues and/or eye-derived cultured cells, such as TM cells, ciliary body epithelial cells, and retinal pigment epithelial cells, have been shown to produce this cytokine in the latent, inactive form. The nonpigmented ciliary epithelium, the microfibrils of the zonule, and the ones surrounding the elastin core in the ECM are the major sites for storage.[82] Activation of TGFβ2 is induced by other proteins, among which plasmin and matricellular thrombospondin-1 (TSP1) are the most important.[166,167] However, membrane receptors are necessary to activate the intracellular signals for production of ECM proteins. CD36 is a receptor present on macrophages that binds TSP1 and activated TGFβ2.[167] The active form of the cytokine is responsible for the fibrotic changes in connective tissues. Only activated TGFβ2 can trigger ECM modifications and collagen deposition. Its activation is not yet well described and likely involves expression, suppression, and modulation of several other proteins. TGFβ2 promotes the formation of ECM components produced by fibroblasts and endothelial cells.[77] The increase in ECM material in the TM has also been positively correlated with a decrease in TM cells. TGFβ2 increases the intraocular expression of the enzyme plasminogen activator inhibitor.[127] Plasminogen activates metalloproteinases that promote collagen proteolysis.[168] Increased levels of TGFβ2 therefore contribute to the decreased permeability of the ECM in the TM.[169] The combination of goniodysgenesis, age-related pigment dispersion and activation of trabecular cells and macrophages, and eventually the fusion of the exposed collagen of the trabecular beams and newly cytokine-induced collagen deposition may all be factors associated with the ciliary cleft collapse that has been seen to progress with age[36,61] and that can eventually lead to clinically apparent increases in IOP in patients with sufficient predisposing factors.

The involvement of resident or recruited macrophages may also lead to different macrophage polarization. A predominance of M2 macrophages is associated with lack of overt inflammation, but with the tendency to tissue scarring and fibrosis as described earlier.[170] However, M1 macrophages increase immune response and induce inflammatory cascades.[170] Macrophages and activated microglia are also the main sources for TNFα and IL-1, IL-2, and IL-6.[171,172] At the same time, they are also highly responsive to TNFα, which is at increased levels in the aqueous humor in glaucoma. Besides TNFα, macrophages express NOS-2 and use NO as a cytotoxic effector to face invaders or foreign proteins. Induced NO contributes to ongoing oxidative damage to trabecular tissues, because RNS leads to the direct activation of macrophages and their production of TNFα and IL-1β.[173]

TNFα, a potent proinflammatory cytokine, orchestrates the inflammatory response in many immune-mediated and autoimmune diseases. Upregulated TNFα is also implicated in other neurodegenerative diseases like Alzheimer and Parkinson.[174,175] Its receptor TNF-R1 is named the death receptor because is also associated with cellular apoptosis. Both TNFα and TNF-R1 are upregulated in glaucoma and they both have a crucial role in GON.[176] TNFα is also upregulated in the aqueous humor in humans and dogs with glaucoma.[177,178] TNFα is upregulated in the vitreous in glaucomatous human patients and TNFα experimentally injected in the vitreous in normal mice can induce the degenerative changes characteristic of GON, without increasing the IOP.[179] Increased TNFα levels activate microglial cells, the retinal and optic nerve macrophages, which produce additional amounts of TNFα, disrupting the homeostatic balance and starting a vicious cycle.

Besides activating inflammatory cascades, TNFα also has an indirect but substantial role in RGC death through transformation of inactive, soluble Fas ligand (FasL) into membrane-bound FasL on RGCs. The binding of FasL to the RGC membrane activates caspases, a series of intracytoplasmic enzymes responsible for inducing apoptosis.[180,181]

SUMMARY

Comprehension of the mechanisms that may cause glaucoma is difficult and extremely complex (see **Figs. 7** and **8**). Structural changes in the anterior and posterior segments occur normally with age and the modulation of subsequent tissue remodeling can be an important event in the pathogenesis of glaucoma in predisposed individuals. The quality of tissue remodeling may be influenced by anatomic, immunologic, and genetic factors. Mechanical and vascular changes are primary triggers for cellular activation leading to ECM modifications and molecular inflammation under oxidative stress. TM cells, glial cells, and macrophages and their associated receptors, cytokines, and growth factors play a prominent role in tissue modifications. Final outcomes are increased resistance to outflow and/or RGC death.

ACKNOWLEDGMENTS

The author would like to acknowledge the terrific help from Dr Stephanie Pumphrey for the editing of the article.

REFERENCES

1. Hernandez MR. The optic nerve head in glaucoma: role of astrocytes in tissue remodeling. Prog Retin Eye Res 2000;19(3):297–321.
2. Gupta V, You Y, Li J, et al. BDNF impairment is associated with age-related changes in the inner retina and exacerbates experimental glaucoma. Biochim Biophys Acta 2014;1842(9):1567–78.
3. Gordon MO, Beiser JA, Brandt JD, et al. The Ocular Hypertension Treatment Study: baseline factors that predict the onset of primary open-angle glaucoma. Arch Ophthalmol 2002;120(6):714–20 [discussion: 829–30].
4. Leske MC, Heijl A, Hussein M, et al. Factors for glaucoma progression and the effect of treatment: the early manifest glaucoma trial. Arch Ophthalmol 2003; 121(1):48–56.
5. Van Veldhuisen PC, Ederer F, Gaasterland DE, et al. The advanced glaucoma intervention study (AGIS): 7. The relationship between control of intraocular pressure and visual field deterioration. Am J Ophthalmol 2000;130(4):429–40.
6. Brusini P, Johnson CA. Staging functional damage in glaucoma: review of different classification methods. Surv Ophthalmol 2007;52(2):156–79.
7. Klein BE, Klein R, Sponsel WE, et al. Prevalence of glaucoma. The Beaver Dam Eye Study. Ophthalmology 1992;99(10):1499–504.
8. Plummer CE, Regnier A, Gelatt KN. The canine glaucomas. In: Gelatt KN, Gilger BC, Kern TJ, editors. Veterinary ophthalmology, vol. 2, 5th edition. Ames (IA): John Wiley, Inc; 2013. p. 1050–145.

9. Ofri R, Dawson WW, Foli K, et al. Primary open-angle glaucoma alters retinal recovery from a thiobarbiturate: spatial frequency dependence. Exp Eye Res 1993;56(4):481–8.
10. Ofri R, Samuelson DA, Strubbe DT, et al. Altered retinal recovery and optic nerve fiber loss in primary open-angle glaucoma in the beagle. Exp Eye Res 1994; 58(2):245–8.
11. Gelatt KN, Miyabayashi T, Gelatt-Nicholson KJ, et al. Progressive changes in ophthalmic blood velocities in Beagles with primary open angle glaucoma. Vet Ophthalmol 2003;6(1):77–84.
12. Kallberg ME, Brooks DE, Gelatt KN, et al. Endothelin-1, nitric oxide, and glutamate in the normal and glaucomatous dog eye. Vet Ophthalmol 2007; 10(Suppl 1):46–52.
13. Quigley HA, Broman AT. The number of people with glaucoma worldwide in 2010 and 2020. Br J Ophthalmol 2006;90(3):262–7.
14. Tektas OY, Lutjen-Drecoll E. Structural changes of the trabecular meshwork in different kinds of glaucoma. Exp Eye Res 2009;88(4):769–75.
15. Pizzirani S, Desai SJ, Pirie CG, et al. Age related changes in the anterior segment of the eye in normal dogs. Vet Ophthalmol 2010;13(6):421.
16. Tian B, Geiger B, Epstein DL, et al. Cytoskeletal involvement in the regulation of aqueous humor outflow. Invest Ophthalmol Vis Sci 2000;41(3):619–23.
17. Alvarado J, Murphy C, Juster R. Trabecular meshwork cellularity in primary open-angle glaucoma and nonglaucomatous normals. Ophthalmology 1984; 91(6):564–79.
18. Grierson I, Hogg P. The proliferative and migratory activities of trabecular meshwork cells. Prog Retin Eye Res 1995;15(1):33–67.
19. Babizhayev MA, Brodskaya MW. Fibronectin detection in drainage outflow system of human eyes in ageing and progression of open-angle glaucoma. Mech Ageing Dev 1989;47(2):145–57.
20. Lutjen-Drecoll E. Morphological changes in glaucomatous eyes and the role of TGFbeta2 for the pathogenesis of the disease. Exp Eye Res 2005;81(1):1–4.
21. Becker B. The decline in aqueous secretion and outflow facility with age. Am J Ophthalmol 1958;46(5 Part 1):731–6.
22. Ekesten B, Torrang I. Age-related changes in ocular distances in normal eyes of Samoyeds. Am J Vet Res 1995;56(1):127–33.
23. Tarongoy P, Ho CL, Walton DS. Angle-closure glaucoma: the role of the lens in the pathogenesis, prevention, and treatment. Surv Ophthalmol 2009;54(2): 211–25.
24. Rudnicka AR, Mt-Isa S, Owen CG, et al. Variations in primary open-angle glaucoma prevalence by age, gender, and race: a Bayesian meta-analysis. Invest Ophthalmol Vis Sci 2006;47(10):4254–61.
25. Alsbirk PH. Anterior chamber depth in Greenland Eskimos. I. A population study of variation with age and sex. Acta Ophthalmol 1974;52(4):551–64.
26. Gelatt KN, MacKay EO. Prevalence of the breed-related glaucomas in purebred dogs in North America. Vet Ophthalmol 2004;7(2):97–111.
27. Tsai S, Almazan A, Lee SS, et al. The effect of topical latanoprost on anterior segment anatomic relationships in normal dogs. Vet Ophthalmol 2013;16(5): 370–6.
28. Slater MR, Erb HN. Effects of risk factors and prophylactic treatment on primary glaucoma in the dog. J Am Vet Med Assoc 1986;188(9):1028–30.
29. Whitacre CC. Sex differences in autoimmune disease. Nat Immunol 2001;2(9): 777–80.

30. Fuse N. Genetic bases for glaucoma. Tohoku J Exp Med 2010;221(1):1–10.
31. Kuchtey J, Olson LM, Rinkoski T, et al. Mapping of the disease locus and identification of ADAMTS10 as a candidate gene in a canine model of primary open angle glaucoma. PLoS Genet 2011;7(2):e1001306.
32. Fan BJ, Wiggs JL. Glaucoma: genes, phenotypes, and new directions for therapy. J Clin Invest 2010;120(9):3064–72.
33. Komáromy AM, Petersen-Jones SM. Genetics of Canine Primary Glaucomas. Vet Clin Small Anim 2015, in press.
34. Ekesten B, Narfstrom K. Correlation of morphologic features of the iridocorneal angle to intraocular pressure in Samoyeds. Am J Vet Res 1991;52(11):1875–8.
35. Wood JL, Lakhani KH, Read RA. Pectinate ligament dysplasia and glaucoma in Flat Coated Retrievers. II. Assessment of prevalence and heritability. Vet Ophthalmol 1998;1(2–3):91–9.
36. Bjerkas E, Ekesten B, Farstad W. Pectinate ligament dysplasia and narrowing of the iridocorneal angle associated with glaucoma in the English Springer Spaniel. Vet Ophthalmol 2002;5(1):49–54.
37. Bedford PG. A gonioscopic study of the iridocorneal angle in the English and American breeds of Cocker Spaniel and the Basset Hound. J Small Anim Pract 1977;18(10):631–42.
38. Pearce WG, Mielke BC, Kulak SC, et al. Histopathology and molecular basis of iridogoniodysgenesis syndrome. Ophthalmic Genet 1999;20(2):83–8.
39. Wyman M, Ketring K. Congenital glaucoma in the basset hound: a biologic model. Trans Sect Ophthalmol Am Acad Ophthalmol Otolaryngol 1976;81(4 Pt 1):OP645–652.
40. van der Linde-Sipman JS. Dysplasia of the pectinate ligament and primary glaucoma in the Bouvier des Flandres dog. Vet Pathol 1987;24(3):201–6.
41. Dubin AJ, Bentley E, Buhr KA, et al. Evaluation and identification of risk factors for primary angle-closure glaucoma (PACG) in Bouvier des Flandres dogs. Paper presented at: 45th Annual Meeting of the American College of Veterinary Ophthalmologists. Ft Worth, TX, October 8–11, 2014.
42. Quigley HA. The iris is a sponge: a cause of angle closure. Ophthalmology 2010;117(1):1–2.
43. Pearl R, Gould D, Spiess B. Progression of pectinate ligament dysplasia over time in two populations of Flat-Coated Retrievers. Vet Ophthalmol 2015;18(1):6–12.
44. Miller PE, Bentley E. Clinical Signs and Diagnosis of the Canine Primary Glaucomas. Vet Clin Small Anim 2015, in press.
45. Kass MA, Heuer DK, Higginbotham EJ, et al. The Ocular Hypertension Treatment Study: a randomized trial determines that topical ocular hypotensive medication delays or prevents the onset of primary open-angle glaucoma. Arch Ophthalmol 2002;120(6):701–13 [discussion: 829–30].
46. Miller PE, Schmidt GM, Vainisi SJ, et al. The efficacy of topical prophylactic antiglaucoma therapy in primary closed angle glaucoma in dogs: a multicenter clinical trial. J Am Anim Hosp Assoc 2000;36(5):431–8.
47. Smith RS, Zabaleta A, Savinova OV, et al. The mouse anterior chamber angle and trabecular meshwork develop without cell death. BMC Dev Biol 2001;1:3.
48. Idrees F, Vaideanu D, Fraser SG, et al. A review of anterior segment dysgeneses. Surv Ophthalmol 2006;51(3):213–31.
49. Gould DB, John SW. Anterior segment dysgenesis and the developmental glaucomas are complex traits. Hum Mol Genet 2002;11(10):1185–93.

50. Kroeber M, Davis N, Holzmann S, et al. Reduced expression of Pax6 in lens and cornea of mutant mice leads to failure of chamber angle development and juvenile glaucoma. Hum Mol Genet 2010;19(17):3332–42.

51. Cvekl A, Tamm ER. Anterior eye development and ocular mesenchyme: new insights from mouse models and human diseases. Bioessays 2004;26(4):374–86.

52. Vasiliou V, Gonzalez FJ. Role of CYP1B1 in glaucoma. Annu Rev Pharmacol Toxicol 2008;48:333–58.

53. Chang TC, Summers CG, Schimmenti LA, et al. Axenfeld-Rieger syndrome: new perspectives. Br J Ophthalmol 2012;96(3):318–22.

54. Mohanty K, Tanwar M, Dada R, et al. Screening of the LTBP2 gene in a north Indian population with primary congenital glaucoma. Mol Vis 2013;19:78–84.

55. Hollander DA, Sarfarazi M, Stoilov I, et al. Genotype and phenotype correlations in congenital glaucoma. Trans Am Ophthalmol Soc 2006;104:183–95.

56. Kulak SC, Kozlowski K, Semina EV, et al. Mutation in the RIEG1 gene in patients with iridogoniodysgenesis syndrome. Hum Mol Genet 1998;7(7):1113–7.

57. Tumer Z, Bach-Holm D. Axenfeld-Rieger syndrome and spectrum of PITX2 and FOXC1 mutations. Eur J Hum Genet 2009;17(12):1527–39.

58. Pumphrey S. Canine Secondary Glaucomas. Vet Clin Small Anim 2015, in press.

59. Ahram DF, Cook AC, Kecova H, et al. Identification of genetic loci associated with primary angle-closure glaucoma in the basset hound. Mol Vis 2014;20: 497–510.

60. Bedford PG. Gonioscopy in the dog. J Small Anim Pract 1977;18(10):615–29.

61. Grozdanic SD, Kecova H, Harper MM, et al. Functional and structural changes in a canine model of hereditary primary angle-closure glaucoma. Invest Ophthalmol Vis Sci 2010;51(1):255–63.

62. Shaffer RN. Primary glaucomas. Gonioscopy, ophthalmoscopy and perimetry. Trans Am Acad Ophthalmol Otolaryngol 1960;64:112–27.

63. Read RA, Wood JL, Lakhani KH. Pectinate ligament dysplasia (PLD) and glaucoma in Flat Coated Retrievers. I. Objectives, technique and results of a PLD survey. Vet Ophthalmol 1998;1(2–3):85–90.

64. Gelatt KN, Peiffer RL Jr, Gwin RM, et al. Glaucoma in the beagle. Trans Sect Ophthalmol Am Acad Ophthalmol Otolaryngol 1976;81(4 Pt 1):OP636–44.

65. Song BJ, Caprioli J. New directions in the treatment of normal tension glaucoma. Indian J Ophthalmol 2014;62(5):529–37.

66. Tripathi RC, Tripathi BJ, Haggerty C. Drug-induced glaucomas: mechanism and management. Drug Saf 2003;26(11):749–67.

67. Salmon JF. Predisposing factors for chronic angle-closure glaucoma. Prog Retin Eye Res 1999;18(1):121–32.

68. Johnson GJ, Foster PJ. Can we prevent angle-closure glaucoma? Eye 2005; 19(10):1119–24.

69. Miller PE, Bentley E, Diehl KA, et al. High resolution ultrasound imaging of the anterior segment of dogs with primary glaucoma prior to and following the topical application of 0.005% latanoprost. Paper presented at: 34th Annual Meeting of the American College of Veterinary Ophthalmologists. Coeur D'Alene, October 22–25, 2003.

70. Pizzirani S, Carroll V, Pirie CG, et al. Pathologic factors involved with the late onset of canine glaucoma associated with goniodysgenesis. Preliminary study. Paper presented at: ACVO 39th Annual Conference. Boston, October 15–18, 2008.

71. Reilly CM, Morris R, Dubielzig RR. Canine goniodysgenesis-related glaucoma: a morphologic review of 100 cases looking at inflammation and pigment dispersion. Vet Ophthalmol 2005;8(4):253–8.

72. Sacca SC, Pulliero A, Izzotti A. The dysfunction of the trabecular meshwork during glaucoma course. J Cell Physiol 2015;230(3):510–25.

73. Grierson I, Howes RC. Age-related depletion of the cell population in the human trabecular meshwork. Eye 1987;1(Pt 2):204–10.

74. Finkel T, Holbrook NJ. Oxidants, oxidative stress and the biology of ageing. Nature 2000;408(6809):239–47.

75. Yang XJ, Ge J, Zhuo YH. Role of mitochondria in the pathogenesis and treatment of glaucoma. Chin Med J 2013;126(22):4358–65.

76. Fuchshofer R, Tamm ER. The role of TGF-beta in the pathogenesis of primary open-angle glaucoma. Cell Tissue Res 2012;347(1):279–90.

77. Tripathi RC, Chan WFA, Li J, et al. Trabecular cells express the TGF-beta2 gene and secrete the cytokine. Exp Eye Res 1994;58(5):523–8.

78. Fuchshofer R, Yu AH, Welge-Lussen U, et al. Bone morphogenetic protein-7 is an antagonist of transforming growth factor beta 2 in human trabecular meshwork cells. Invest Ophthalmol Vis Sci 2007;48(2):715–26.

79. Maatta M, Tervahartiala T, Harju M, et al. Matrix metalloproteinases and their tissue inhibitors in aqueous humor of patients with primary open-angle glaucoma, exfoliation syndrome, and exfoliation glaucoma. J Glaucoma 2005;14(1):64–9.

80. Alexander JP, Samples JR, Van Buskirk EM, et al. Expression of matrix metalloproteinases and inhibitor by human trabecular meshwork. Invest Ophthalmol Vis Sci 1991;32(1):172–80.

81. Samuelson DA, Gum GG, Gelatt KN. Ultrastructural changes in the aqueous outflow apparatus of beagles with inherited glaucoma. Invest Ophthalmol Vis Sci 1989;30(3):550–61.

82. Kuchtey J, Kuchtey RW. The microfibril hypothesis of glaucoma: implications for treatment of elevated intraocular pressure. J Ocul Pharmacol Ther 2014; 30(2–3):170–80.

83. Flammer J, Mozaffarieh M. What is the present pathogenetic concept of glaucomatous optic neuropathy? Surv Ophthalmol 2007;52(Suppl 2):S162–173.

84. Quigley HA, Nickells RW, Kerrigan LA, et al. Retinal ganglion cell death in experimental glaucoma and after axotomy occurs by apoptosis. Invest Ophthalmol Vis Sci 1995;36(5):774–86.

85. Garcia-Valenzuela E, Gorczyca W, Darzynkiewicz Z, et al. Apoptosis in adult retinal ganglion cells after axotomy. J Neurobiol 1994;25(4):431–8.

86. Cullen SP, Henry CM, Kearney CJ, et al. Fas/CD95-induced chemokines can serve as "find-me" signals for apoptotic cells. Mol Cell 2013;49(6):1034–48.

87. Davidovich P, Kearney CJ, Martin SJ. Inflammatory outcomes of apoptosis, necrosis and necroptosis. Biol Chem 2014;395(10):1163–71.

88. Burgoyne CF. A biomechanical paradigm for axonal insult within the optic nerve head in aging and glaucoma. Exp Eye Res 2011;93(2):120–32.

89. Brooks DE, Komaromy AM, Kallberg ME. Comparative optic nerve physiology: implications for glaucoma, neuroprotection, and neuroregeneration. Vet Ophthalmol 1999;2(1):13–25.

90. Almasieh M, Wilson AM, Morquette B, et al. The molecular basis of retinal ganglion cell death in glaucoma. Prog Retin Eye Res 2012;31(2):152–81.

91. Johnson JE, Barde YA, Schwab M, et al. Brain-derived neurotrophic factor supports the survival of cultured rat retinal ganglion cells. J Neurosci 1986;6(10): 3031–8.

92. Mey J, Thanos S. Intravitreal injections of neurotrophic factors support the survival of axotomized retinal ganglion cells in adult rats in vivo. Brain Res 1993; 602(2):304–17.

93. Morgan JE. Optic nerve head structure in glaucoma: astrocytes as mediators of axonal damage. Eye 2000;14(Pt 3B):437–44.
94. Alyahya K, Chen CT, Mangan BG, et al. Microvessel loss, vascular damage and glutamate redistribution in the retinas of dogs with primary glaucoma. Vet Ophthalmol 2007;10(Suppl 1):70–7.
95. Sacca SC, Izzotti A, Rossi P, et al. Glaucomatous outflow pathway and oxidative stress. Exp Eye Res 2007;84(3):389–99.
96. Izzotti A, Bagnis A, Sacca SC. The role of oxidative stress in glaucoma. Mutat Res 2006;612(2):105–14.
97. Chrysostomou V, Trounce IA, Crowston JG. Mechanisms of retinal ganglion cell injury in aging and glaucoma. Ophthalmic Res 2010;44(3):173–8.
98. Yan DB, Coloma FM, Metheetrairut A, et al. Deformation of the lamina cribrosa by elevated intraocular pressure. Br J Ophthalmol 1994;78(8):643–8.
99. Quigley HA, Hohman RM, Addicks EM, et al. Morphologic changes in the lamina cribrosa correlated with neural loss in open-angle glaucoma. Am J Ophthalmol 1983;95(5):673–91.
100. Flammer J, Orgul S, Costa VP, et al. The impact of ocular blood flow in glaucoma. Prog Retin Eye Res 2002;21(4):359–93.
101. Flammer J, Pache M, Resink T. Vasospasm, its role in the pathogenesis of diseases with particular reference to the eye. Prog Retin Eye Res 2001;20(3):319–49.
102. Tezel G. Oxidative stress in glaucomatous neurodegeneration: mechanisms and consequences. Prog Retin Eye Res 2006;25(5):490–513.
103. Bechetoille A, Bresson-Dumont H. Diurnal and nocturnal blood pressure drops in patients with focal ischemic glaucoma. Graefes Arch Clin Exp Ophthalmol 1994;232(11):675–9.
104. Flammer J. The vascular concept of glaucoma. Surv Ophthalmol 1994;38(Suppl):S3–6.
105. Gelatt-Nicholson KJ, Gelatt KN, MacKay EO, et al. Comparative Doppler imaging of the ophthalmic vasculature in normal Beagles and Beagles with inherited primary open-angle glaucoma. Vet Ophthalmol 1999;2(2):97–105.
106. Hayreh SS. The ophthalmic artery: III. Branches. Br J Ophthalmol 1962;46(4):212–47.
107. Brooks DE, Samuelson DA, Gelatt KN, et al. Scanning electron microscopy of corrosion casts of the optic nerve microcirculation in dogs. Am J Vet Res 1989;50(6):908–14.
108. Mayordomo-Febrer A, Lopez-Murcia M, Morales-Tatay JM, et al. Metabolomics of the aqueous humor in the rat glaucoma model induced by a series of intra-camerular sodium hyaluronate injection. Exp Eye Res 2015;131:84–92.
109. Osborne NN. Pathogenesis of ganglion "cell death" in glaucoma and neuroprotection: focus on ganglion cell axonal mitochondria. Prog Brain Res 2008;173:339–52.
110. Lin WJ, Kuang HY. Oxidative stress induces autophagy in response to multiple noxious stimuli in retinal ganglion cells. Autophagy 2014;10(10):1692–701.
111. Anderson DR, Hendrickson A. Effect of intraocular pressure on rapid axoplasmic transport in monkey optic nerve. Invest Ophthalmol 1974;13(10):771–83.
112. Cui H, Kong Y, Zhang H. Oxidative stress, mitochondrial dysfunction, and aging. J Signal Transduct 2012;2012:646354.
113. Osborne NN, Alvarez CN, del Olmo Aguado S. Targeting mitochondrial dysfunction as in aging and glaucoma. Drug Discov Today 2014;19(10):1613–22.

114. Boveris A, Navarro A. Brain mitochondrial dysfunction in aging. IUBMB Life 2008;60(5):308–14.

115. Malinin NL, West XZ, Byzova TV. Oxidation as "the stress of life". Aging (Albany NY) 2011;3(9):906–10.

116. Chrysostomou V, Rezania F, Trounce IA, et al. Oxidative stress and mitochondrial dysfunction in glaucoma. Curr Opin Pharmacol 2013;13(1):12–5.

117. El Assar M, Angulo J, Rodriguez-Manas L. Oxidative stress and vascular inflammation in aging. Free Radic Biol Med 2013;65:380–401.

118. Wang JY, Wen LL, Huang YN, et al. Dual effects of antioxidants in neurodegeneration: direct neuroprotection against oxidative stress and indirect protection via suppression of glia-mediated inflammation. Curr Pharm Des 2006;12(27): 3521–33.

119. Chung HY, Sung B, Jung KJ, et al. The molecular inflammatory process in aging. Antioxid Redox Signal 2006;8(3–4):572–81.

120. Haefliger IO, Dettmann E, Liu R, et al. Potential role of nitric oxide and endothelin in the pathogenesis of glaucoma. Surv Ophthalmol 1999;43(Suppl 1): S51–58.

121. Chen T, Gionfriddo JR, Tai PY, et al. Oxidative stress increases in retinas of dogs in acute glaucoma but not in chronic glaucoma. Vet Ophthalmol 2015;18(4): 261–70.

122. Hernandez MR, Miao H, Lukas T. Astrocytes in glaucomatous optic neuropathy. Prog Brain Res 2008;173:353–73.

123. Waniewski RA, Martin DL. Exogenous glutamate is metabolized to glutamine and exported by rat primary astrocyte cultures. J Neurochem 1986;47(1): 304–13.

124. Goss JR, O'Malley ME, Zou L, et al. Astrocytes are the major source of nerve growth factor upregulation following traumatic brain injury in the rat. Exp Neurol 1998;149(2):301–9.

125. Neumann C, Yu A, Welge-Lussen U, et al. The effect of TGF-beta2 on elastin, type VI collagen, and components of the proteolytic degradation system in human optic nerve astrocytes. Invest Ophthalmol Vis Sci 2008;49(4):1464–72.

126. Pena JD, Netland PA, Vidal I, et al. Elastosis of the lamina cribrosa in glaucomatous optic neuropathy. Exp Eye Res 1998;67(5):517–24.

127. Zode GS, Sethi A, Brun-Zinkernagel AM, et al. Transforming growth factor-beta2 increases extracellular matrix proteins in optic nerve head cells via activation of the Smad signaling pathway. Mol Vis 2011;17:1745–58.

128. Yafai Y, Iandiev I, Lange J, et al. Muller glial cells inhibit proliferation of retinal endothelial cells via TGF-beta2 and Smad signaling. Glia 2014;62(9):1476–85.

129. Perry VH, Nicoll JA, Holmes C. Microglia in neurodegenerative disease. Nat Rev Neurol 2010;6(4):193–201.

130. Neufeld AH. Microglia in the optic nerve head and the region of parapapillary chorioretinal atrophy in glaucoma. Arch Ophthalmol 1999;117(8):1050–6.

131. Agarwal R, Agarwal P. Glaucomatous neurodegeneration: an eye on tumor necrosis factor-alpha. Indian J Ophthalmol 2012;60(4):255–61.

132. Shen Y, Liu XL, Yang XL. N-methyl-D-aspartate receptors in the retina. Mol Neurobiol 2006;34(3):163–79.

133. Lucas DR, Newhouse JP. The toxic effect of sodium L-glutamate on the inner layers of the retina. AMA Arch Ophthalmol 1957;58(2):193–201.

134. Vorwerk CK, Gorla MS, Dreyer EB. An experimental basis for implicating excitotoxicity in glaucomatous optic neuropathy. Surv Ophthalmol 1999;43(Suppl 1): S142–150.

135. Dreyer EB, Zurakowski D, Schumer RA, et al. Elevated glutamate levels in the vitreous body of humans and monkeys with glaucoma. Arch Ophthalmol 1996;114(3):299–305.
136. McIlnay TR, Gionfriddo JR, Dubielzig RR, et al. Evaluation of glutamate loss from damaged retinal cells of dogs with primary glaucoma. Am J Vet Res 2004;65(6):776–86.
137. Brooks DE, Garcia GA, Dreyer EB, et al. Vitreous body glutamate concentration in dogs with glaucoma. Am J Vet Res 1997;58(8):864–7.
138. Siliprandi R, Canella R, Carmignoto G, et al. N-methyl-D-aspartate-induced neurotoxicity in the adult rat retina. Vis Neurosci 1992;8(6):567–73.
139. Kemp JA, McKernan RM. NMDA receptor pathways as drug targets. Nat Neurosci 2002;5(Suppl):1039–42.
140. Madl JE, McIlnay TR, Powell CC, et al. Depletion of taurine and glutamate from damaged photoreceptors in the retinas of dogs with primary glaucoma. Am J Vet Res 2005;66(5):791–9.
141. Kwon YH, Rickman DW, Baruah S, et al. Vitreous and retinal amino acid concentrations in experimental central retinal artery occlusion in the primate. Eye 2005;19(4):455–63.
142. Ullian EM, Barkis WB, Chen S, et al. Invulnerability of retinal ganglion cells to NMDA excitotoxicity. Mol Cell Neurosci 2004;26(4):544–57.
143. Lotery AJ. Glutamate excitotoxicity in glaucoma: truth or fiction? Eye 2005;19(4):369–70.
144. Findings of scientific misconduct. In: Services DoHH, editor. Available at: http://grants.nih.gov/grants/guide/notice-files/NOT-OD-01-006.html. Accessed July 25, 2015.
145. Dalton R. Private investigations. Nature 2001;411(6834):129–30.
146. Olmos G, Llado J. Tumor necrosis factor alpha: a link between neuroinflammation and excitotoxicity. Mediators Inflamm 2014;2014:861231.
147. Wax MB, Tezel G. Immunoregulation of retinal ganglion cell fate in glaucoma. Exp Eye Res 2009;88(4):825–30.
148. Grus FH, Joachim SC, Wuenschig D, et al. Autoimmunity and glaucoma. J Glaucoma 2008;17(1):79–84.
149. Yang X, Luo C, Cai J, et al. Neurodegenerative and inflammatory pathway components linked to TNF-alpha/TNFR1 signaling in the glaucomatous human retina. Invest Ophthalmol Vis Sci 2011;52(11):8442–54.
150. Maggio M, Guralnik JM, Longo DL, et al. Interleukin-6 in aging and chronic disease: a magnificent pathway. J Gerontol A Biol Sci Med Sci 2006;61(6):575–84.
151. Xu H, Chen M, Forrester JV. Para-inflammation in the aging retina. Prog Retin Eye Res 2009;28(5):348–68.
152. Keller KE, Aga M, Bradley JM, et al. Extracellular matrix turnover and outflow resistance. Exp Eye Res 2009;88(4):676–82.
153. Ueda J, Wentz-Hunter K, Yue BY. Distribution of myocilin and extracellular matrix components in the juxtacanalicular tissue of human eyes. Invest Ophthalmol Vis Sci 2002;43(4):1068–76.
154. Tamm ER. Myocilin and glaucoma: facts and ideas. Prog Retin Eye Res 2002;21(4):395–428.
155. Hart H, Samuelson DA, Tajwar H, et al. Immunolocalization of myocilin protein in the anterior eye of normal and primary open-angle glaucomatous dogs. Vet Ophthalmol 2007;10(Suppl 1):28–37.
156. Mackay EO, Kallberg ME, Gelatt KN. Aqueous humor myocilin protein levels in normal, genetic carriers, and glaucoma Beagles. Vet Ophthalmol 2008;11(3):177–85.

157. MacKay EO, Kallberg ME, Barrie KP, et al. Myocilin protein levels in the aqueous humor of the glaucomas in selected canine breeds. Vet Ophthalmol 2008;11(4): 234–41.

158. Tripathi BJ, Tripathi RC, Chen J, et al. Trabecular cell expression of fibronectin and MMP-3 is modulated by aqueous humor growth factors. Exp Eye Res 2004;78(3):653–60.

159. Pizzirani S, Desai SJ, Pirie CG, et al. Age related changes in the anterior segment of the eye in normal dogs. Paper presented at: 41st Annual Meeting of the American College of Veterinary Ophthalmologists. San Diego, CA, October 6–9, 2010.

160. Oppenheim JJ, Yang D. Alarmins: chemotactic activators of immune responses. Curr Opin Immunol 2005;17(4):359–65.

161. Cruise LJ, McClure R. Posterior pathway for aqueous humor drainage in the dog. Am J Vet Res 1981;42(6):992–5.

162. Watson P, Grierson I, Hitchings RA, et al. Pathological dilemmas in the outflow system in primary open-angle glaucoma - Discussion. Acta Ophthalmol Scand 1997;75:13–4.

163. Sethi A, Mao W, Wordinger RJ, et al. Transforming growth factor-beta induces extracellular matrix protein cross-linking lysyl oxidase (LOX) genes in human trabecular meshwork cells. Invest Ophthalmol Vis Sci 2011;52(8):5240–50.

164. Hogg P, Calthorpe M, Ward S, et al. Migration of cultured bovine trabecular meshwork cells to aqueous humor and constituents. Invest Ophthalmol Vis Sci 1995;36(12):2449–60.

165. Hasegawa M, Sato S, Takehara K. Augmented production of transforming growth factor-beta by cultured peripheral blood mononuclear cells from patients with systemic sclerosis. Arch Dermatol Res 2004;296(2):89–93.

166. Rhee DJ, Haddadin RI, Kang MH, et al. Matricellular proteins in the trabecular meshwork. Exp Eye Res 2009;88(4):694–703.

167. Yehualaeshet T, O'Connor R, Green-Johnson J, et al. Activation of rat alveolar macrophage-derived latent transforming growth factor beta-1 by plasmin requires interaction with thrombospondin-1 and its cell surface receptor, CD36. Am J Pathol 1999;155(3):841–51.

168. Davis GE, Pintar Allen KA, Salazar R, et al. Matrix metalloproteinase-1 and -9 activation by plasmin regulates a novel endothelial cell-mediated mechanism of collagen gel contraction and capillary tube regression in three-dimensional collagen matrices. J Cell Sci 2001;114(Pt 5):917–30.

169. Fuchshofer R, Welge-Lussen U, Lütjen-Drecoll E. The effect of TGF-β2 on human trabecular meshwork extracellular proteolytic system. Exp Eye Res 2003; 77(6):757–65.

170. Mantovani A. Macrophage diversity and polarization: in vivo veritas. Blood 2006; 108(2):408–9.

171. Baatz H, Puchta J, Reszka R, et al. Macrophage depletion prevents leukocyte adhesion and disease induction in experimental melanin-protein induced uveitis. Exp Eye Res 2001;73(1):101–9.

172. Parameswaran N, Patial S. Tumor necrosis factor-alpha signaling in macrophages. Crit Rev Eukaryot Gene Expr 2010;20(2):87–103.

173. Merry HE, Phelan P, Doaks M, et al. Functional roles of tumor necrosis factor-alpha and interleukin 1-Beta in hypoxia and reoxygenation. Ann Thorac Surg 2015;99(4):1200–5.

174. Perry RT, Collins JS, Wiener H, et al. The role of TNF and its receptors in Alzheimer's disease. Neurobiol Aging 2001;22(6):873–83.

175. Nagatsu T, Sawada M. Inflammatory process in Parkinson's disease: role for cytokines. Curr Pharm Des 2005;11(8):999–1016.

176. Tezel G, Li LY, Patil RV, et al. TNF-alpha and TNF-alpha receptor-1 in the retina of normal and glaucomatous eyes. Invest Ophthalmol Vis Sci 2001;42(8):1787–94.

177. Sawada H, Fukuchi T, Tanaka T, et al. Tumor necrosis factor-alpha concentrations in the aqueous humor of patients with glaucoma. Invest Ophthalmol Vis Sci 2010;51(2):903–6.

178. Durieux P, Etchepareborde S, Fritz D, et al. Tumor necrosis factor-alpha concentration in the aqueous humor of healthy and diseased dogs: a preliminary pilot study. J Fr Ophtalmol 2015;38(4):288–94.

179. Nakazawa T, Nakazawa C, Matsubara A, et al. Tumor necrosis factor-alpha mediates oligodendrocyte death and delayed retinal ganglion cell loss in a mouse model of glaucoma. J Neurosci 2006;26(49):12633–41.

180. Tezel G. TNF-alpha signaling in glaucomatous neurodegeneration. Prog Brain Res 2008;173:409–21.

181. Gregory MS, Hackett CG, Abernathy EF, et al. Opposing roles for membrane bound and soluble Fas ligand in glaucoma-associated retinal ganglion cell death. PLoS One 2011;6(3):e17659.

Genetics of Canine Primary Glaucomas

András M. Komáromy, DrMedVet, PhD*, Simon M. Petersen-Jones, DVetMed, PhD

KEYWORDS

- *ADAMTS10* • *ADAMTS17* • Canine • Genetics • Glaucoma • Open-angle
- Closed-angle • Lens luxation

KEY POINTS

- Primary angle-closure glaucoma (PACG) is the most common form of canine primary glaucoma and is a complex trait with multiple genetic and possibly environmental risk factors.
- Five susceptibility genes or loci have been identified as possible contributors to canine PACG.
- Primary open-angle glaucoma (POAG) is a monogenic, autosomal-recessively inherited disease, and it has recently been associated with primary lens luxation (PLL).
- Discoveries of disease mutations in *ADAMTS10* and *ADAMTS17* suggest that canine POAG and PLL are homologous to the human connective tissue disorders Weill-Marchesani and Marfan syndromes.
- Identification of canine glaucoma disease genes and development of genetic tests will help to avoid the breeding of affected dogs and enable earlier diagnosis and potentially more effective therapy.

INTRODUCTION

Glaucoma is a leading cause of incurable vision loss in dogs.[1,2] It is defined as an optic neuropathy with characteristic damage of the optic nerve head, retinal ganglion cell death, and resulting loss of sight.[3] In most affected dogs, abnormal intraocular pressure (IOP) elevation leads to degeneration of the optic nerve and retina.[3] Compared with healthy eyes, in which physiologic IOP is maintained by a tight regulation of aqueous humor production and drainage, in glaucomatous eyes the outflow of

This work was supported in part by Michigan State University Startup Funds, Glaucoma Research Foundation, Edward Sheppard and family, and Myers-Dunlap Endowment for Canine Health. The authors have no conflict of interest regarding the content presented in this article. Department of Small Animal Clinical Sciences, Veterinary Medical Center, College of Veterinary Medicine, Michigan State University, 736 Wilson Road, Room D-208, East Lansing, MI 48824, USA
* Corresponding author.
E-mail address: komaromy@cvm.msu.edu

aqueous humor through the iridocorneal angle (ICA) is impaired, resulting in an IOP increase.[4,5] In primary glaucomas, both eyes are typically affected by an increased resistance along the aqueous outflow pathways, resulting from primary abnormalities, rather than secondary to other pathologic intraocular processes, as in secondary glaucoma.[1,3] Based on the specific breed predilection for primary glaucomas, genetic factors are suspected to be major contributors to the cellular and molecular disease mechanisms resulting in impaired aqueous humor outflow.[1] Both the American and European Colleges of Veterinary Ophthalmologists recommend against the breeding of dogs affected by primary glaucomas (**Table 1**).[6,7] Despite the high prevalence of primary glaucomas in dogs,[1] their genetics has been studied in only a relatively small number of breeds. This review serves as a comprehensive summary of the current knowledge of the genetics of primary glaucomas in dogs. Because of their close association with either primary angle-closure glaucoma (PACG) or primary open-angle glaucoma (POAG),[8–13] the genetics of pectinate ligament dysplasia (PLD) and primary lens luxation (PLL) are also discussed. Recent advances in the genetics of canine glaucomas have provided a better understanding of molecular and cellular

Table 1	
Breeds affected by primary glaucomas or primary lens luxation according to the American College of Veterinary Ophthalmologists and the European College of Veterinary Ophthalmologists	
Primary Glaucoma	**Primary Lens Luxation**
Alaskan malamute	Australian cattle dog[a]
American cocker spaniel	Border collie
Australian cattle dog[a]	Brittany
Basset hound (PLD)	Brussels griffon
Beagle	Bull terrier
Boston terrier	Chinese crested dog
Bouvier des Flandres (PLD)	Chinese shar-pei[a]
Bullmastiff	Greyhound
Chinese shar-pei[a]	Italian greyhound
Chow Chow	Jack Russell terrier[a]
Dalmatian	Lancashire heeler
English cocker spaniel	Miniature bull terrier
English springer spaniel	Parson Russell terrier
Entlebucher	Petit basset griffon vendéen[a]
Eurasier	Pyrenean shepherd
Flat-coated retriever (PLD)	Rat terrier
Golden retriever	Sealyham terrier
Great Dane	Smooth fox terrier[a]
Jack Russell terrier (PLD)[a]	Spanish water dog
Labrador retriever	Tibetan terrier
Newfoundland (PLD)	Toy fox terrier
Norwegian elkhound	Welsh terrier[a]
Petit basset griffon vendéen[a]	Wire fox terrier[a]
Poodle (PLD)	Yorkshire terrier
Samoyed	
Shiba inu (PLD)	
Siberian husky	
Smooth fox terrier[a]	
Welsh springer spaniel (PLD)	
Welsh terrier[a]	
Wire fox terrier[a]	

[a] Breeds affected by both primary glaucomas and PLL.

disease mechanisms as well as the resulting clinical signs. Despite these advances, there is a need to identify additional genetic risk factors for glaucoma to avoid breeding affected dogs in the future. Furthermore, identifying these risk factors may also allow for earlier diagnosis and more effective application of traditional and novel treatments before disease onset.

TECHNIQUES USED TO STUDY GENETIC DISORDERS

A genetic cause or predisposition is suspected when there is an increased prevalence of glaucoma within a particular canine breed or family. By compiling a pedigree of affected and unaffected animals that are related, the mode of inheritance may be determined, especially if the disease is caused by mutations in a single gene, resulting in a simple Mendelian trait rather than a complex trait that results from the interaction of several genes and possible environmental factors.[14] An important and often difficult part of such a pedigree analysis, as well as of other genetic methods, is the thorough examination and phenotyping of all the animals included in order to make sure that unaffected animals are truly free of the disease of interest and that all affected animals have the same disease phenotype. Particularly in diseases such as primary glaucomas, which often do not occur until later in life, a minimal age needs to be established based on the typical disease history, when one can confirm with confidence that an animal is unaffected.

In addition to pedigree analysis, molecular techniques are being used to identify genetic mutations that contribute to the disease phenotype.[14–16] If the clinical signs of an inherited canine disease is comparable to an analogous human disease and if the genes responsible for the human disease are known, then these particular genes can be screened for mutations in the affected dogs. Alternatively, the gene loci can be screened for association with the canine disease. Although this candidate gene approach was initially not successful in the study of canine primary glaucomas,[17–20] it led to the discovery of the SRBD1 glaucoma susceptibility gene in the Shiba inu and Shih Tzu (**Table 2**).[21]

With the availability of improved canine genomic resources, approaches for discovering disease-causing mutations have evolved from a candidate gene approach, which focuses only on small genomic regions, to whole-genome linkage analyses and genome-wide association studies (GWAS).[14,15,22,23] With the latter methods, the whole genome is evaluated using genetic markers such as microsatellites or single-nucleotide polymorphisms (SNPs) to look for markers correlated to the disease status and therefore closely linked to the disease mutations. In a linkage analysis, markers are evaluated across a pedigree in which the disease is segregating.[14–16] For GWAS, cases and controls are compared.[14–16] The genomic region around the identified markers/variations linked to the disease can then be examined in more detail in order to find the DNA variant responsible for the disease. These methods have been used to identify risk loci, linked chromosomal regions, or causal DNA mutations for primary glaucoma in the basset hound, beagle, Dandie Dinmont terrier, and Norwegian elkhound (**Figs. 1** and **2**) as well as for PLL in multiple canine breeds (see **Table 2**).[24–30] As molecular technologies continue to evolve, the next-generation sequencing of the entire genome of affected animals and the search for disease mutations will become more efficient and economical.

Once a genetic disease marker has been identified, it can be used for genetic testing, even before the specific disease-causing DNA mutation has been identified. The reliability of such a marker-based test depends on how closely the marker is linked to the disease-causing DNA mutation; the closer the marker and mutation,

Table 2
Breeds affected by primary glaucoma or primary lens luxation with identified disease or susceptibility genes or loci

Disease	Breeds	Disease/Susceptibility Gene/Locus	Genetic Testing[a]	References
PACG	Basset hound	3 susceptibility genes: COL1A2, RAB22A, and NEB	No	Ahram et al,[26] 2014 Ahram et al,[27] 2015
	Dandie Dinmont terrier	9.5-Mb susceptibility locus on canine chromosome 8	No	Ahonen et al,[28] 2013
	Shiba inu	SRBD1 susceptibility gene	No	Kanemaki et al,[21] 2013
	Shih Tzu	SRBD1 susceptibility gene	No	Kanemaki et al,[21] 2013
POAG	Beagle	ADAMTS10 disease gene: Gly661Arg missense mutation	OptiGen	Kuchtey et al,[24] 2011
	Norwegian elkhound	ADAMTS10 disease gene: Ala387Thr missense mutation	No	Ahonen et al,[25] 2014
	Petit basset griffon vendéen	Pending	AHT	Pending
PLL	American Eskimo dog American hairless (rat) terrier Australian cattle dog Chinese crested dog Chinese foo dog Jack Russell terrier Jagdterrier Lakeland terrier Lancashire heeler Lucas terrier Miniature bull terrier Norfolk terrier Norwich terrier Parson Russell terrier Patterdale terrier Rat terrier Russell terrier Sealyham terrier Teddy Roosevelt terrier Tenterfield terrier Tibetan terrier Toy fox terrier Volpino Italiano Welsh terrier Wire-haired fox terrier Yorkshire terrier	ADAMTS17 disease gene: c.1473+1G>A splice donor site mutation	AHT, OFA, OptiGen, VetGen	Sargan et al,[30] 2007 Farias et al,[29] 2010 Gould et al,[77] 2011

[a] Animal Health Trust (AHT): www.aht.org.uk; http://www.ahtdnatesting.co.uk; OFA: http://www.offa.org/dnatesting/kits.html; OptiGen: www.optigen.com; VetGen: www.vetgen.com.

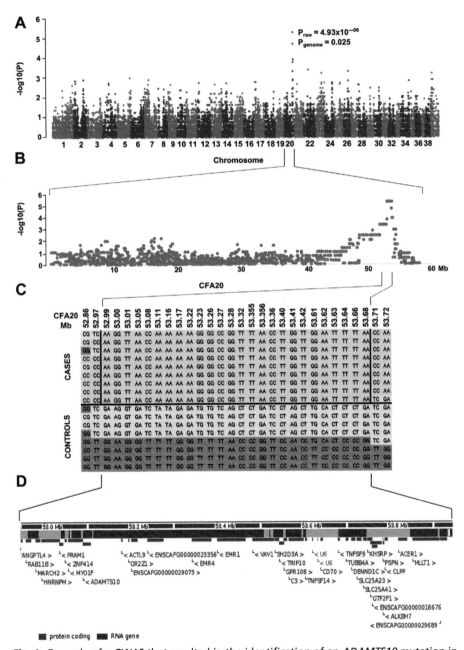

Fig. 1. Example of a GWAS that resulted in the identification of an *ADAMTS10* mutation in Norwegian elkhound POAG. (*A*) A Manhattan plot of genome-wide case-control association analysis indicates the most highly associated region in chromosome 20. (*B*) The glaucoma associated region on chromosome 20 spans from 53.1 to 53.8 Mb. (*C*) Genotypes at the associated region; all cases share a 750-kb homozygous block. (*D*) The associated region harbors 35 genes, of which only *ADAMTS10* has been associated with POAG. (*From* Ahonen SJ, Kaukonen M, Nussdorfer FD, et al. A novel missense mutation in ADAMTS10 in Norwegian elkhound primary glaucoma. PLoS One 2013;9:e111941.)

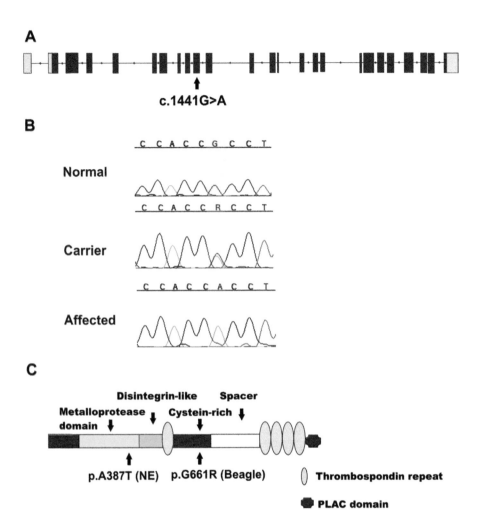

Fig. 2. Identification of the *ADAMTS10* missense mutation responsible for Norwegian elkhound POAG. (*A*) A schematic representation of the *ADAMTS10* gene structure. The gene is composed of 24 coding exons (*dark blue*), and the c.1441G.A variant/mutation is positioned in the exon 9 (not to scale). (*B*) Chromatograms of the nonsynonymous variant position in an affected, a carrier, and a wild-type dog. (*C*) The Ala387Thr (p.A387T) missense mutation is positioned in the catalytic metalloprotease domain. The location of the Gly661Arg (p.G661R) responsible for POAG in the beagle is also shown. NE, Norwegian elkhound. (*From* Ahonen SJ, Kaukonen M, Nussdorfer FD, et al. A novel missense mutation in ADAMTS10 in Norwegian elkhound primary glaucoma. PLoS One 2013;9:e111941.)

the less likely they will be separated by a recombination event, and the more reliable the test.[14] The reliability of a marker-based test to identify normals or affecteds also depends on how common the disease-associated allele is in the general population, as discussed later in this text when describing the *NEB* risk allele for PACG in the basset hound.[14,27] Once the specific disease-causing DNA mutation has been identified, the marker-based test can be replaced by the more reliable mutation detection test. **Table 2** lists the currently known markers and mutations for primary glaucoma in dogs and the availability of any commercial genetic tests.

GENETICS OF HUMAN GLAUCOMA AND ITS RELEVANCE TO CANINE GLAUCOMA STUDIES

Because the genetics of primary glaucomas is being studied more intensely in humans than in dogs, there are many lessons that can be learned from human glaucoma that aid in the investigation of canine glaucoma genetics. Many glaucoma-related genes identified in human patients have been investigated as candidate genes in dogs.[17–19] The genetics of most forms of human primary glaucoma is complex and still not completely understood because most are not monogenic but rather polygenic, with a complex inheritance and interacting environmental factors.[16]

Juvenile open-angle glaucoma (JOAG), which is diagnosed before 20 years of age, is more commonly a monogenic trait.[16] The investigation of JOAG led to the discovery of the first glaucoma-related gene in 1997: Mutations in *myocilin* (*MYOC*), or *TIGR* (*trabecular meshwork-induced glucocorticoid response*) gene, are responsible for 10% of juvenile and 3% to 5% of adult-onset POAG.[31–34] To date, no *MYOC* mutations have been identified in dogs.[18,19] MYOC protein concentrations were shown to be elevated in the aqueous humor of several canine breeds with primary glaucoma,[35,36] but the function of MYOC and its role in the molecular disease process resulting in increased IOP remain unknown.

Other prominent human glaucoma genes include *OPTN* (*optineurin*),[37] cytochrome P450 1B1 (*CYP1B1*),[38] *NTF4* (*neurotrophin 4*),[39,40] *TBK1* (*TANK-binding kinase 1*),[41,42] and *WDR36* (*WD repeat domain 36*).[43] In addition to these specific glaucoma genes, large-scale GWAS have led to the identification of genetic loci that contribute to the development of POAG[44–50] and PACG.[51,52] GWAS were also performed to identify genetic variants associated with quantitative risk factors for glaucoma, such as IOP,[53–55] central corneal thickness,[56–58] optic nerve head area, and optic cup-to-disc ratio.[59–64]

GENETICS OF EXTRACELLULAR MATRIX ABNORMALITIES ASSOCIATED WITH PRIMARY GLAUCOMA

There are currently no indications that any of the prominent glaucoma genes associated with human POAG and PACG contribute to the development of canine primary glaucomas. Instead, genes involved in the normal extracellular matrix (ECM) metabolism have recently emerged as important players in the canine glaucoma pathogenesis. There are strong indications in both humans and dogs that changes in the ECM composition along the aqueous humor outflow pathways are responsible for increased resistance and IOP elevation.[65–68] Abnormalities in the ECM and the biomechanics of the optic nerve head's lamina cribrosa and the sclera also contribute to greater susceptibility of retinal ganglion cells to variations in IOP.[69–75]

The recent discoveries of *ADAMTS10* mutations responsible for POAG in beagles and Norwegian elkhounds,[25,76] as well as a mutation in *ADAMTS17* causing canine PLL in many breeds,[29,77] and ongoing studies of canine POAG by the authors and others,[8,10] revealed that many forms of primary canine glaucoma are closely related to a group of connective tissue disorders resulting from abnormal microfibril formation. These so-called microfibrillopathies include Weill-Marchesani syndrome (WMS) and Marfan syndrome (MS) and are caused by mutations in genes responsible for normal microfibril formation, most importantly *ADAMTS10*, *ADAMTS17*, and *fibrillin-1* (*FBN1*), resulting in defective microfibrils.[78–84] Similar to variations of canine POAG and PLL, the ocular phenotype of WMS/MS in human patients is characterized by ectopia lentis/PLL, which can occur in combination with either POAG or PACG, the latter caused by a shallow anterior chamber and pupillary block from anterior dislocation of the lens.[78,80–82,84–88] The accumulation of plaques within the trabecular meshwork has been well documented in eyes of humans and beagles with POAG; these plaques may contain *FBN1* and are likely responsible for increased aqueous humor outflow resistance.[67,70,89–93] To the best of the authors' knowledge, POAG- and PLL-affected dogs do not show any of the systemic changes seen in human patients with WMS/MS, such as skeletal abnormalities and cardiovascular defects.[78,80,85,94,95]

Microfibrils are fiberlike strands formed by chains of FBN1 beads.[78,96–98] ADAMTS10 and ADAMTS17 are secreted metalloproteinases that are located in the ECM and aid in the proper assembly of FBN1 to microfibrils.[78,82,83,99–101] Microfibrils play an important role in connective tissue biology.[78] They are common components of elastic fibers and also a main part of the lens zonules, the fine ligaments that attach the lens to the ciliary body,[82,102] which explains why zonular dysplasia and ectopia lentis are the most common ocular abnormalities in WMS/MS patients with mutations in *ADAMTS10*, *ADAMTS17*, or *FBN1*.[78] The authors recently reported that zonular dysplasia is also part of the ocular disease phenotype in *ADAMTS10*-mutant beagles with POAG.[8] In their experience, these animals may be presented to the clinician with primary signs of either POAG or PLL. The same is true for other POAG-/PLL-affected breeds, such as the petit basset griffon vendéen.[10] In addition to their mechanical function, microfibrils also play an important role in ECM metabolism, such as in the trabecular meshwork, through binding/storage and activation of transforming growth factor-β (TGF-β), a growth factor that contributes to increased trabecular outflow resistance and IOP when up-regulated in glaucomatous eyes.[68,78,82,103–121]

It should be noted that mutations in the gene encoding for the *LTBP2* (latent transforming growth factor-β binding protein 2), which is another ECM component associated with microfibrils, have been associated with primary congenital glaucoma in both humans and cats as well as human POAG.[122–126]

GENETICS OF CANINE PRIMARY ANGLE-CLOSURE GLAUCOMA

PACG is the most common form of canine primary glaucomas, and it is characterized by a narrowing and collapse of the ICA and ciliary cleft, resulting in blockage of the conventional aqueous humor outflow and increase in IOP that is more extreme and more abrupt than in POAG.[3,9,127–129] If not treated quickly and effectively, the acute IOP elevation results in rapid, irreversible vision loss due to the widespread death of retinal neurons by necrosis or apoptosis.[129] At the time of disease onset, most affected dogs are middle-aged (4–10 years) when the progressive narrowing of the ICA and ciliary cleft reaches a critical threshold, resulting in decreased aqueous humor drainage and IOP elevation.[1,3,9,130] Welsh springer spaniels and Great Danes can be affected at much younger ages of less than 2 years.[131,132] The condition usually begins in one eye, and the fellow eye typically becomes affected within 1 year.[133,134] Similar to human PACG, and in contrast to the tendency in POAG, female dogs are twice as likely to be affected as male dogs.[1,3,9,131,134–140] The reasons for this difference are not well understood; it is possible that a shorter axial globe length in female compared with male dogs may result in a higher susceptibility for IOP to increase.[141] Furthermore, female dogs tend to have a narrower ICA opening, which may predispose them to angle closure.[138]

The pathogenesis of canine PACG is still not well understood. A narrow ICA and ciliary cleft are considered to be the prerequisite structural abnormality and are related to PLD.[9,128,130,132,142,143] The pectinate ligament is the most anterior and visible part of the ICA in dogs; it projects from the base of the iris to the peripheral Descemet membrane of the cornea.[127,144] The genetics of PLD has been studied independently from the genetics of PACG and are discussed in the next section.

A large number of breeds are predisposed to PACG, with the highest prevalences found in breeds such as the American cocker spaniel, basset hound, Chow Chow, Siberian husky, Shiba inu, Shih Tzu, Magyar Vizsla, and Newfoundland.[1,3,134,139,145] The disease has been studied most thoroughly in American and English cocker spaniels,[128,129,146–152] basset hound,[26,27,127–129,146,150–154] English and Welsh springer spaniels,[9,131] Bouvier des Flandres,[142,149] Chow Chow,[152,155] Siberian husky,[152] Great Dane,[132] flat-coated retriever,[143,156,157] Samoyed,[11–13] Shiba inu,[19,21,130,145] Shih Tzu,[21,145] Eurasier dog (created from Chow Chow and Samoyed),[141] Dandie Dinmont terrier,[28] and golden retriever.[158]

Despite the proposed autosomal-dominant and autosomal-recessive inheritance of PACG in the Welsh springer spaniel[131] and Siberian husky,[159] respectively, PACG generally appears to be a complex trait with multiple genetic and possibly environmental risk factors; the investigation of its genetics has been challenging, and much work remains to be done. Thanks to the establishment of informative pedigrees in a colony setting, the genetics of canine PACG has been studied in the greatest detail in the basset hound.[26,27,127] Three genetic loci have recently been implicated by GWAS as possible contributors to the PACG phenotype in this breed and contain the positional candidate genes COL1A2, RAB22A, and NEB.[26,27] All 3 of these genes are expressed in the anterior segment of the eye and may play a role in the regulation of aqueous humor outflow.[26,27] Because of the suspected function of collagen and other ECM components in the development of glaucoma,[51,57] COL1A2 (encoding the pro-alpha2 chain of type I collagen) is a promising PACG candidate gene. NEB encodes for nebulin, a protein that regulates muscle contractility, and it has been found to be expressed in the ciliary muscle.[27,160] It is conceivable that altered Nebulin function may contribute to PACG development through a muscle-related mechanism.[27]

SRBD1 was identified as a PACG risk gene in Shiba inus and Shih Tzus.[21] Its function remains unknown; the gene encodes for S1 RNA-binding domain and also has been associated with primary glaucoma in human patients.[161–163] Another susceptibility locus for canine PACG was mapped to a 9.5-Mb region on canine chromosome 8 in the Dandie Dinmont terriers, but no specific disease gene could be identified by screening positional candidate genes.[28]

Although individual genetic risk factors for PACG may be inherited as an autosomal-recessive trait, PACG as a whole is still considered a complex trait. For example, 88% of PACG-affected basset hounds are homozygous for the NEB risk allele; the remaining 12% are heterozygous.[27] When evaluating PACG-unaffected basset hounds, 33% and 44% of them are homozygous and heterozygous for the NEB risk allele, respectively.[27] Only 22% of PACG-unaffected basset hounds are homozygous for the nonrisk allele.[27] In other words, the disease-associated NEB allele appears to be quite common in the basset hound population,[27] but not all of the homozygous and heterozygous animals develop PACG; additional genetic and environmental factors likely contribute.

GENETICS OF PECTINATE LIGAMENT DYSPLASIA AND CILIARY CLEFT OPENING

Combined with the narrowing of the ICA and ciliary cleft, an abnormal development of the pectinate ligament, also called goniodysgenesis or PLD, is considered a risk factor for the development of PACG.[9,13,130,132,142,143,153] However, it is important to keep in mind that not all dogs with PLD develop glaucoma. PLD results from an insufficient resorption of mesenchymal tissue within the anterior aspect of the ciliary cleft during ocular development; this resorption is completed in normal puppies by 19 to 28 days of age.[11,142,144,146,164] The term dysplasia is controversial because the prevalence and severity of PLD appear to progress with age, along with a narrowing of the ICA, the latter being associated with an age-related increased size of the lens.[9,11,128,141,143,157,158,165] Similar to PACG, a higher prevalence and severity of PLD as well as a narrower ICA opening are generally observed in female dogs.[131,138,141,148,158] In some breeds, such as the English springer spaniel, flat-coated retriever, Great Dane, Samoyed, and Shiba Inu, no predisposition for PLD and ICA opening based on sex was documented.[9,12,130,132,156]

The inheritance of PLD and the width of the ciliary cleft opening were documented in several breeds, including English springer spaniel,[9] flat-coated retriever,[143,156] Great Dane,[132] and Samoyed.[165] Both the severity of PLD and the narrowing of the ciliary cleft worsen with the degree of kinship with PACG-affected animals, suggesting a quantitative polygenic, rather than monogenic, trait.[9,165] In the English springer spaniel, mating of dogs with normal ICAs appears to reduce the presence and degree of an abnormal appearance of the ICA in the offspring.[9] However, breeding only dogs with normal ICAs without considering their relationship to dogs with glaucoma is not a guarantee that the offspring will not develop glaucoma.[9] The Bouvier des Flandres appears to be an exception, with pedigree analysis suggesting a recessive inheritance of PLD.[166]

Recommendations to examine the ICA by gonioscopy as part of the genetic eye screening and in giving breeding advice for dogs with PLD differ between the American College of Veterinary Ophthalmologists (ACVO) and the European College of Veterinary Ophthalmologists (ECVO).[6,7] The ECVO has stricter guidelines regarding the need for gonioscopy and the exclusion of PLD-affected animals from breeding.[7] Gonioscopy is advised by the ECVO in the following breeds: American cocker spaniel, all types of bassets, Bouvier des Flandres, Chow Chow, border collie, Dandy Dinmont terrier, rough-haired Dutch shepherd, English springer spaniel, Entlebucher mountain dog, flat-coated retriever, Siberian husky, Leonberger, Magyar Vizsla, Samoyed, and Tatra.[7] PLD is classified by the ECVO, based on severity, as free, fibrae latae (abnormally broad and thickened pectinate ligament fibers), laminae (solid plates or sheets of pectinate ligament tissue), and occlusio (persistence of an embryonic sheet of ICA tissue and the absence of intraligamentary spaces, except for flow holes).[7,141,158] Fibrae latae, laminae, and occlusio are associated with a narrow ICA.[13,142,158,165] With mild changes affecting less than 25% of the pectinate ligament circumference, the animal can still be considered unaffected; however, a diagnosis of laminae and occlusio will prompt a recommendation against breeding.[7,158]

Despite the recent issue of a special form by the ACVO Genetics Committee and the Orthopedic Foundation for Animals (OFA) for information gathering and tracking information related to PLD, performing a gonioscopy as part of the genetic eye screening remains optional.[6] Furthermore, there are no ACVO guidelines against the breeding of PLD-affected dogs.[6] The looser ACVO recommendations were justified by the poor predictive value of gonioscopy findings for PACG development in individual dogs and their offspring. Furthermore, without the additional assessment of the ciliary cleft width by high-resolution ultrasonography or ultrasound biomicroscopy, the examination of the ICA by gonioscopy alone may not provide a full picture about the status of the aqueous humor outflow pathways.[3,127,138]

GENETICS OF PRIMARY OPEN-ANGLE GLAUCOMA

Most of the recent advances in canine glaucoma genetics have been made on POAG, even though this form of glaucoma is less prevalent in the canine population than

PACG.[3] The study on canine POAG genetics was facilitated by (1) the availability of a well-established POAG beagle colony, and (2) the monogenic, autosomal-recessive inheritance of all investigated forms of canine POAG.[3,25,76,167] The disease is characterized by the gradual bilateral increase in aqueous humor outflow resistance and IOP over months or years despite normal-appearing ICA and pectinate ligament.[3] In contrast to PACG, vision loss occurs more slowly, and there is no apparent sex predisposition.[3,24,25,168]

The autosomal-recessive inheritance of beagle POAG has been well known for years.[167] Initial candidate gene studies failed to detect mutations in the classic human glaucoma genes *MYOC*, *CYP1B1*, and *NTF4*.[17,18,20] A Gly661Arg missense mutation (the amino acid glycine has been replaced by arginine at position 661) in *ADAMTS10* was identified by a family-based mapping approach as the probable cause of beagle POAG.[76] *ADAMTS10* is strongly expressed in the trabecular meshwork, supporting its role in aqueous humor outflow.[76] However, the molecular and cellular disease mechanisms leading from the *ADAMTS10* missense mutation to plaque formation and increased aqueous humor outflow resistance within the trabecular meshwork still need to be determined.[24,67] The discovery of *ADAMTS10* as a POAG gene in the beagle resulted in the microfibril hypothesis of glaucoma.[82] (The genetics of ECM abnormalities associated with primary glaucoma was discussed in an earlier section.)

The Gly661Arg missense mutation in *ADAMTS10* described in POAG-affected beagles was excluded as a cause of primary glaucoma in the American cocker spaniel, Australian cattle dog, Chihuahua, Jack Russell terrier, Jindo, Siberian husky, Shiba inu, Shih Tzu, and Yorkshire terrier.[76] However, the authors have recently described a novel Ala387Thr missense mutation in *ADAMTS10* of POAG-affected Norwegian elkhounds (see **Figs. 1** and **2**); this alanine-to-threonine change mutation interrupts a highly conserved residue in the ADAMTS10 metalloprotease domain.[25]

As discussed in a previous section, the discovery of *ADAMTS10* as a disease gene, combined with the finding of zonular dysplasia and lens zonule rupture in mutant beagles before the onset of clinical POAG,[8] suggests that beagle POAG is analogous to human WMS/MS, a group of ECM diseases with the ocular phenotype consisting of ectopia lentis/PLL and glaucoma.[77,79–81,83–87] Consistent with the human disease phenotype, it is the authors' clinical experience that *ADAMTS10*-mutant beagles can present to the veterinary ophthalmologist because of primary clinical signs of either primary glaucoma or PLL.

The authors are not aware of any reports of zonular dysplasia or PLL in *ADAMTS10*-mutant Norwegian elkhounds. However, several other breeds affected by both POAG and PLL are currently being evaluated by the authors and others for mutations in WMS/MS candidate genes, including the basset fauve de Bretagne, Chinese sharpei,[77,169] and petit basset griffon vendéen.[10] A genetic POAG test is already available for the petit basset griffon vendéen, but the disease gene has not yet been published (see **Table 2**).

Interestingly, the *ADAMTS10* mutations in the beagle and Norwegian elkhound do not appear to result in the skeletal or cardiovascular changes observed in human WMS/MS patients.[78,80,85,94,95] In support of the proposition that an abnormal ECM metabolism results from mutations in *ADAMTS10*, the authors observed that the sclera of mutant beagles is weaker and has biochemical differences compared with wild-type tissue.[75] They posit that the altered biomechanical properties of the *ADAMTS10*-mutant sclera has a neuroprotective effect and may partially explain their clinical observation that POAG-affected beagles maintain vision longer at high IOPs than PACG-affected dogs without an *ADAMTS10* mutation.

GENETICS OF PRIMARY LENS LUXATION

Based on what has been learned in recent years about canine POAG and PLL and the close/overlapping relationship between the 2 disorders, a discussion of PLL genetics is included in this review on canine primary glaucoma, despite the previous classification of glaucoma as being a secondary phenomenon. Canine PLL is a painful and blinding inherited condition (when glaucoma arises) and is defined as the spontaneous displacement of the crystalline lens due to zonular dysplasia rather than damage of the lens zonule by another disease process such as trauma or inflammation.[170–173] The lens may be partially luxated/subluxated or completely displaced either into the anterior chamber or into the vitreous.[170] PLL tends to affect dogs 3 to 8 years of age, and it typically manifests in both eyes within weeks or months.[169,170,173–178] No sex predisposition has been documented. PLL has been reported in more than 45 breeds, and it predominantly affects smaller western terriers as well as the Tibetan terrier and other breeds that may or may not have terrier coancestry, such as the Australian cattle dog, border collie, and Chinese shar-pei.[169–172,175,176,178] Both the ACVO and the ECVO advise against breeding dogs affected by PLL; the ECVO also recommends excluding parents and offspring of affected animals (see **Table 1**).[6,7]

There is a general consensus that glaucoma seen commonly in dogs with PLL occurs secondary to the dislocation of the lens, especially following lens luxation into the anterior chamber.[2,170] The mechanisms for the often acute IOP increase are not well understood; they may include inhibition of aqueous humor flow through the pupil by the dislocated lens or vitreous as well as the obstruction of the ICA by vitreous prolapsed into the anterior chamber or by inflammatory cells.[170] However, there are strong indications that at least some of the PLL-affected dogs also suffer from primary glaucoma. This association is supported by the observation of high IOP in some PLL-affected dogs with posterior lens luxation and lens subluxation, rather than anterior lens luxation.[173,179] Furthermore, POAG-affected dogs can clinically present with PLL before the onset of IOP elevation, as the authors and others have observed in the petit basset griffon vendéen and the *ADAMTS10*-mutant beagle.[8,10]

The major PLL-causing mutation was mapped by a combination of microsatellite mapping, SNP GWAS mapping, and SNP fine mapping in the Jack Russell terrier, Lancashire heeler, and miniature bull terrier: sequencing of a strong positional candidate gene led to the identification of a splice donor site mutation in *ADAMTS17* (*ADAMTS17c.1473+1G>A*), which resulted in exon-skipping with a resulting frameshift and premature stop codon.[29,30] Subsequently, the c.1473+1G>A mutation in *ADAMTS17* was found in PLL-affected dogs of an additional 14 breeds, not all of them with terrier coancestry: Australian cattle dog, Chinese crested dog, Jagdterrier, Parson Russell terrier, Patterdale terrier, rat terrier, Sealyham terrier, Tenterfield terrier, Tibetan terrier, toy fox terrier, Volpino Italiano, Welsh terrier, wire-haired fox terrier, and Yorkshire terrier.[77] Genetic testing for this *ADAMTS17* mutation is currently available for 26 breeds (see **Table 2**). PLL-affected dogs from other breeds, such as the border collie,[180] Brittany, and shar-pei,[169] tested negative for the *ADAMTS17* mutation, indicating that at least one more genetically distinct form of canine PLL exists.[77] The presence of the same *ADAMTS17* mutation in many canine breeds with diverse origins suggests that this genetic defect is ancient and developed in a founder dog for all of these breeds.[77]

Based on the well-documented autosomal inheritance of canine PLL,[169,173,174,176,177,181] the large majority of dogs that are heterozygous for the *ADAMTS17* mutation remain clinically unaffected.[29,77] However, it is estimated that nearly 5% of heterozygous miniature bull terriers, but also a few heterozygous dogs of other breeds, such as the Parson Russell terrier, Chinese crested dog, and Tenterfield terrier, might develop PLL.[29,77] The investigators speculate that this finding could be attributed to haploinsufficiency, a dominant-negative effect of the mutant ADAMTS17 protein, or additional mutations in *ADAMTS17* or elsewhere in the genome.[29,77] The Animal Health Trust recommends that carriers of the *ADAMTS17* mutation be regularly screened for signs of PLL.

As discussed in previous sections, *ADAMTS17*, together with *ADAMTS10* and *FBN1*, plays an important role in the formation of microfibrils, and in humans, mutation in any of these genes results in WMS/MS.[78–84] In contrast to ADAMTS17-mutant human patients with short stature and ocular signs, such as ectopia lentis/PLL and glaucoma,[80,182,183] the canine disease phenotype is limited to ocular symptoms.[80]

STRATEGIES TO TARGET PRIMARY GLAUCOMA IN CANINE POPULATIONS

Because of the large number of dogs affected by primary glaucoma,[1] a painful, blinding disease without a cure, there is a strong desire to find improved strategies to eliminate this condition from the canine population. Despite the higher disease prevalence compared with inherited retinopathy,[1,15] progress has been much slower to identify disease genes and genetic markers, mostly because many forms of primary glaucoma are complex traits with several genetic and environmental risk factors. Based on the quality of available scientific data, suggested breeding strategies may vary, as shown by the different approaches developed by the ACVO and ECVO to address PLD.[6,7]

The availability of a mutation detection test is an optimal tool to tackle monogenic, autosomal-recessive diseases such as POAG in the beagle, Norwegian elkhound, and petit basset griffon vendéen or PLL in many breeds (see **Table 2**). Nevertheless, breeding recommendations should be carefully developed in order not to cause harm by inbreeding. It is especially true for genetic diseases with a high prevalence within a breed; breeding of affected and carrier dogs may need to be permitted in order to avoid serious limitations of the available gene pool that can result in the emergence of other hereditary diseases or loss of desirable traits.[14] However, these affected and carrier dogs should only be bred to homozygous normals in order to ensure that the puppies are not affected. Such a breeding strategy may not be ideal if heterozygous animals also potentially develop the disease, such as in the case of PLL in the miniature bull terrier and other breeds.[29,77]

When dealing with a polygenic condition with a late disease onset, such as canine PACG, the development of breeding strategies is more challenging. Both the ACVO and the ECVO advise against breeding glaucoma-affected dogs (see **Table 1**). For quantitative traits such as PLD that affect a large number of animals within a breed, the exclusion of only the most severely affected animals, as recommended by the ECVO, may result in a gradual reduction of PLD severity and it is hoped will make glaucoma far less prevalent.[7]

If genetic tests for glaucoma risk alleles should become available, their results will have to be interpreted with great caution and considered alongside other genetic or clinical information. For the *NEB* risk allele, which is quite common in the basset hound population, a considerable number of PACG-unaffected dogs are homozygous or heterozygous for the *NEB* risk allele.[27]

The identification of glaucoma-affected animals by genetic testing before disease onset has several advantages: The animal can potentially be treated earlier and more effectively in order to prevent vision loss, and breeding pairs can be selected so as to avoid the birth of affected animals.

SUMMARY

Considering the high prevalence of canine primary glaucomas, advances in the understanding of their genetics have been slow and challenging, mostly because PACG, the most common form of canine primary glaucomas, is a complex trait with multiple genetic and possibly environmental risk factors. Five susceptibility genes or loci have been identified so far as possible contributors to canine PACG. In addition, the 2 disease genes *ADAMTS10* and *ADAMTS17* have been identified as causes for canine POAG and PLL in several breeds; they are autosomal-recessive traits that have some phenotypic overlap in dogs and are homologous to the human connective tissue disorders WMS/MS. It is hoped the identification of canine glaucoma disease genes and the development of genetic tests will help to avoid the breeding of affected dogs in the future and may allow for earlier diagnosis and potentially more effective therapy.

ACKNOWLEDGMENTS

The authors thank Ms Elizabeth Gratch and Mr Gabriel Stewart for their assistance with the writing of this article.

REFERENCES

1. Gelatt KN, MacKay EO. Prevalence of the breed-related glaucomas in purebred dogs in North America. Vet Ophthalmol 2004;7(2):97–111.
2. Gelatt KN, MacKay EO. Secondary glaucomas in the dog in North America. Vet Ophthalmol 2004;7(4):245–59.
3. Plummer CE, Regnier A, Gelatt KN. The canine glaucomas. In: Gelatt KN, Gilger BC, Kern TJ, editors. Veterinary ophthalmology. 5th edition. Hoboken (NJ): John Wiley & Sons, Inc; 2013. p. 1050–145.
4. Gelatt KN, Gum GG, Mackay EO, et al. Estimations of aqueous humor outflow facility by pneumatonography in normal, genetic carrier and glaucomatous beagles. Vet Comp Ophthalmol 1996;6(3):148–51.
5. Peiffer RL Jr, Gum GG, Grimson RC, et al. Aqueous humor outflow in beagles with inherited glaucoma: constant pressure perfusion. Am J Vet Res 1980; 41(11):1808–13.
6. American College of Veterinary Ophthalmologists' Genetics Committee. Ocular disorders presumed to be inherited in purebred dogs. 5th edition. Meridian (ID): American College of Veterinary Ophthalmologists; 2010.
7. European College of Veterinary Ophthalmologists' Hereditary Eye Disease Committee. Manual for presumed inherited eye diseases in dogs and cats. Utrecht (The Netherlands): European College of Veterinary Ophthalmologists; 2013.
8. Teixeira LB, Scott EM, Iwabe S, et al. Zonular ligament dysplasia in beagles with hereditary primary open angle glaucoma (POAG) [abstract 3564]. In: Annual Meeting of the Association for Research in Vision and Ophthalmology (ARVO). Seattle (WA), May 5–9, 2013.
9. Bjerkas E, Ekesten B, Farstad W. Pectinate ligament dysplasia and narrowing of the iridocorneal angle associated with glaucoma in the English Springer Spaniel. Vet Ophthalmol 2002;5(1):49–54.
10. Bedford P. Primary open angle glaucoma (POAG) in the Petit Basset Griffon Vendéen (PBGV) [abstract 66]. In: European College of Veterinary Ophthalmologists (ECVO) Annual Scientific Meeting. London (UK), May 15–18, 2014.

11. Ekesten B. Correlation of intraocular distances to the iridocorneal angle in Samoyeds with special reference to angle-closure. Prog Vet Comp Ophthalmol 1992; 2:67–73.

12. Ekesten B, Narfsrom K. Age-related changes in intraocular pressure and iridocorneal angle in Samoyeds. Prog Vet Comp Ophthalmol 1991;1:37–40.

13. Ekesten B, Narfstrom K. Correlation of morphologic features of the iridocorneal angle to intraocular pressure in Samoyeds. Am J Vet Res 1991;52(11):1875–8.

14. Petersen-Jones SM. Ophthalmic genetics and DNA testing. In: Gelatt KN, Gilger BC, Kern TJ, editors. Veterinary ophthalmology. 5th edition. Hoboken (NJ): John Wiley & Sons, Inc; 2013. p. 524–32.

15. Miyadera K, Acland GM, Aguirre GD. Genetic and phenotypic variations of inherited retinal diseases in dogs: the power of within- and across-breed studies. Mamm Genome 2012;23(1–2):40–61.

16. Wang R, Wiggs JL. Common and rare genetic risk factors for glaucoma. Cold Spring Harb Perspect Med 2014;4(12):a017244.

17. Kato K, Kamida A, Sasaki N, et al. Evaluation of the CYP1B1 gene as a candidate gene in beagles with primary open-angle glaucoma (POAG). Mol Vis 2009; 15:2470–4.

18. Kato K, Sasaki N, Gelatt KN, et al. Autosomal recessive primary open angle glaucoma (POAG) in beagles is not associated with mutations in the myocilin (MYOC) gene. Graefes Arch Clin Exp Ophthalmol 2009;247(10):1435–6.

19. Kato K, Sasaki N, Matsunaga S, et al. Cloning of canine myocilin cDNA and molecular analysis of the myocilin gene in Shiba Inu dogs. Vet Ophthalmol 2007;10(Suppl 1):53–62.

20. Kato K, Sasaki N, Shastry BS. Retinal ganglion cell (RGC) death in glaucomatous beagles is not associated with mutations in p53 and NTF4 genes. Vet Ophthalmol 2012;15(Suppl 2):8–12.

21. Kanemaki N, Tchedre KT, Imayasu M, et al. Dogs and humans share a common susceptibility gene SRBD1 for glaucoma risk. PLoS One 2013;8(9):e74372.

22. Kirkness EF, Bafna V, Halpern AL, et al. The dog genome: survey sequencing and comparative analysis. Science 2003;301(5641):1898–903.

23. Lindblad-Toh K, Wade CM, Mikkelsen TS, et al. Genome sequence, comparative analysis and haplotype structure of the domestic dog. Nature 2005;438(7069): 803–19.

24. Kuchtey J, Olson LM, Rinkoski T, et al. Mapping of the disease locus and identification of ADAMTS10 as a candidate gene in a canine model of primary open angle glaucoma. PLoS Genet 2011;7(2):e1001306.

25. Ahonen SJ, Kaukonen M, Nussdorfer FD, et al. A novel missense mutation in ADAMTS10 in Norwegian Elkhound primary glaucoma. PLoS One 2014;9(11): e111941.

26. Ahram DF, Cook AC, Kecova H, et al. Identification of genetic loci associated with primary angle-closure glaucoma in the basset hound. Mol Vis 2014;20: 497–510.

27. Ahram DF, Grozdanic SD, Kecova H, et al. Variants in nebulin (NEB) are linked to the development of familial primary angle closure glaucoma in basset hounds. PLoS One 2015;10(5):e0126660.

28. Ahonen SJ, Pietila E, Mellersh CS, et al. Genome-wide association study identifies a novel canine glaucoma locus. PLoS One 2013;8(8):e70903.

29. Farias FH, Johnson GS, Taylor JF, et al. An ADAMTS17 splice donor site mutation in dogs with primary lens luxation. Invest Ophthalmol Vis Sci 2010;51(9): 4716–21.

30. Sargan DR, Withers D, Pettitt L, et al. Mapping the mutation causing lens luxation in several terrier breeds. J Hered 2007;98(5):534–8.
31. Wiggs JL, Allingham RR, Vollrath D, et al. Prevalence of mutations in TIGR/Myocilin in patients with adult and juvenile primary open-angle glaucoma. Am J Hum Genet 1998;63(5):1549–52.
32. Fingert JH, Heon E, Liebmann JM, et al. Analysis of myocilin mutations in 1703 glaucoma patients from five different populations. Hum Mol Genet 1999;8(5):899–905.
33. Stone EM, Fingert JH, Alward WL, et al. Identification of a gene that causes primary open angle glaucoma. Science 1997;275(5300):668–70.
34. Kubota R, Noda S, Wang Y, et al. A novel myosin-like protein (myocilin) expressed in the connecting cilium of the photoreceptor: molecular cloning, tissue expression, and chromosomal mapping. Genomics 1997;41(3):360–9.
35. MacKay EO, Kallberg ME, Barrie KP, et al. Myocilin protein levels in the aqueous humor of the glaucomas in selected canine breeds. Vet Ophthalmol 2008;11(4):234–41.
36. Mackay EO, Kallberg ME, Gelatt KN. Aqueous humor myocilin protein levels in normal, genetic carriers, and glaucoma beagles. Vet Ophthalmol 2008;11(3):177–85.
37. Rezaie T, Child A, Hitchings R, et al. Adult-onset primary open-angle glaucoma caused by mutations in optineurin. Science 2002;295(5557):1077–9.
38. Stoilov I, Akarsu AN, Sarfarazi M. Identification of three different truncating mutations in cytochrome P4501B1 (CYP1B1) as the principal cause of primary congenital glaucoma (buphthalmos) in families linked to the GLC3A locus on chromosome 2p21. Hum Mol Genet 1997;6(4):641–7.
39. Pasutto F, Matsumoto T, Mardin CY, et al. Heterozygous NTF4 mutations impairing neurotrophin-4 signaling in patients with primary open-angle glaucoma. Am J Hum Genet 2009;85(4):447–56.
40. Vithana EN, Nongpiur ME, Venkataraman D, et al. Identification of a novel mutation in the NTF4 gene that causes primary open-angle glaucoma in a Chinese population. Mol Vis 2010;16:1640–5.
41. Morton S, Hesson L, Peggie M, et al. Enhanced binding of TBK1 by an optineurin mutant that causes a familial form of primary open angle glaucoma. FEBS Lett 2008;582(6):997–1002.
42. Fingert JH, Robin AL, Stone JL, et al. Copy number variations on chromosome 12q14 in patients with normal tension glaucoma. Hum Mol Genet 2011;20(12):2482–94.
43. Monemi S, Spaeth G, DaSilva A, et al. Identification of a novel adult-onset primary open-angle glaucoma (POAG) gene on 5q22.1. Hum Mol Genet 2005;14(6):725–33.
44. Burdon KP, Macgregor S, Hewitt AW, et al. Genome-wide association study identifies susceptibility loci for open angle glaucoma at TMCO1 and CDKN2B-AS1. Nat Genet 2011;43(6):574–8.
45. Wiggs JL, Yaspan BL, Hauser MA, et al. Common variants at 9p21 and 8q22 are associated with increased susceptibility to optic nerve degeneration in glaucoma. PLoS Genet 2012;8(4):e1002654.
46. Thorleifsson G, Walters GB, Hewitt AW, et al. Common variants near CAV1 and CAV2 are associated with primary open-angle glaucoma. Nat Genet 2010;42(10):906–9.
47. Li Z, Allingham RR, Nakano M, et al. A common variant near TGFBR3 is associated with primary open angle glaucoma. Hum Mol Genet 2015;24(13):3880–92.

48. Loomis SJ, Kang JH, Weinreb RN, et al. Association of CAV1/CAV2 genomic variants with primary open-angle glaucoma overall and by gender and pattern of visual field loss. Ophthalmology 2014;121(2):508–16.

49. Wiggs JL, Howell GR, Linkroum K, et al. Variations in COL15A1 and COL18A1 influence age of onset of primary open angle glaucoma. Clin Genet 2013;84(2): 167–74.

50. Pasquale LR, Loomis SJ, Weinreb RN, et al. Estrogen pathway polymorphisms in relation to primary open angle glaucoma: an analysis accounting for gender from the United States. Mol Vis 2013;19:1471–81.

51. Vithana EN, Khor CC, Qiao C, et al. Genome-wide association analyses identify three new susceptibility loci for primary angle closure glaucoma. Nat Genet 2012;44(10):1142–6.

52. Awadalla MS, Thapa SS, Hewitt AW, et al. Association of genetic variants with primary angle closure glaucoma in two different populations. PLoS One 2013; 8(6):e67903.

53. Hysi PG, Cheng CY, Springelkamp H, et al. Genome-wide analysis of multi-ancestry cohorts identifies new loci influencing intraocular pressure and susceptibility to glaucoma. Nat Genet 2014;46(10):1126–30.

54. Ozel AB, Moroi SE, Reed DM, et al. Genome-wide association study and meta-analysis of intraocular pressure. Hum Genet 2014;133(1):41–57.

55. van Koolwijk LM, Ramdas WD, Ikram MK, et al. Common genetic determinants of intraocular pressure and primary open-angle glaucoma. PLoS Genet 2012; 8(5):e1002611.

56. Ulmer M, Li J, Yaspan BL, et al. Genome-wide analysis of central corneal thickness in primary open-angle glaucoma cases in the NEIGHBOR and GLAUGEN consortia. Invest Ophthalmol Vis Sci 2012;53(8):4468–74.

57. Vithana EN, Aung T, Khor CC, et al. Collagen-related genes influence the glaucoma risk factor, central corneal thickness. Hum Mol Genet 2011;20(4):649–58.

58. Toh T, Liew SH, MacKinnon JR, et al. Central corneal thickness is highly heritable: the twin eye studies. Invest Ophthalmol Vis Sci 2005;46(10):3718–22.

59. Springelkamp H, Hohn R, Mishra A, et al. Meta-analysis of genome-wide association studies identifies novel loci that influence cupping and the glaucomatous process. Nat Commun 2014;5:4883.

60. Springelkamp H, Mishra A, Hysi PG, et al. Meta-analysis of genome-wide association studies identifies novel loci associated with optic disc morphology. Genet Epidemiol 2015;39(3):207–16.

61. Macgregor S, Hewitt AW, Hysi PG, et al. Genome-wide association identifies ATOH7 as a major gene determining human optic disc size. Hum Mol Genet 2010;19(13):2716–24.

62. Ramdas WD, van Koolwijk LM, Ikram MK, et al. A genome-wide association study of optic disc parameters. PLoS Genet 2010;6(6):e1000978.

63. Axenovich T, Zorkoltseva I, Belonogova N, et al. Linkage and association analyses of glaucoma related traits in a large pedigree from a Dutch genetically isolated population. J Med Genet 2011;48(12):802–9.

64. Fan BJ, Wang DY, Pasquale LR, et al. Genetic variants associated with optic nerve vertical cup-to-disc ratio are risk factors for primary open angle glaucoma in a US Caucasian population. Invest Ophthalmol Vis Sci 2011;52(3): 1788–92.

65. Gum GG, Gelatt KN, Knepper PA. Histochemical localization of glycosaminoglycans in the aqueous outflow pathways in normal beagles and beagles with inherited glaucoma. Prog Vet Comp Ophthalmol 1993;3(2):52–7.

66. Gum GG, Samuelson DA, Gelatt KN. Effect of hyaluronidase on aqueous outflow resistance in normotensive and glaucomatous eyes of dogs. Am J Vet Res 1992; 53(5):767–70.

67. Samuelson DA, Gum GG, Gelatt KN. Ultrastructural changes in the aqueous outflow apparatus of beagles with inherited glaucoma. Invest Ophthalmol Vis Sci 1989;30(3):550–61.

68. Acott TS, Kelley MJ. Extracellular matrix in the trabecular meshwork. Exp Eye Res 2008;86(4):543–61.

69. Crawford Downs J, Roberts MD, Sigal IA. Glaucomatous cupping of the lamina cribrosa: a review of the evidence for active progressive remodeling as a mechanism. Exp Eye Res 2011;93(2):133–40.

70. Ueda J, Wentz-Hunter K, Yue BY. Distribution of myocilin and extracellular matrix components in the juxtacanalicular tissue of human eyes. Invest Ophthalmol Vis Sci 2002;43(4):1068–76.

71. Pijanka JK, Coudrillier B, Ziegler K, et al. Quantitative mapping of collagen fiber orientation in non-glaucoma and glaucoma posterior human sclerae. Invest Ophthalmol Vis Sci 2012;53(9):5258–70.

72. Downs JC. Optic nerve head biomechanics in aging and disease. Exp Eye Res 2015;133:19–29.

73. Coudrillier B, Tian J, Alexander S, et al. Biomechanics of the human posterior sclera: age- and glaucoma-related changes measured using inflation testing. Invest Ophthalmol Vis Sci 2012;53(4):1714–28.

74. Girard MJ, Suh JK, Bottlang M, et al. Biomechanical changes in the sclera of monkey eyes exposed to chronic IOP elevations. Invest Ophthalmol Vis Sci 2011;52(8):5656–69.

75. Palko JR, Iwabe S, Pan X, et al. Biomechanical properties and correlation with collagen solubility profile in the posterior sclera of canine eyes with an ADAMTS10 mutation. Invest Ophthalmol Vis Sci 2013;54(4):2685–95.

76. Kuchtey J, Kunkel J, Esson D, et al. Screening ADAMTS10 in dog populations supports Gly661Arg as the glaucoma-causing variant in beagles. Invest Ophthalmol Vis Sci 2013;54(3):1881–6.

77. Gould D, Pettitt L, McLaughlin B, et al. *ADAMTS17* mutation associated with primary lens luxation is widespread among breeds. Vet Ophthalmol 2011;14(6): 378–84.

78. Hubmacher D, Apte SS. Genetic and functional linkage between ADAMTS superfamily proteins and fibrillin-1: a novel mechanism influencing microfibril assembly and function. Cell Mol Life Sci 2011;68(19):3137–48.

79. Le Goff C, Cormier-Daire V. The ADAMTS(L) family and human genetic disorders. Hum Mol Genet 2011;20(R2):R163–7.

80. Morales J, Al-Sharif L, Khalil DS, et al. Homozygous mutations in ADAMTS10 and ADAMTS17 cause lenticular myopia, ectopia lentis, glaucoma, spherophakia, and short stature. Am J Hum Genet 2009;85(5):558–68.

81. Dagoneau N, Benoist-Lasselin C, Huber C, et al. ADAMTS10 mutations in autosomal recessive Weill-Marchesani syndrome. Am J Hum Genet 2004;75(5): 801–6.

82. Kuchtey J, Kuchtey RW. The microfibril hypothesis of glaucoma: implications for treatment of elevated intraocular pressure. J Ocul Pharmacol Ther 2014; 30(2–3):170–80.

83. Kutz WE, Wang LW, Bader HL, et al. ADAMTS10 protein interacts with fibrillin-1 and promotes its deposition in extracellular matrix of cultured fibroblasts. J Biol Chem 2011;286(19):17156–67.

84. Kutz WE, Wang LW, Dagoneau N, et al. Functional analysis of an ADAMTS10 signal peptide mutation in Weill-Marchesani syndrome demonstrates a long-range effect on secretion of the full-length enzyme. Hum Mutat 2008;29(12): 1425–34.
85. Wright KW, Chrousos GA. Weill-Marchesani syndrome with bilateral angle-closure glaucoma. J Pediatr Ophthalmol Strabismus 1985;22(4):129–32.
86. Chu BS. Weill-Marchesani syndrome and secondary glaucoma associated with ectopia lentis. Clin Exp Optom 2006;89(2):95–9.
87. Izquierdo NJ, Traboulsi EI, Enger C, et al. Glaucoma in the Marfan syndrome. Trans Am Ophthalmol Soc 1992;90:111–7 [discussion: 118–22].
88. Faivre L, Collod-Beroud G, Loeys BL, et al. Effect of mutation type and location on clinical outcome in 1,013 probands with Marfan syndrome or related phenotypes and FBN1 mutations: an international study. Am J Hum Genet 2007;81(3): 454–66.
89. Ueda J, Yue BY. Distribution of myocilin and extracellular matrix components in the corneoscleral meshwork of human eyes. Invest Ophthalmol Vis Sci 2003; 44(11):4772–9.
90. Rohen JW, Futa R, Lutjen-Drecoll E. The fine structure of the cribriform meshwork in normal and glaucomatous eyes as seen in tangential sections. Invest Ophthalmol Vis Sci 1981;21(4):574–85.
91. Lutjen-Drecoll E, Futa R, Rohen JW. Ultrahistochemical studies on tangential sections of the trabecular meshwork in normal and glaucomatous eyes. Invest Ophthalmol Vis Sci 1981;21(4):563–73.
92. Lutjen-Drecoll E, Shimizu T, Rohrbach M, et al. Quantitative analysis of 'plaque material' in the inner- and outer wall of Schlemm's canal in normal- and glaucomatous eyes. Exp Eye Res 1986;42(5):443–55.
93. Rohen JW, Lutjen-Drecoll E, Flugel C, et al. Ultrastructure of the trabecular meshwork in untreated cases of primary open-angle glaucoma (POAG). Exp Eye Res 1993;56(6):683–92.
94. Robinson PN, Arteaga-Solis E, Baldock C, et al. The molecular genetics of Marfan syndrome and related disorders. J Med Genet 2006;43(10):769–87.
95. Faivre L, Dollfus H, Lyonnet S, et al. Clinical homogeneity and genetic heterogeneity in Weill-Marchesani syndrome. Am J Med Genet A 2003;123A(2):204–7.
96. Wright DW, Mayne R. Vitreous humor of chicken contains two fibrillar systems: an analysis of their structure. J Ultrastruct Mol Struct Res 1988;100(3):224–34.
97. Keene DR, Maddox BK, Kuo HJ, et al. Extraction of extendable beaded structures and their identification as fibrillin-containing extracellular matrix microfibrils. J Histochem Cytochem 1991;39(4):441–9.
98. Cain SA, Morgan A, Sherratt MJ, et al. Proteomic analysis of fibrillin-rich microfibrils. Proteomics 2006;6(1):111–22.
99. Sengle G, Tsutsui K, Keene DR, et al. Microenvironmental regulation by fibrillin-1. PLoS Genet 2012;8(1):e1002425.
100. Hollister DW, Godfrey M, Sakai LY, et al. Immunohistologic abnormalities of the microfibrillar-fiber system in the Marfan syndrome. N Engl J Med 1990;323(3): 152–9.
101. Somerville RP, Jungers KA, Apte SS. Discovery and characterization of a novel, widely expressed metalloprotease, ADAMTS10, and its proteolytic activation. J Biol Chem 2004;279(49):51208–17.
102. Wheatley HM, Traboulsi EI, Flowers BE, et al. Immunohistochemical localization of fibrillin in human ocular tissues. Relevance to the Marfan syndrome. Arch Ophthalmol 1995;113(1):103–9.

103. Ramirez F, Rifkin DB. Extracellular microfibrils: contextual platforms for TGFbeta and BMP signaling. Curr Opin Cell Biol 2009;21(5):616–22.

104. Horiguchi M, Ota M, Rifkin DB. Matrix control of transforming growth factor-beta function. J Biochem 2012;152(4):321–9.

105. Chaudhry SS, Cain SA, Morgan A, et al. Fibrillin-1 regulates the bioavailability of TGFbeta1. J Cell Biol 2007;176(3):355–67.

106. Massam-Wu T, Chiu M, Choudhury R, et al. Assembly of fibrillin microfibrils governs extracellular deposition of latent TGF beta. J Cell Sci 2010;123(Pt 17):3006–18.

107. Tripathi RC, Li J, Chan WF, et al. Aqueous humor in glaucomatous eyes contains an increased level of TGF-beta 2. Exp Eye Res 1994;59(6):723–7.

108. Inatani M, Tanihara H, Katsuta H, et al. Transforming growth factor-beta 2 levels in aqueous humor of glaucomatous eyes. Graefes Arch Clin Exp Ophthalmol 2001;239(2):109–13.

109. Ochiai Y, Ochiai H. Higher concentration of transforming growth factor-beta in aqueous humor of glaucomatous eyes and diabetic eyes. Jpn J Ophthalmol 2002;46(3):249–53.

110. Picht G, Welge-Luessen U, Grehn F, et al. Transforming growth factor beta 2 levels in the aqueous humor in different types of glaucoma and the relation to filtering bleb development. Graefes Arch Clin Exp Ophthalmol 2001;239(3):199–207.

111. Schlotzer-Schrehardt U, Zenkel M, Kuchle M, et al. Role of transforming growth factor-beta1 and its latent form binding protein in pseudoexfoliation syndrome. Exp Eye Res 2001;73(6):765–80.

112. Ozcan AA, Ozdemir N, Canataroglu A. The aqueous levels of TGF-beta2 in patients with glaucoma. Int Ophthalmol 2004;25(1):19–22.

113. Yamamoto N, Itonaga K, Marunouchi T, et al. Concentration of transforming growth factor beta2 in aqueous humor. Ophthalmic Res 2005;37(1):29–33.

114. Min SH, Lee TI, Chung YS, et al. Transforming growth factor-beta levels in human aqueous humor of glaucomatous, diabetic and uveitic eyes. Korean J Ophthalmol 2006;20(3):162–5.

115. Fuchshofer R, Tamm ER. The role of TGF-beta in the pathogenesis of primary open-angle glaucoma. Cell Tissue Res 2012;347(1):279–90.

116. Gottanka J, Chan D, Eichhorn M, et al. Effects of TGF-beta2 in perfused human eyes. Invest Ophthalmol Vis Sci 2004;45(1):153–8.

117. Fleenor DL, Shepard AR, Hellberg PE, et al. TGFbeta2-induced changes in human trabecular meshwork: implications for intraocular pressure. Invest Ophthalmol Vis Sci 2006;47(1):226–34.

118. Robertson JV, Golesic E, Gauldie J, et al. Ocular gene transfer of active TGF-beta induces changes in anterior segment morphology and elevated IOP in rats. Invest Ophthalmol Vis Sci 2010;51(1):308–18.

119. Shepard AR, Millar JC, Pang IH, et al. Adenoviral gene transfer of active human transforming growth factor-{beta}2 elevates intraocular pressure and reduces outflow facility in rodent eyes. Invest Ophthalmol Vis Sci 2010;51(4):2067–76.

120. Robertson JV, Siwakoti A, West-Mays JA. Altered expression of transforming growth factor beta 1 and matrix metalloproteinase-9 results in elevated intraocular pressure in mice. Mol Vis 2013;19:684–95.

121. Johnson M. What controls aqueous humour outflow resistance? Exp Eye Res 2006;82(4):545–57.

122. Jelodari-Mamaghani S, Haji-Seyed-Javadi R, Suri F, et al. Contribution of the latent transforming growth factor-beta binding protein 2 gene to etiology of primary open angle glaucoma and pseudoexfoliation syndrome. Mol Vis 2013;19: 333–47.

123. Narooie-Nejad M, Paylakhi SH, Shojaee S, et al. Loss of function mutations in the gene encoding latent transforming growth factor beta binding protein 2, LTBP2, cause primary congenital glaucoma. Hum Mol Genet 2009;18(20):3969–77.

124. Ali M, McKibbin M, Booth A, et al. Null mutations in LTBP2 cause primary congenital glaucoma. Am J Hum Genet 2009;84(5):664–71.

125. Kuehn MH, McLellan GJ, Pfleging A, et al. Spontaneous mutations in LTBP2 are associated with congenital glaucoma in cats [abstract 2424]. In: Annual Meeting of the Association for Research in Vision and Ophthalmology (ARVO). Fort Lauderdale (FL), May 1–5, 2011.

126. Lim SH, Tran-Viet KN, Yanovitch TL, et al. CYP1B1, MYOC, and LTBP2 mutations in primary congenital glaucoma patients in the United States. Am J Ophthalmol 2013;155(3):508–17.e5.

127. Grozdanic SD, Kecova H, Harper MM, et al. Functional and structural changes in a canine model of hereditary primary angle-closure glaucoma. Invest Ophthalmol Vis Sci 2010;51(1):255–63.

128. Bedford PG. The aetiology of primary glaucoma in the dog. J Small Anim Pract 1975;16(4):217–39.

129. Whiteman AL, Klauss G, Miller PE, et al. Morphologic features of degeneration and cell death in the neurosensory retina in dogs with primary angle-closure glaucoma. Am J Vet Res 2002;63(2):257–61.

130. Kato K, Sasaki N, Matsunaga S, et al. Possible association of glaucoma with pectinate ligament dysplasia and narrowing of the iridocorneal angle in Shiba Inu dogs in Japan. Vet Ophthalmol 2006;9(2):71–5.

131. Cottrell BD, Barnett KC. Primary glaucoma in the Welsh springer spaniel. J Small Anim Pract 1988;29(3):185–99.

132. Wood JL, Lakhani KH, Mason IK, et al. Relationship of the degree of goniodysgenesis and other ocular measurements to glaucoma in Great Danes. Am J Vet Res 2001;62(9):1493–9.

133. Miller PE, Schmidt GM, Vainisi SJ, et al. The efficacy of topical prophylactic antiglaucoma therapy in primary closed angle glaucoma in dogs: a multicenter clinical trial. J Am Anim Hosp Assoc 2000;36(5):431–8.

134. Strom AR, Hassig M, Iburg TM, et al. Epidemiology of canine glaucoma presented to University of Zurich from 1995 to 2009. Part 1: congenital and primary glaucoma (4 and 123 cases). Vet Ophthalmol 2011;14(2):121–6.

135. Foster PJ. The epidemiology of primary angle closure and associated glaucomatous optic neuropathy. Semin Ophthalmol 2002;17(2):50–8.

136. Congdon N, Wang F, Tielsch JM. Issues in the epidemiology and population-based screening of primary angle-closure glaucoma. Surv Ophthalmol 1992;36(6):411–23.

137. Quigley HA, Broman AT. The number of people with glaucoma worldwide in 2010 and 2020. Br J Ophthalmol 2006;90(3):262–7.

138. Tsai S, Bentley E, Miller PE, et al. Gender differences in iridocorneal angle morphology: a potential explanation for the female predisposition to primary angle closure glaucoma in dogs. Vet Ophthalmol 2012;15(Suppl 1):60–3.

139. Slater MR, Erb HN. Effects of risk factors and prophylactic treatment on primary glaucoma in the dog. J Am Vet Med Assoc 1986;188(9):1028–30.

140. Vajaranant TS, Nayak S, Wilensky JT, et al. Gender and glaucoma: what we know and what we need to know. Curr Opin Ophthalmol 2010;21(2):91–9.

141. Boillot T, Rosolen SG, Dulaurent T, et al. Determination of morphological, biometric and biochemical susceptibilities in healthy Eurasier dogs with suspected inherited glaucoma. PLoS One 2014;9(11):e111873.

142. van der Linde-Sipman JS. Dysplasia of the pectinate ligament and primary glaucoma in the Bouvier des Flandres dog. Vet Pathol 1987;24(3):201–6.
143. Wood JL, Lakhani KH, Read RA. Pectinate ligament dysplasia and glaucoma in Flat Coated Retrievers. II. Assessment of prevalence and heritability. Vet Ophthalmol 1998;1(2–3):91–9.
144. Martin CL. Development of pectinate ligament structure of the dog: study by scanning electron microscopy. Am J Vet Res 1974;35(11):1433–9.
145. Kato K, Sasaki N, Matsunaga S, et al. Incidence of canine glaucoma with goniodysplasia in Japan : a retrospective study. J Vet Med Sci 2006;68(8):853–8.
146. Bedford PG. A gonioscopic study of the iridocorneal angle in the English and American breeds of cocker spaniel and the basset hound. J Small Anim Pract 1977;18(10):631–42.
147. Magrane WG. Canine glaucoma. II. Primary classification. J Am Vet Med Assoc 1957;131(8):372–4.
148. Lovekin LG. Primary glaucoma in dogs. J Am Vet Med Assoc 1964;145:1081–91.
149. Boeve MH, Stades FC. Glaucoma in dogs and cats. Review and retrospective evaluation of 421 patients. I. Pathobiological background, classification and breed predisposition. Tijdschr Diergeneeskd 1985;110(6):219–27.
150. Alyahya K, Chen CT, Mangan BG, et al. Microvessel loss, vascular damage and glutamate redistribution in the retinas of dogs with primary glaucoma. Vet Ophthalmol 2007;10(Suppl 1):70–7.
151. Mangan BG, Al-Yahya K, Chen CT, et al. Retinal pigment epithelial damage, breakdown of the blood-retinal barrier, and retinal inflammation in dogs with primary glaucoma. Vet Ophthalmol 2007;10(Suppl 1):117–24.
152. Reilly CM, Morris R, Dubielzig RR. Canine goniodysgenesis-related glaucoma: a morphologic review of 100 cases looking at inflammation and pigment dispersion. Vet Ophthalmol 2005;8(4):253–8.
153. Martin CL, Wyman M. Glaucoma in the basset hound. J Am Vet Med Assoc 1968;153(10):1320–7.
154. Wyman M, Ketring K. Congenital glaucoma in the basset hound: a biologic model. Trans Sect Ophthalmol Am Acad Ophthalmol Otolaryngol 1976;81(4 Pt 1):OP645–52.
155. Corcoran KA, Koch SA, Peiffer RL Jr. Primary glaucoma in the chow chow. Vet Comp Ophthalmol 1994;4(4):193–7.
156. Read RA, Wood JL, Lakhani KH. Pectinate ligament dysplasia (PLD) and glaucoma in flat coated retrievers. I. Objectives, technique and results of a PLD survey. Vet Ophthalmol 1998;1(2–3):85–90.
157. Pearl R, Gould D, Spiess B. Progression of pectinate ligament dysplasia over time in two populations of flat-coated retrievers. Vet Ophthalmol 2015;18(1):6–12.
158. Spiess BM, Bolliger J, Borer-Germann SE, et al. Untersuchung zur Dysplasie des Ligamentum Pectinatum beim Golden Retriever in der Schweiz. Schweiz Arch Tierheilkd 2014;156(6):279–84.
159. Nell B, Walde I, Stur I. Kammerwinkelbefunde bei Siberian Huskies im Hinblick auf Glaukompradisposition. Kleintierpraxis 1993;38:353–62.
160. McElhinny AS, Kazmierski ST, Labeit S, et al. Nebulin: the nebulous, multifunctional giant of striated muscle. Trends Cardiovasc Med 2003;13(5):195–201.
161. Writing Committee for the Normal Tension Glaucoma Genetic Study Group of Japan Glaucoma, Meguro A, Inoko H, et al. Genome-wide association study of normal tension glaucoma: common variants in SRBD1 and ELOVL5 contribute to disease susceptibility. Ophthalmology 2010;117(7):1331–8.e5.

162. Liu Y, Garrett ME, Yaspan BL, et al. DNA copy number variants of known glaucoma genes in relation to primary open-angle glaucoma. Invest Ophthalmol Vis Sci 2014;55(12):8251–8.

163. Mabuchi F, Sakurada Y, Kashiwagi K, et al. Involvement of genetic variants associated with primary open-angle glaucoma in pathogenic mechanisms and family history of glaucoma. Am J Ophthalmol 2015;159(3):437–44.e2.

164. Samuelson DA, Gelatt KN. Aqueous outflow in the beagle. I. Postnatal morphologic development of the iridocorneal angle: pectinate ligament and uveal trabecular meshwork. Curr Eye Res 1984;3(6):783–94.

165. Ekesten B, Torrang I. Heritability of the depth of the opening of the ciliary cleft in Samoyeds. Am J Vet Res 1995;56(9):1138–43.

166. Ruhli MB, Spiess BM. Goniodysplasia in the Bouvier des Flandres. Schweiz Arch Tierheilkd 1996;138(6):307–11.

167. Gelatt KN, Gum GG. Inheritance of primary glaucoma in the beagle. Am J Vet Res 1981;42(10):1691–3.

168. Gelatt KN, Gum GG, Gwin RM, et al. Primary open angle glaucoma: inherited primary open angle glaucoma in the beagle. Am J Pathol 1981; 102(2):292–5.

169. Lazarus JA, Pickett JP, Champagne ES. Primary lens luxation in the Chinese Shar Pei: clinical and hereditary characteristics. Vet Ophthalmol 1998;1(2–3): 101–7.

170. Davidson MG, Nelms SR. Diseases of the lens and cataract formation. In: Gelatt KN, Gilger BC, Kern TJ, editors. Veterinary ophthalmology. 5th edition. Hoboken (NJ): John Wiley & Sons, Inc; 2013. p. 1199–233.

171. Alario AF, Pizzirani S, Pirie CG. Histopathologic evaluation of the anterior segment of eyes enucleated due to glaucoma secondary to primary lens displacement in 13 canine globes. Vet Ophthalmol 2013;16(Suppl 1):34–41.

172. Morris RA, Dubielzig RR. Light-microscopy evaluation of zonular fiber morphology in dogs with glaucoma: secondary to lens displacement. Vet Ophthalmol 2005;8(2):81–4.

173. Curtis R, Barnett KC, Lewis SJ. Clinical and pathological observations concerning the aetiology of primary lens luxation in the dog. Vet Rec 1983;112(11): 238–46.

174. Curtis R. Lens luxation in the dog and cat. Vet Clin North Am Small Anim Pract 1990;20(3):755–73.

175. Curtis R, Barnett KC. Primary lens luxation in the dog. J Small Anim Pract 1980; 21(12):657–68.

176. Willis MB, Curtis R, Barnett KC, et al. Genetic aspects of lens luxation in the Tibetan terrier. Vet Rec 1979;104(18):409–12.

177. Curtis R, Barnett KC, Startup FG. Primary lens luxation in the miniature bull terrier. Vet Rec 1983;112(14):328–30.

178. Strom AR, Hassig M, Iburg TM, et al. Epidemiology of canine glaucoma presented to University of Zurich from 1995 to 2009. Part 2: secondary glaucoma (217 cases). Vet Ophthalmol 2011;14(2):127–32.

179. Glover TL, Davidson MG, Nasisse MP, et al. The intracapsular extraction of displaced lenses in dogs: a retrospective study of 57 cases (1984–1990). J Am Anim Hosp Assoc 1995;31(1):77–81.

180. Foster SJ, Curtis R, Barnett KC. Primary lens luxation in the border collie. J Small Anim Pract 1986;27(1):1–6.

181. Ketteritzsch K, Hamann H, Brahm R, et al. Genetic analysis of presumed inherited eye diseases in Tibetan Terriers. Vet J 2004;168(2):151–9.

182. Khan AO, Aldahmesh MA, Al-Ghadeer H, et al. Familial spherophakia with short stature caused by a novel homozygous ADAMTS17 mutation. Ophthalmic Genet 2012;33(4):235–9.

183. Shah MH, Bhat V, Shetty JS, et al. Whole exome sequencing identifies a novel splice-site mutation in ADAMTS17 in an Indian family with Weill-Marchesani syndrome. Mol Vis 2014;20:790–6.

Clinical Signs and Diagnosis of the Canine Primary Glaucomas

Paul E. Miller, DVM*, Ellison Bentley, DVM

KEYWORDS

- Glaucoma • Canine • Tonometry • Optic neuropathy • Intraocular pressure
- Ocular imaging

KEY POINTS

- Early diagnosis is critical in primary angle closure glaucoma (PACG) in dogs.
- Risk factors include breed, age, gender, presence of disease in related dogs, an abnormally formed iridocorneal angle, increased intraocular pressure, and a narrowed or closed ciliary cleft.
- Diagnosis depends on careful ophthalmic examination, particularly of the optic nerve and iridociliary angle if possible, tonometry, and other forms of imaging, such as anterior-segment ultrasound.
- PACG is a bilateral disease, so prophylactic therapy should be initiated immediately after diagnosis in the fellow, nonaffected eye of dogs with PACG.

DEFINITION OF PRIMARY GLAUCOMA

A clinician's working definition of glaucoma determines which clinical signs and diagnostic values are considered important and pivotal in directing therapy. Unfortunately, there is no clear consensus on the definition of glaucoma or its various forms in human or veterinary medicine.[1,2] For more than 100 years, glaucoma has been thought of as a "disease of elevated intraocular pressure (IOP)" and this parameter has been emphasized as the defining clinical sign, diagnostic variable, and therapeutic guide. This remains true for the vast majority of patients with glaucoma in veterinary medicine. Recent advances in both human and veterinary medicine, however, have demonstrated

This work was supported in part by the Core Grant for Vision Research from the NIH to the University of Wisconsin-Madison (P30 EY016665).
The authors have nothing to disclose.
Department of Surgical Sciences, School of Veterinary Medicine, University of Wisconsin-Madison, 2015 Linden Drive, Madison, WI 53706-1102, USA
* Corresponding author.
E-mail address: millerp@svm.vetmed.wisc.edu

that damage to the optic nerve or associated tissues, such as the retinal nerve fiber layer (RNFL) can occur before IOP increases are documented or even after IOP has returned to normal values. This indicates that IOP alone is not the sole characteristic that defines the presence or absence of glaucoma and this fact has caused vision scientists to focus on the anatomic and molecular mechanisms that lead to the characteristic optic disc and visual field changes resulting in glaucomatous vision loss. The evolution of the definition of glaucoma to essentially a specific type of optic neuropathy has led to the proliferation of other diagnostic techniques that evaluate the posterior segment in more detail and tend to de-emphasize the role that IOP plays in this disorder.

For the purpose of this article, "primary glaucoma" is defined as a group of disorders that are typically bilateral, have a strong breed predisposition, are associated with increasing age, are documented or believed to have a genetic basis,[3–5] result in characteristic changes to the optic nerve, and have no readily identifiable secondary ocular or systemic cause on routine ophthalmic examination. IOP is an important risk factor but not the sole risk factor for glaucomatous damage. The gonioscopic appearance of the iridocorneal angle (ICA) further categorizes primary glaucoma into "open" and "closed" forms. The term "primary angle closure glaucoma" (PACG) is used to reflect that the gonioscopic appearance of the ICA changes over time and eventually this structure appears closed.[6,7] In clinical practice, PACG is many times more frequent than primary open angle glaucoma (POAG) in dogs and as such will be emphasized here.

PRIMARY OPEN ANGLE GLAUCOMA

This clinically rare disorder typically occurs in the beagle, where the ADAMTS10 gene has been implicated (**Figs. 1** and **2**).[4,5] POAG is also sporadically observed in other breeds, including the Norwegian elkhound, which also has a mutation in the ADAMTS10 gene but at a different location from that in beagles.[8,9] Because the clinical signs of this form of glaucoma mimic key elements of human POAG, dogs with this form of glaucoma have been used as a model of human POAG for more than 4 decades, resulting in a robust literature base even though the disease is clinically rare.[8]

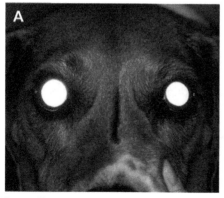 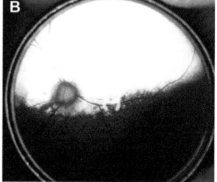

Fig. 1. Chronic POAG in a beagle. (*A*) Both pupils are dilated and IOP is increased in both eyes to approximately 50 mm Hg. (*B*) Fundus photograph of the same dog. The optic disc is depressed from the surface of the fundus (cupped), has little myelin and is darker than normal. The area surrounding the disc has altered reflectivity. (*From* Miller PE. The glaucomas. In: Maggs DJ, Miller PE, Ofri R, editors. Slatter's fundamentals of veterinary ophthalmology. 5th edition. St Louis (MO): Elsevier; 2013. p. 259; with permission.)

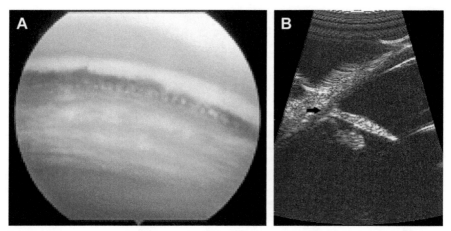

Fig. 2. Primary open angle glaucoma in the beagle (same dog as in **Fig. 1**). (*A*) The iridocorneal angle is gonioscopically relatively open. (*B*) High-resolution ultrasound image of the anterior segment. Note that the iris does not have the same configuration as in PACG (see **Fig. 3**) and that the ciliary cleft is still open (*arrow*). (*From* Miller PE. The glaucomas. In: Maggs DJ, Miller PE, Ofri R, editors. Slatter's fundamentals of veterinary ophthalmology. 5th edition. St Louis (MO): Elsevier; 2013. p. 259; with permission.)

Clinical signs in beagles include an initially open ICA that narrows as the disease progresses, slowly progressive increases in IOP that occur over months to years, mydriasis, lens luxation (which may be part of this genetic mutation), optic nerve atrophy, and vision loss.[8] The disease is similar in Norwegian elkhounds, although it frequently is not diagnosed until the dog is middle-aged or older.[9] With these distinct clinical features in mind, the remaining clinical signs and diagnostic evaluation is similar to that for dogs with PACG.

PRIMARY ANGLE CLOSURE GLAUCOMA

Figs. 3 and **4** demonstrate the typical clinical presentation of this disorder. This entity is typically associated with gonioscopically visible pectinate ligament dysplasia (PLD) in a large number of breeds (**Figs. 5** and **6**).[7,8] In dandie dinmont terriers, it has been associated with a novel genetic locus on CFA8, although it is likely that multiple genes are involved in this disorder.[3] Two genetic loci have been suggested as possible PACG risk-conferring variants in basset hounds.[10] In one study of almost 100 bouvier des Flandres dogs in the United States, a single male dog was the father or grandfather of all affected dogs, even though affected dogs had 5 different mothers.[11] Although the vast majority of dogs who develop PACG have PLD, only a small fraction of dogs with PLD will develop PACG in their lifetime.[11] This strongly suggests that other factors are involved in the genesis of PACG and that the presence or absence of these factors is sufficiently important to determine whether an individual develops PACG or not.

Reverse Pupillary Block

A reverse pupillary block mechanism has been proposed by the authors as the pathophysiologic mechanism of PACG (**Fig. 7**).[7] This hypothesis appears consistent with all known epidemiologic, anatomic, physiologic, and histologic features of PACG in dogs and can explain many of the clinical signs seen in this disorder. In brief, PLD

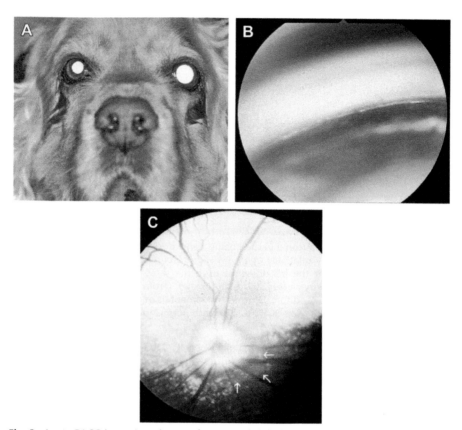

Fig. 3. Acute PACG in an American cocker spaniel. (*A*) This disorder first manifests as a unilateral disease, but both eyes are typically ultimately affected. (*B*) A closed iridocorneal angle on gonioscopy. (*C*) In the acute stages, the optic disc is pale (poorly perfused) and there is subtle peripapillary edema (*arrows*). In the latter stages, it looks similar to that seen in **Fig. 1**. (*From* Miller PE. The glaucomas. In: Maggs DJ, Miller PE, Ofri R, editors. Slatter's fundamentals of veterinary ophthalmology. 5th edition. St Louis (MO): Elsevier; 2013. p. 258; with permission.)

is proposed to the be the first "hit" in a multistep process in which the dysplastic ligament functions as a form of peripheral anterior synechia and holds the peripheral iris in close contact with the inner surface of the cornea. Stress or excitement puts the pupil into a midrange to dilated position and increases pulse pressure amplitudes in the choroid, thereby expanding and contracting the choroid in a pulsatile fashion to a greater degree than what occurs normally. These pulsatile forces are transmitted through the vitreous as a fluid wave to the posterior chamber where small aliquots of aqueous humor are forced through the pupil into the anterior chamber. In humans, it has been calculated that a 5% change in the volume of the choroid would displace 25 µL of aqueous, which is more than enough to raise IOP outside of the normal range.[12] This fluid movement results in slightly higher pressure in the anterior chamber than in the posterior chamber/vitreous (based on calculations in the human eye IOP in the posterior chamber is normally 1 to 2 mm Hg greater than that in the anterior chamber[12]). Normally this increased pressure would force the ICA open,[13] but this compensatory mechanism is abrogated by PLD, which prevents the angle from opening

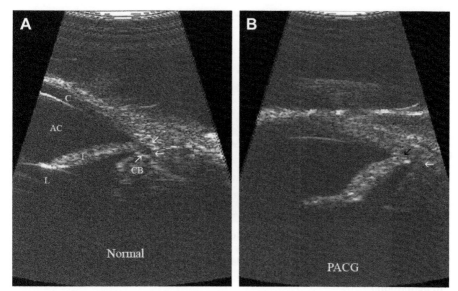

Fig. 4. (*A*) High-resolution ultrasound image of a normal eye. AC, anterior chamber; C, cornea; CB, ciliary body; I, iris; L, lens. White arrows outline the ciliary cleft. (*B*) An eye with acute PACG. Note the sigmoidal shape of the iris, increased contact of the peripheral iris with the cornea (*black arrow*) and collapse of the ciliary cleft (*white arrow*). (*From* Miller PE. The glaucomas. In: Maggs DJ, Miller PE, Ofri R, editors. Slatter's fundamentals of veterinary ophthalmology. 5th edition. St Louis (MO): Elsevier; 2013. p. 258; with permission.)

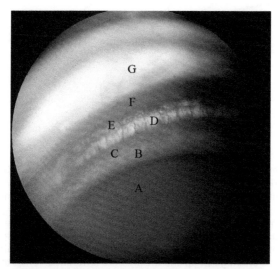

Fig. 5. Goniophotograph of a normal dog. A, pupil; B, iris; C, pectinate ligament strands (*thin brown lines*); D, bluish-white zone of the trabecular meshwork; E, deep pigmented zone; F, superficial pigmented zone; G, cornea. (*From* Miller PE. The glaucomas. In: Maggs DJ, Miller PE, Ofri R, editors. Slatter's fundamentals of veterinary ophthalmology. 5th edition. St Louis (MO): Elsevier; 2013. p. 250; with permission.)

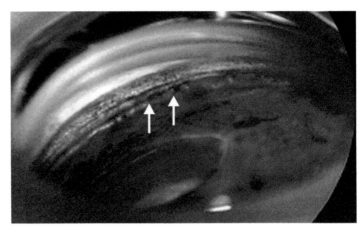

Fig. 6. Marked PLD characterized by broad sheets of tissue. Although IOP was within normal limits, aqueous humor can exit the eye only via a few small "flow holes" (*arrows*) in the sheets. (*From* Miller PE. The glaucomas. In: Maggs DJ, Miller PE, Ofri R, editors. Slatter's fundamentals of veterinary ophthalmology. 5th edition. St Louis (MO): Elsevier; 2013. p. 251; with permission.)

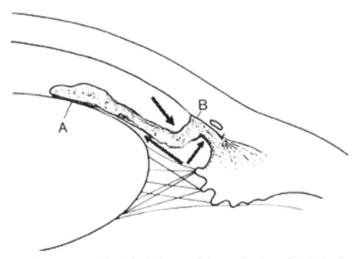

Fig. 7. Proposed reverse pupillary block theory of the mechanism of PACG in dogs. See text for complete description. PLD holds the peripheral iris in close contact with the peripheral cornea and prevents the angle from opening farther when anterior chamber pressures increase. Stress or excitement puts the pupil into the midrange to dilated position and also increases the choroidal pulse pressure. The increase in choroidal pulse pressure forces small aliquots of aqueous humor into the anterior chamber, which results in slightly higher pressure in the anterior chamber than in the posterior chamber (*arrows*). This additional fluid cannot escape via the drainage angle and the pressure differential forces the iris into tighter contact with the anterior lens capsule creating pupil block (A), which prevents aqueous from returning to the posterior chamber. Prolonged increases in IOP lead to peripheral anterior synechia (B) and a further impediment to aqueous outflow. (*From* Miller PE. The glaucomas. In: Maggs DJ, Miller PE, Ofri R, editors. Slatter's fundamentals of veterinary ophthalmology. 5th edition. St Louis (MO): Elsevier; 2013. p. 260; with permission.)

further allowing the additional aqueous to escape. Progressive closure of the ICA over time due to a variety of factors may further facilitate angle closure. The increased pressure in the anterior chamber presses the pupillary zone of the iris more tightly against the anterior lens capsule and creates a "ball-valve" effect at the pupil, which prevents the increased volume of aqueous in the anterior chamber escaping backward to the posterior chamber and normalizing anterior chamber IOP. Mid-range pupils (as seen with dim light and increased sympathetic tone) are more susceptible to pupil block, as they have greater contact with the anterior lens capsule than maximally dilated or very miotic pupils.[12,14] This may be appreciated clinically on detailed slit-lamp biomicroscopy or on high-resolution ultrasonography in which the anterior iris surface assumes a sigmoid appearance and the area of contact between the posterior iris and anterior lens is increased. With subsequent systoles, additional aliquots of aqueous are forced through the pupil and entrapped in the anterior chamber, thereby further increasing IOP until it is counterbalanced by uveal/corneal/scleral resistance to compression/distention, usually in the 50 to 80 mm Hg range. This entire process can occur in the span of minutes and subsequently initiates posterior segment changes affecting the retina and optic nerve that can create a vicious cycle of glaucomatous degeneration.

CLINICAL FORMS OF PRIMARY ANGLE CLOSURE GLAUCOMA

The proposed reverse pupillary block mechanism can explain the various recognized clinical forms of PACG and their associated clinical signs.

Latent

In the *latent* (*occluded angle*) phase, the animal appears asymptomatic, but on gonioscopy the ICA is partially occluded by PLD (primary angle closure, see **Fig. 6**); however, IOP is within the normal range and glaucomatous damage to the optic disc is absent. The vast majority of animals with PLD fall into this category and only a small percentage will go on to develop glaucomatous damage in their lifetimes.[11] The pectinate ligament itself, even if dysplastic, may offer relatively little resistance to outflow. In one study of bouvier des Flandres dogs, aqueous outflow through the ICA of eyes affected with PLD was normal.[15] Additionally, significant differences in IOP were not found in samoyeds with varying degrees of PLD.[16] These studies and the common clinical observation of normal IOP even in the face of severe PLD strongly suggests that PLD itself typically offers relatively little resistance to outflow and that the location of the resistance to outflow (and hence the cause of the increased IOP) is likely located deeper within the ciliary cleft. However, sectioning of normal pectinate ligament fibers considerably opens the ICA and substantially increases outflow, indicating that they serve as a "strut" that prevents the ICA from excessively opening or closing during normal physiologic changes in IOP.[17]

The appearance of PLD is not static and may change over time without an overtly detected increase in IOP.[6] It is unclear, however, whether this change represents progressive thickening of the PLD with age, which is unusual for true dysplasias, or if this represents a form of peripheral anterior synechia that is occurring secondary to chronic apposition between the pectinate ligament and peripheral iris against the trabecular meshwork. In humans, frictional contact between the peripheral iris and the trabecular meshwork degrades the architecture and function of the trabecular meshwork, both in areas with overt peripheral anterior synechia and, more importantly, in areas without overt PAS.[18] In another study, contact between the iris and trabecular meshwork and the peripheral anterior synechia were related to the degree of angle closure on gonioscopy.[19]

This suggests that this contact attenuates aqueous flow through the trabecular meshwork, which in turn results in progressive dysfunction of the endothelium of the Schlemm canal, reduced trabecular meshwork mitochondrial function, fusion of trabecular beams, and eventual occlusion of the iridocorneal angle.[19] Such a process may be involved in the apparent progression of PLD over time in dogs.

Intermittent

In this phase of the disease, the ICA becomes occluded (primary angle closure), resulting in transient increases in IOP that may or may not become overtly symptomatic or result in glaucomatous damage to the posterior segment (PACG). Often owners will comment that at night or under stressful conditions, the conjunctiva becomes hyperemic, the pupil may dilate, and the cornea may become somewhat hazy. Acute vision loss is not a prominent feature of this phase, although with chronic intermittent angle closure, episodic or persistent alterations in vision may occur, indicating that the dog has overt PACG and not just angle closure. It is hypothesized that in this phase a reverse pupillary block is established, but as the pupil dilates, this block is spontaneously broken as the iris slides down the more steeply curved peripheral lens and aqueous humor can once again more freely move through the pupil between the anterior and posterior chambers.[7] Clinically this phase is manifested by acute increases in IOP that spontaneously resolve. However, repeated episodes of intermittent closure may be responsible for the ICA progressing to complete closure and sustained increases in IOP. Histologically (and clinically), evidence for this frictional change is seen as stripping of pigmented epithelial cells from the posterior iris (especially in the pupillary zone) and pigment on the anterior lens capsule and in the ICA, especially inferiorly.[20] In some instances the only means of identifying dogs affected with intermittent primary angle closure is to perform tonometry repeatedly over the course of the day and often evening and demonstrating an intermittent increase in IOP. The presence of notable amounts of pigment in the inferior angle or on the anterior lens surface is also very suggestive of intermittent primary angle closure. Dogs with this form often progress to acute congestive PACG.

Acute Congestive

This phase has the most florid symptoms and is the greatest threat to the maintenance of vision (see **Fig. 3**; **Fig. 8**). This may be the result of a single acute episode of pupil

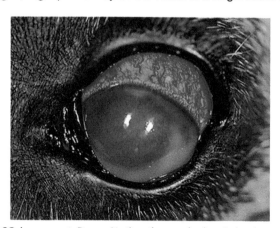

Fig. 8. Acute PACG in a great Dane. Notice the marked episcleral vascular congestion, diffuse corneal edema, and midrange to dilated pupil.

block, although histologically and clinically there is often a suggestion that intermittent but spontaneously resolving rises in IOP may have occurred. Vision alterations are rapid in onset and common in this phase.

Post Congestive

This phase represents animals that have had an attack of acute congestive glaucoma that has resolved, usually through medical or surgical intervention. Clinical signs can be quite variable. IOP is within normal limits and in some instances the eye appears otherwise normal with no detectable vision loss or changes in the appearance of the optic disc. More frequently, however, there are residual signs of an acute attack that can range from mild episcleral injection to a grossly enlarged eye with massive intraocular changes.

Chronic Primary Angle Closure Glaucoma

This end-stage phase is common in dogs. Usually all of the ICA has become permanently closed by peripheral anterior synechia, the ciliary cleft is collapsed, and IOP is chronically elevated. This form may be the result of a prolonged attack of acute congestive glaucoma or repeated intermittent attacks. The latter form is the most common in eyes that are being treated with antiglaucoma drugs. as these tend to blunt the larger IOP spikes but do not completely eliminate the progressive damage to the ICA through frictional contact among the iris, dysplastic pectinate ligament, and trabecular meshwork. These patients tend to exhibit variable IOP measurements on serial examinations, often with sporadic instances of grossly abnormal values. In very advanced instances in which the eye is blind and typically buphthalmic, IOP may decline to normal or subnormal values (despite persistence of angle closure) as the ciliary body becomes atrophic. Severe reductions in aqueous humor production via this mechanism may lead to phthisis bulbi.

CLINICAL SIGNS OF PRIMARY ANGLE CLOSURE GLAUCOMA

Signalment is one of the most useful clinical features in the diagnosis of PACG in dogs. Although numerous breeds are at risk, and the major breeds affected vary by region of the United States and by country, some at-risk breeds dominate large-scale surveys more than others.[21] These include American and English cocker spaniels, basset hound, miniature and toy poodles, great Dane, flat-coated retriever, chow chow, shar-pei, Welsh springer spaniel, and bouvier des Flandres.[21] These breed predispositions are believed to have a genetic basis. Additionally, in most breeds PACG has a significant female predisposition,[21] perhaps due to a significantly smaller angle opening distance than male dogs[22] or a shorter axial length as reported for Eurasier dogs.[23] Both a smaller angle opening distance and shorter axial length would lead to crowding of the ICA. Even small changes in angle opening distance are important, as aqueous humor flow through the trabecular meshwork is related to the radius of the opening distance to the fourth power in accordance with Poiseuille's law. Although any age can be affected, most dogs are middle to older aged,[21] indicating that PLD (which is present at birth) is not, in and of itself, a common cause of PACG.

Historical features are also important factors in the diagnosis of PACG. Many intermittent and acute congestive attacks occur in dim light or under stressful circumstances, such as being groomed or kenneled, moving to a new home, or the arrival of a new baby in the home. This is significant because these stressors result in a midrange pupil, which greatly increases its susceptibility to pupil block.[14] Other historical features of intermittent angle closure also may be present on careful questioning of the client.

EARLY TO MIDSTAGE CLINICAL SIGNS
Pain

Although very mild increases in IOP (5–15 mm Hg) may not be associated with any ocular pain, severe pain is a common feature of most phases of PACG in dogs in which the IOP increase is marked. Owners, and occasionally veterinarians, frequently underestimate the degree of discomfort the animal is experiencing. Pain in acute PACG is often rapidly progressive and may be initially confined to the eye, but, as in humans, it appears to rapidly spread around the orbit and to be associated with frontal or generalized headaches that some humans liken to a migraine. Some dogs will in fact demonstrate blepharospasm in both eyes even though only one eye is affected, likely due to this generalized migraine sensation. This can mistakenly lead to a diagnosis of acute PACG in both eyes if a careful examination is not performed. The degree of pain is likely related to the magnitude of the IOP rise as well as its duration, and it should be assumed that all significant IOP elevations in dogs are associated with ocular pain until proven otherwise. The vast majority of owners will comment that the pet appears more energetic, lively, and youthful when an eye with chronically elevated IOP is enucleated, supporting the view that IOP elevations are painful in dogs.

Systemic Malaise

Dogs with acute congestive PACG appear unwell and may vomit or appear nauseous. Others may sleep more, hide in unusual locations, eat less, or have reduced tolerance for disturbances.

Alterations in Vision

Humans with PACG report colored halos around lights and blurred vision often at night, suggesting mild subacute attacks. These alterations rapidly progress to loss of peripheral vision and eventually complete vision loss if the attack does not spontaneously resolve. Once IOP is lowered, it may take several days to weeks for vision to return, if it returns at all.[24] Progressive vision loss due to an ongoing apoptotic cascade (see Definition, Classification, and Pathophysiology of Canine Glaucoma by Stefano Pizzirani, elsewhere in this issue, for more detailed discussion) is very common and even with successful IOP control vision is frequently lost over the ensuing months to years due to this process.[25]

Episcleral Injection

Episcleral vascular congestion is a common clinical sign in PACG (see **Fig. 8**). It is not simply the result of increased IOP, as it frequently does not accompany postoperative IOP spikes in which comparably high levels of IOP lasting for hours are achieved or when IOP is experimentally increased by infusing saline into the anterior chamber.[26–28] This suggests that episcleral vascular congestion is associated with poorly described vasodilatory factors or intraocular inflammatory pathways that are activated in acute congestive PACG. Episcleral vascular congestion also can occur as drainage of aqueous humor and blood from the scleral venous plexus and vortex venous system is impaired, resulting in blood being shunted through the more superficial episcleral and conjunctival vessels.

Corneal Edema

As noted for episcleral congestion, corneal edema is a common clinical sign of PACG (see **Fig. 8**); however, it is also typically not observed in eyes with acute postoperative IOP spikes or with manometrically controlled marked IOP elevations, suggesting that it is not simply the result of increased IOP driving more aqueous humor into the cornea.[26–28] With normal corneal endothelial function, increased IOP may initially compress the corneal stroma rather than making it edematous; however, persistently elevated IOP drives fluid across the corneal endothelium, creating edema of both the epithelium and stroma. Corneal microcystic changes (subepithelial corneal edema) may initially be observed without gross increases in corneal thickness. Although increased IOP alone does not disrupt the barrier function, a greater pressure gradient forces more fluid across an intact barrier and decreases the efficiency of the endothelial pump.[29] In chronic cases, the corneal endothelium may be damaged to the point that it can no longer maintain normal corneal clarity, even if IOP is restored to normal values.

Mild Aqueous Flare and Cell

These findings are regularly observed in dogs and humans[20,30] and are attributable to pressure-associated anterior-segment ischemia. Flare and cell may worsen after a dramatic reduction in IOP as previously hypoxic tissues become reperfused. Anecdotally, the authors have observed a number of animals in which aqueous flare/cell were absent on detailed slit-lamp biomicroscopy when the eye was normotensive, only to observe mild to moderate flare/cell 1 to 3 days later during an acute attack of PACG. This strongly suggests that, like humans with PACG, not all canine eyes with aqueous flare and cell have secondary glaucoma.[30] This understanding becomes important when assessing the risk to the fellow eye in dogs with unilateral PACG and considering whether prophylactic therapy is warranted,[31] as one should not mistake an eye with mild aqueous flare/cell and acute congestive PACG as having secondary glaucoma.

Pupil Alterations

Pupil abnormalities, such as midrange to dilated, sluggish to fixed, and irregularly shaped pupils, are common signs of primary glaucoma in dogs (see **Figs. 1**, **3**, and **8**). Peripheral anterior synechia can form rapidly (distorting the shape of the iris), and IOP-induced ischemia may produce sectorial or diffuse atrophy of the iris, especially the iris sphincter muscle. This results in a permanently fixed and midrange to dilated pupil. Such atrophy releases pigment and causes pigmentary dusting of the iris surface and corneal endothelium, which are observable both clinically and histologically.[20]

The authors have noted the responsiveness of the pupil to miosis with latanoprost has prognostic value in dogs with acute PACG.[32] Eyes that rapidly develop miosis (indicating relatively mild ischemia may be present) will typically have better short-term outcomes than eyes that do not develop miosis when exposed to fresh latanoprost, presumably because the latter is indicative of greater anterior-segment ischemia, which likely indicates greater posterior segment ischemia as well. Additionally, on detailed slit-lamp biomicroscopy, it may be possible to appreciate the sigmoid appearance of the anterior iris surface (especially seen in the peripheral iris), suggesting reverse pupillary block is present.

Lens Changes

Age-related changes in lens thickness in samoyeds has been suggested to result in anterior chamber shallowing and an increased risk of pupil block in PACG.[33] These changes, however, are difficult to appreciate with slit-lamp biomicroscopy and are best detected on ultrasonography. Glaukomflecken are characteristic small anterior subcapsular lens opacities that occur secondary to lens epithelial cell necrosis in humans with PACG. Similar opacities may also develop as a result of ischemia, but are not routinely recognized in dogs.

Vitreous Alterations

Clinically useful clinical signs involving the vitreous are not recognized in dogs. The vitreous may elongate on ultrasonography, but this is not clinically appreciable.[33]

Retina

During an acute attack, IOP may be high enough to cause retinal or choroidal vascular occlusion and ischemic retinal damage resulting in irregular wedge-shaped retinal lesions that have their apex directed toward the optic disc. Nerve fiber layer defects commonly seen in human PACG are typically difficult to clinically appreciate in dogs, but may be best appreciated by use of red-free (green) light and magnification (see later in this article).

Optic Disc Changes

Optic disc cupping occurs only in glaucoma (see **Fig. 1**; **Fig. 9**); however, early detection of optic disc changes in PACG in dogs is extremely difficult and confounded by the presence of potentially large amounts of myelin over the disc surface. This myelin can obscure the relationship between the optic cup and the surrounding neuroretinal rim and alter the typical cup/disc ratio (typically 0.3 in normal dogs) that is used to evaluate the optic disc for glaucomatous changes in humans. The authors have found that examination of the optic disc by indirect ophthalmoscopy alone is often insufficient in evaluating the disc for potential glaucomatous changes and prefer to use a pediatric gonioprism in which the center lens allows one to view the optic disc with a slit-lamp biomicroscope.

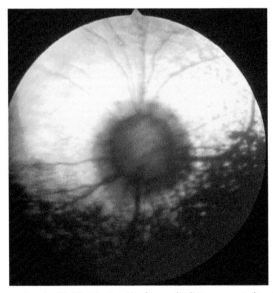

Fig. 9. Optic disc cupping in PACG. Most retinal vessels disappear at the disc edge. The center of the disc is in focus below the level of the retinal surface and is grayish in color. There is also a peripapillary ring of altered retinal reflectivity. (*Courtesy of* Christopher J. Murphy, DVM, PhD, University of California, Davis, Davis, CA.)

In the initial stages of acute congestive PACG, the optic disc often appears swollen with an adjacent peripapillary ring of retinal edema (see **Fig. 3**). The optic disc also may appear paler than normal, suggesting poor perfusion of disc tissue itself. With time, focal areas of disc atrophy may appear, although a more generalized concentric atrophy is more common in dogs. The "laminar dot sign," in which the pores of the lamina cribrosa become visible, may develop in chronic cases, indicating loss of neuronal tissue. In advanced stages, myelin is completely lost, the entire disc is cupped, and the disc is often surrounded by a peripapillary ring of altered reflectivity that extends for one-third to one-half disc diameter around the disc (see **Figs. 1** and **9**).

Changes in the Lateral Geniculate Nucleus and Visual Cortex

There is accumulating evidence that glaucomatous damage to retinal ganglion cells also results in degenerative changes in the brain, including the lateral geniculate and the visual cortex.[34,35] Histopathologic findings are even present in lateral geniculate layers driven by the unaffected fellow eye.[34,35] This has significant implications on the therapy for glaucoma, especially those directed toward neuroprotection or neuro-regeneration, and indicates that this disorder affects more than the eye.

CHRONIC CLINICAL SIGNS

Most of these signs are poor prognostic indicators for vision (**Fig. 10**); however, animals with low scleral rigidity, such as very young dogs or the shar-pei breed, may retain some degree of vision despite the presence of Haab striae and buphthalmia.

Haab Striae

These linear corneal lesions represent breaks in Descemet membranes that occur secondary to stretching of the globe. On detailed examination, the edge of these breaks are thickened and curled, and secondarily proliferate, whereas the area between the breaks is thin and smooth. If the cornea is clear, these breaks usually do not result in surrounding corneal edema despite the endothelial damage, presumably because epithelial fibrotic changes tightly seal the Descemet fracture.

Buphthalmos

Literally meaning "cow" or "ox" eye, this term refers to enlargement of the globe that occurs secondary to chronically elevated IOP (see **Fig. 10**). It is generally an indicator

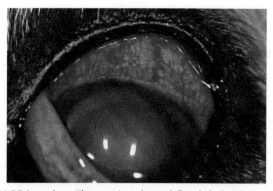

Fig. 10. Chronic PACG in a dog. The eye is enlarged (buphthalmic), irreversibly blind, and has a subluxated lens.

that vision is completely lost. In some instances, clients may comment that the eye appears to grossly change in size, indicating that this finding may fluctuate to some degree with changes in IOP, although once it has occurred, it tends to remain present. This disorder frequently leads to exposure keratitis, corneal ulceration, and other alterations, such as subluxation of the lens and occasionally scleral ectasia. Lens subluxation due to buphthalmia needs to be carefully differentiated from primary lens luxation that leads to secondary glaucoma. History and patient signalment usually readily allow this distinction to be made.

Reduced Episcleral Injection

With time, episcleral vascular injection tends to become less apparent in eyes with chronic glaucoma. The reason for this is unclear but may relate to shifts in blood flow within the eye or a reduction in ischemia-associated damage.

Phthisis Bulbi

This disorder may result in advanced cases of glaucoma, as the ciliary body ceases to produce aqueous humor. It is also a common sequelae to many antiglaucoma therapies that are directed at destroying aqueous humor production. It is also occasionally observed after gonio-implantation with excessive filtration.

DIAGNOSIS OF PRIMARY ANGLE CLOSURE GLAUCOMA

There are several diagnostic aides in addition to the presence of the previously described clinical signs and vision changes that can assist with the diagnosis of PACG in dogs. These techniques can generally be categorized by which aspect of glaucoma pathophysiology they seek to further define (ie, IOP, the iridocorneal angle, visual capabilities of the eye, optic disc, or nerve fiber layer).

TECHNIQUES THAT EVALUATE INTRAOCULAR PRESSURE
Tonometry

All currently available tonometers do not actually measure IOP but instead measure a physical feature of the cornea and use these measurements to *estimate* true IOP (**Fig. 11**). Therefore, all tonometers only provide approximations of IOP and these vary in accordance with a variety of anatomic and physiologic factors.

Indentation tonometry
With Schiotz tonometry, the parameter measured is the extent to which the cornea is indented by a known weight (see **Fig. 11**). Because of the gross distortion of the cornea and the requirement for perpendicular positioning, this instrument has the largest number of potential errors and is the most difficult to use correctly. Nevertheless, with careful adherence to manufacturer's recommendations, accurate estimates of IOP are possible in cooperative animals. Use of the human calibration table that comes with the instrument more closely mimics IOP estimates acquired with the applanation tonometers than canine-specific conversion tables.[36]

Applanation tonometry
With the Tono-Pen XL, Tono-Pen Vet, or Avia (see **Fig. 11**) devices (Reichert Inc, Buffalo, NY, USA), the parameter measured is the force required to flatten (applanate) the corneal surface. The underlying physical principles for applanation tonometers, however, require that the surface be perfectly spherical, flexible, infinitely thin, and dry; features that the cornea only roughly approximates.[28] Corneal drying (after application of a topical anesthetic) or increased tear film viscosity (from mucoid ocular discharge

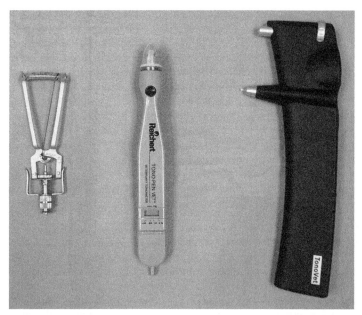

Fig. 11. Tonometers commonly used in the diagnosis of PACG. Far left, Schiotz indentation tonometer; middle, Tono-Pen Vet applanation tonometer; far right, TonoVet rebound tonometer.

or artificial tears/gels) can alter readings with these devices, although applanation tonometers are generally the least affected by abnormalities in the cornea itself.

Rebound tonometry
With the TonoVet (see **Fig. 11**), a blunted pinlike probe is bounced off of the corneal surface.[27] The motion parameters of the probe are then measured and converted by species-specific algorithms (that were derived by comparison to manometric measurements of IOP) to estimates of IOP.[27] The user can select between settings for cat/dog = d, horse = h, and other = p.[27]

By careful calibration to manometrically determined IOP, the measurements obtained with any tonometer can be converted to estimates of IOP by the use of tables (in the case of the Schiotz) or by the use of on-board microprocessors (in the case of the Tono-Pen and TonoVet). Each of these methods has their pros and cons, although when used correctly, all are sufficiently accurate to document elevated IOP in dogs. The authors prefer the Tono-Pen Vet or the TonoVet rebound tonometer because of their ease of use.

There are 3 main sources of error with all tonometers, and it is critical that the clinician fully understand these sources of potential errors.

Tonometer factors Each device has an inherent 1 to 2 mm Hg variability according to the manufacturer, although in manometric studies, the authors have noted that all tonometers can occasionally provide IOP estimates that vary by 3 to 4 mm Hg when they are applied at exactly the same location at exactly the same manometrically controlled IOP. Therefore, the clinician should not overinterpret small (few mm Hg) changes in IOP over time as indicative of a trend in IOP.

It is also important to recognize that most tonometers (with the exception of the TonoVet rebound tonometer) are optimized and calibrated for the human eye. This means that the instruments tend to underestimate true IOP when used in animals.[27,28,36] This error, however, is of limited clinical significance because the underestimation is generally linear over the range of IOP encountered in the clinics and so it is unnecessary to convert these tonometric values to true IOP values by corrective equations. It is critical, however, to recognize that because of this potential underestimation, normal values for one instrument cannot be transferred to another.[27,28,36,37] For example, in one study, mean IOP with the TonoVet was 16.9 ± 3.7 mm Hg, whereas it was 11.6 ± 2.7 mm Hg with the Tono-Pen XL in the same set of dogs.[37] Therefore, it is imperative that normal values be determined for each tonometer, species, and potentially tonometrist.[27,28,36,37] In general, however, if the instrument is properly maintained and instrument-specific normal values are used, instrument-related error has the least impact on IOP estimates in a clinical setting.

Tonometrist-controlled factors This is often the greatest source of error in estimating IOP. Proper application of the device to the cornea is essential. The Schiotz tonometer must be placed perpendicular to the cornea and ground so that the full force of the attached weight is available to indent the cornea. The TonoVet must impact the cornea with the probe parallel to the ground to avoid the effects of gravity on the probe's reverberation characteristics. It also is critical to avoid confounding results secondary to technical errors, such as compressing the globe while holding the eyelids apart (**Figs. 12** and **13**), compressing the jugular veins with a tight collar,[38] corneal drying, or viscous materials present on the corneal surface. IOP estimates in eyes that have had intraocular surgery are also especially prone to erroneous overestimations of IOP because of reductions in ocular rigidity. In the authors' experience, tonometrist-controlled factors are the most frequent and largest source of error in a clinical setting. Corneal changes, such as thinning, neovascularization, and fibrosis, also can affect IOP readings, although typically to a lesser degree than errors in technique do.

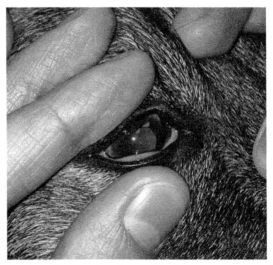

Fig. 12. Incorrect technique for opening the eyelids for tonometry. The lids are being held open with pressure on the globe, thereby artificially increasing IOP.

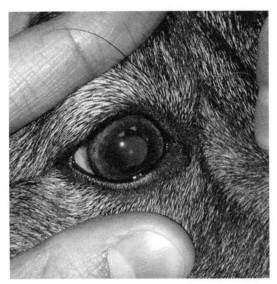

Fig. 13. Proper technique for holding the eyelids open. The lids are opened from over the boney orbital rim thereby avoiding pressure on the globe.

Animal factors IOP is essentially a physiologic parameter and as such it is influenced by the animal's ocular and systemic physiology (especially that related to the respiratory and cardiovascular system). Ideally, the animal should be resting quietly and its head should be the same distance above the heart at each interval.[39] Resisting application of the tonometer by nervous or excited dogs, or dogs that are moving, often results in inaccurate readings and may cause the clinician to believe that increased IOP is present when in fact it is absent. In stressed or uncooperative animals, these errors can be very large.

The Effect of Corneal Thickness on Intraocular Pressure Measurements

Although not a major factor in a clinical setting, corneal thickness plays a role in tonometric estimates of IOP in animals. In a recent study in dogs, it was found that for every 100-μm increase in corneal thickness, the IOP estimate was increased by 1 mm Hg for the Tono-Pen XL and 2 mm Hg for the TonoVet.[37]

TECHNIQUES THAT EVALUATE THE IRIDOCORNEAL ANGLE
Gonioscopy

Because the sclera extends anteriorly in dogs, it is difficult to impossible to view the normal ICA directly. Although it sometimes is possible to visualize the ICA with an indirect ophthalmoscope and a condensing lens held at an extremely oblique angle to the eye, these structures can be more fully and consistently examined by use of a specialized goniolens. Careful evaluation of the iridocorneal angle plays an important role in identifying the type of glaucoma that is present and the likely location of the impediments to outflow. Gonioscopy requires specialized training to properly perform and interpret, and, as such, cases requiring gonioscopy should be referred to a specialist, if possible, to confirm the diagnosis of primary glaucoma and to localize where the impediment to outflow is. Identification and correction of all impediments to outflow are critical to the effective treatment of glaucoma. Because gonioscopy can alter IOP by compressing the cornea, tonometry should be performed before gonioscopy.

A number of goniolenses are commercially available and can be broken down into those that directly view the iridocorneal angle by using the principle of total internal reflection (Koeppe or Barkan, for example) and those that indirectly visualize it by use of one or more reflecting mirrors ("gonioprism," such as a Goldmann single-mirror or 3-mirror or Zeiss 4-mirror [Ocular Instruments Inc, Bellevue, WA, USA]; **Fig. 14**). The latter examines the angle opposite to where the mirror is located. The authors prefer use of indirect gonioscopy with a 3-mirror Goldmann-type diagnostic lens designed for infants, as it allows examination of the entire iridocorneal angle with a slit-lamp biomicroscope and much higher magnification than that achieved with a direct goniolens (which does not allow use of a slit-lamp biomicroscope). Many of the mirrored goniolenses also have a central viewing lens that permits the optic disc to also be examined with a slit-lamp biomicroscope, thereby facilitating identification of subtle glaucomatous changes to the optic disc. The examiner must be careful to avoid indentation of the cornea, as this will make the ICA appear narrower. In the early stages of glaucoma, it is possible to identify compaction of the anterior aspect of the ciliary cleft (seen as a posterior "slanting" of the trabecular meshwork).

Indentation gonioscopy uses a lens in which the area of contact with the cornea is smaller than the corneal diameter (such as a Zeiss 4-mirror goniolens). With this technique, gentle pressure on the cornea will force the peripheral iris posteriorly. If the angle is closed because of simple apposition between the iris and cornea, the angle will be forced open, allowing visualization of the pectinate ligament and trabecular meshwork, whereas if it is closed by adhesions between the iris and cornea (peripheral anterior synechia), it will remained closed. In the authors' experience, appositional closure is uncommon in dogs and the vast majority of angles do not open with indentation gonioscopy. Indentation gonioscopy cannot be performed with lenses that cover most of the corneal surface.

The authors have found the grading scheme proposed by Ekesten and Narfström,[16] which evaluates both the width of the of the iridocorneal angle and the presence or absence of PLD, to be the most useful system (**Fig. 15**). The authors have further

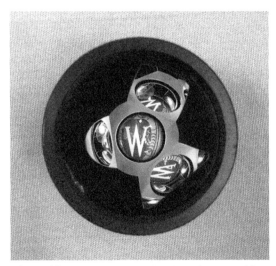

Fig. 14. View through a Goldmann 3-mirror gonioprism. The central lens allows for viewing of the fundus with a slit-lamp biomicroscope. The 3 surrounding mirrors have different degrees of angulation so as to facilitate examination of different structures within the iridocorneal angle.

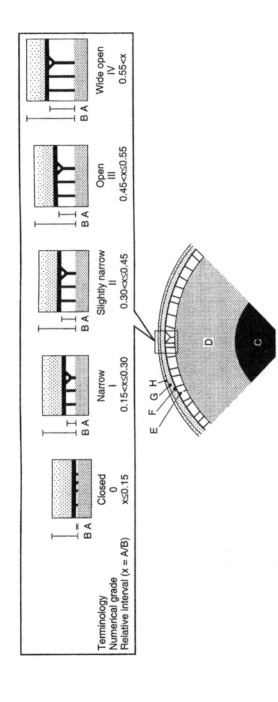

Fig. 15. Schematic drawing of a grading scheme for the width of the iridocorneal angle. The ratio of the width of the anterior opening of the ciliary cleft (A) and the distance from the origin of the pectinate ligaments to the anterior surface of the cornea (B) is estimated. Also shown are the pupil (C), iris (D), pectinate ligament (E), deep pigmented zone (F), superficial pigmented zone (G), and cornea (H). (*From* Ekesten B, Narfström K. Correlation of morphologic features of the iridocorneal angle to intraocular pressure in Samoyeds. Am J Vet Res 1991;52:1875; with permission.)

modified this scheme by calculating an "angle index," which factors in the width of the ICA and the degree of sheeting of the angle.[11] With this technique, the width of the ICA and the extent of sheeting are evaluated and scored separately according to the scheme published by Ekesten and Narfström.[16] These 2 values are then combined into 1 number that is related to the estimated overall capacity for outflow through the iridocorneal angle. This standardized value can be used for statistical analysis and for comparisons between eyes with varying percentages of angle width and PLD, but with different or similar restrictions on the apparent capacity for outflow through the ICA. The angle index is calculated by giving a closed angle a value of 0, a very narrow angle a value of 1, a mildly narrowed angle a value of 2, an open angle a value of 3, and a wide open angle a value of 4, per the previously described criteria.[11,16] For scoring PLD, the percentage of the iridocorneal angle (for 360°) affected by sheeting is visually estimated. The angle index is then calculated by multiplying the angle width score by (1 − the percentage of sheeting). For example, if the iridocorneal angle width is scored as a "2" and 80% of the iridocorneal angle is sheeted closed by PLD, the angle index is 2 × (1 − 0.80) = 2 × 0.20 = 0.40. With this scheme, the maximal angle index value is 4.0 and the minimum value is 0. Therefore, in the preceding example, an eye with an iridocorneal angle width of "2" and PLD sheeting affecting 80% of the circumference of the iridocorneal angle has only 0.4/4 or 10% of the estimated outflow capacity of a fully open iridocorneal angle with no PLD sheeting.

In an almost 9-year longitudinal study of approximately 100 bouvier des Flandres dogs, it was found that there was a strong association between the development of glaucoma and the sheeting corrected angle index ($P<.001$) with the odds of glaucoma doubling for each 0.20-unit decrease in the angle index value.[11] Dogs with an angle index of less than or equal to 1 had a 21% risk of developing PACG compared with a risk of 1.9% for other dogs.[11] Additionally, in this study, all dogs who developed PACG over an approximately 9-year period had PLD at the initial examination.[11]

Ultrasonography

High-frequency ultrasound probes with frequencies ranging from 20 MHz (high-resolution ultrasound [HRUS]) to 60 MHz (ultrasound biomicroscopy [UBM]) have been developed that allow imaging at resolutions that are comparable to low-power microscopic views (20–80 μm). These techniques were developed to improve the visualization of anterior-segment structures and have significantly contributed to our understanding of the pathogenic mechanisms involved in glaucoma and in glaucoma management. They have led to the theory of reverse pupillary block in PACG and have highlighted the critical prognostic and diagnostic role the ciliary cleft plays in glaucoma.

On HRUS imaging of patients with overt PACG or in the normotensive fellow eye that is at risk of PACG, the most striking features are substantial contact between the posterior iris and anterior lens capsule, a sigmoidally shaped iris, and the status of the ciliary cleft (see **Figs. 2** and **4**). The latter may be open (roughly interpreted as the outer and inner walls diverge), narrowed (roughly interpreted as the outer and inner walls are parallel or the overall volume of the cleft is less than normal), or closed (the cleft is not visible). This increased iridolenticular contact is believed to allow for a reversal of the pressure gradients between the anterior and posterior chambers (reverse pupillary block) and is correlated with pigment loss from the posterior iris surface and its deposition in the inferior iridocorneal angle. The authors have come to regard this iris configuration and the presence of ciliary cleft abnormalities to be important diagnostic features of glaucoma.[11] In a recent study of almost 100 bouvier des Flandres dogs, it was determined that the rate of development of glaucoma in dogs with at least one eye with a narrow or closed cleft was 24% (8/33) compared with 1.8% (1/57) in dogs with bilaterally open clefts.[11]

Anterior-Segment Optical Coherence Tomography

This technique uses light instead of sound (in contrast to the HRUS and UBM) to obtain cross-sectional in vivo images of the anterior (or with modifications the posterior segment, see **Fig. 16**). Near-infrared light with a wavelength of 830 nm was first used to acquire images of the anterior segment, but recently this technology has been adapted to use a longer wavelength (1310 nm), which allows for increased penetration of nontransparent tissues such as sclera and iris. Image acquisition is fast and comfortable for the patient (as there is no contact with the eye), and is comparable to those acquired with a UBM. However, as the technique involves light transmission through optically opaque tissues, such as iris and sclera, visualization of the lens and structures posterior to the iris is decreased compared with HRUS or UBM. Due to the large diameter the canine eye, anterior-segment optical coherence tomography (AS-OCT) images also do not span from limbus-to-limbus as they do in humans. The lack of contact with the ocular surface (and hence reduced chance for indentation of the cornea) with AS-OCT versus HRUS and UBM may offer a less distorted view of the ICA than other modalities; however, the UBM and HRUS are the only devices that allow for imaging of the ciliary cleft, and this tissue plays a major role in evaluating the risk for PACG in dogs.

TECHNIQUES THAT EVALUATE THE VISUAL CAPABILITIES OF THE EYE
Visual Field

In theory, directly assessing the patient's full range of vision is the ideal clinical technique for estimating the functional impact of glaucoma on the patient's vision.[40] Manual or automated perimetry tests the light-difference sensitivity across the visual field by asking patients to push a button when they observe a variably sized white target on a white background (so-called standard achromatic perimetry). Although automated perimetry (Humphrey Field Analyzer, for example) is the current gold standard for assessing visual field defects and disease progression in humans, its

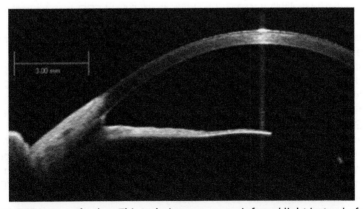

Fig. 16. AS-OCT image of a dog. This technique uses near-infrared light instead of sound to image the iridocorneal angle. As such, visualization of the ciliary body and lens are not as apparent as that observed on high-resolution ultrasound (see **Figs. 2** and **4** for comparison). (*Courtesy of* Carol Rasmussen, MS, University of Wisconsin-Madison, Madison, WI.)

requirement for the patient to follow verbal instructions, maintain fixation on one point in space, and to push a button when the target is observed renders it unsuitable for use in veterinary medicine. Clinicians may be able to crudely estimate a dog's visual field by covering one eye and attempting to get the animal to fixate on a single point in space. A novel and interesting target (such as a food treat) is then introduced from the periphery of the animal's visual field and it is noted when the dog first responds to the presence of the treat. Such techniques, however, are very crude and at best detect only massive changes in the animal's vision. Furthermore, confounding factors, such as scent, may confuse such an evaluation. However, even with standard automated perimetry in humans, visual field defects become apparent only after a substantial number of ganglion cells have been lost, indicating that it is missing early stages of the disease.[41]

In an effort to increase the ability of perimetry to detect glaucomatous changes in the visual field, variations on this technique also have been explored in humans. Although almost all ganglion cells can respond to white light, more specific functions of ganglion cells, such as contrast sensitivity, motion perception, and color vision, are encoded by different subsets of ganglion cells.[42] It is theorized that by "teasing" out these subsets of ganglion cells, so-called function-specific perimetry may be more sensitive at detecting visual field changes before large numbers of ganglion cells are lost. Short-wavelength automated perimetry, which isolates the blue cone visual pathway (a pathway shown to be abnormal in early glaucoma), can be performed with most of the automated achromatic perimetry units. This technique differs from standard achromatic perimetry in that it uses a narrow-band blue-light stimulus on a yellow background, but it still requires the patient to cooperate with the procedure in the same was as for standard automated perimetry.[42] Although this technique may allow detection of visual field changes before standard white-light automated perimetry, further study is required to confirm this.

Electrophysiologic Testing

Electrophysiologic testing is another method for trying to understand the effect of glaucoma on a patient's visual function.[43] The standard *full-field electroretinogram* (ERG), which is predominately driven by the outer retina, is generally not helpful in the diagnosis or treatment of glaucoma, especially PACG, in which the IOP increase may be very sudden.[43–45] If IOP is very high, the full-field ERG may be extinguished, and although this has negative prognostic significance, in the authors' experience it is still possible for vision to be temporarily regained once IOP returns to normal and adequate perfusion to the retina is returned.[24,43–45]

The *pattern ERG* (PERG) is thought to originate from the inner retina in response to patterned stimuli (instead of a white flash of light in standard electroretinography), and is considered one of the best electrophysiological tools for assessing retinal ganglion cell function in a clinical setting.[43–45] Initial testing in humans and dogs suggests that the PERG is more sensitive than the full-field ERG to IOP increases.[43–45]

Another component of electrophysiologic testing, the *visual evoked potential* (VEP) is also generally agreed to be abnormal in glaucoma, either in terms of its amplitude or its latency.[43] Standard white light, pattern, or flicker-based VEPs have been investigated but the results are variable enough across studies to indicate that VEP does not perform well enough to be useful clinically.[43]

Multifocal electroretinogram/visual evoked potential

With this instrumentation, very discrete stimuli (usually a preset number of hexagons that may flash or show a pattern) are projected onto the retina, and the local response of that region of retina is recorded.[43] The great advantage of this technique is that it one can record a detailed multifocal ERG (mfERG) that shows a topographic distribution of the signal amplitudes instead of just a single mass response representing the average response across the entire retina. This technique allows for the detection of regional midperipheral retinal damage that occurs in the earlier stages of glaucoma and these correspond to regions of visual field loss.[43] In a sense, this is a more objective method for estimating visual field loss in animals than standard perimetry that requires the patient's cooperation. However, the application of mfERG testing to human glaucoma has thus far met with limited clinical success.[43] By changing the stimulus from white light to an alternating pattern of black and white triangular checks it becomes possible to record a pattern multifocal VEP.

TECHNIQUES THAT EVALUATE THE OPTIC DISC
Optic Disc Photography

Because changes to the optic disc are a hallmark of glaucoma, much effort has been spent on carefully evaluating the optic disc, especially over time. Photography of the disc offers a number of clinical advantages, and the recent introduction of simple fundus cameras and fundus adaptors for smart phones may facilitate identification of alterations in the optic disc in dogs with glaucoma (see **Figs. 1, 3**, and **9**). This is especially true in dogs, in which a high variation in the amount of myelin exists in normal dogs of different breeds at the level of the optic nerve head. Images should include the optic disc and the adjacent peripapillary region. Images are very useful because the magnification is relatively high, the animal is not moving, the images are in full color, and they can be examined for an unlimited amount of time or compared across time. Evaluation of disc photos should include the size and shape of the optic disc, color of the optic disc, configuration and depth of the optic cup, the cup/disc-diameter ratio, the presence or absence of the laminar dot sign (small dark dots on the optic disc representing pores of the lamina cribrosa), the presence or absence of peripapillary chorioretinal atrophy, the visibility of the RNFL, the appearance of retinal blood vessels and those over the surface of the disc, and the nature of the myelin on the surface of the disc.

Advanced Optic Disc Imaging

These instruments provide the clinician with reproducible objective measurements of the optic nerve head that may be useful in detecting glaucomatous damage or progression over time. However, any one of these tests is limited in its ability to detect glaucomatous damage and therefore they should be used in conjunction with careful clinical examination and ideally functional vision testing. This technology is rapidly evolving, and with additional studies over time they may demonstrate great utility in the diagnosis and treatment of patients with glaucoma.

Confocal Scanning Laser Ophthalmoscopy (Heidelberg Retina Tomograph)

This instrument uses a confocal scanning laser (670-nm diode laser) to obtain multiple measures of retinal height at various points on the fundus (**Fig. 17**).[46,47] Multiple confocal slices are acquired at different focal planes, allowing for a detailed 3-dimensional reconstruction of the optic disc and adjacent peripapillary retina. Three consecutive scans are acquired in approximately 2 seconds, making this a very rapid method for evaluation of the optic disc. Once the image is acquired, a number of automated methods for data evaluation are possible.[46]

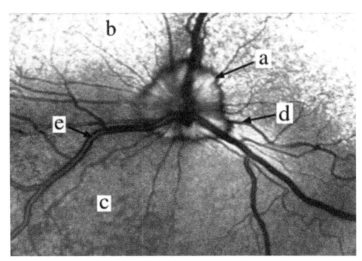

Fig. 17. Confocal Scanning Laser Ophthalmoscopy of a dog. A laser is used to image the optic disc (a), tapetum lucidum (b), nontapetal zone (c), retinal arterioles (d), and retina venules (e). (*From* Rosolen SG, Saint-Macary G, Gautier V, et al. Ocular fundus images with confocal scanning laser ophthalmoscopy in the dog, monkey and minipig. Vet Ophthalmol 2001;4(1):42; with permission.)

Optical Coherence Tomography

This technology differs from confocal scanning laser ophthalmoscopy in that it provides a histologic representation of the tissues and is not subject to some of the polarization artifacts stemming from the anterior segment (**Fig. 18**). With some changes in configuration, this device also can examine the posterior segment as well as the anterior segment.[48–50] It provides high-resolution cross-sectional images of the fundus, and the distances and sizes of tissues in the fundus are determined by the amount of time it takes for light to reflect from the different structures. In this sense, it functions much like an ultrasound unit but it uses light instead of sound waves and it provides a level of resolution that approximates histopathology.

Time-Domain Optical Coherence Tomography

Time-domain OCT assessment of the optic nerve head consists of 6 scans centered on the optic disc that radiate from the disc in a spokelike manner. With this technology, each data point in each A-scan is obtained by moving the reference mirror for each depth, a process that is relatively slow and creates practical problems due to eye movement. Tissues between these scans are interpolated between the 6 radial scans. A topographic image of the optic disc is constructed and this can be automatically analyzed in detail. The advantage of this technique is that it allows for not only evaluation of the optic disc but also for cross-sectional analysis of the RNFL(ie, its thickness) and the macula with a single instrument.[48,50]

Spectral-Domain Optical Coherence Tomography

There are a number of commercially available units (unlike only a single unit for time-domain OCT), and these have largely replaced time-domain OCT.[48–50] This technology is similar to that of time-domain OCT but keeps the reference mirror fixed and obtains the entire A-scan at once using spectrally (color) separated detectors. The

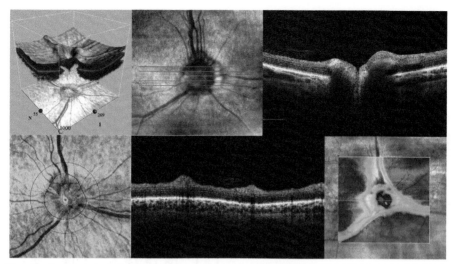

Fig. 18. Spectral-domain OCT image of a normal dog. This instrument provides high-resolution images of the posterior segment and includes an adjustable 3-dimensional view of the optic disc and surrounding retina (*upper left*), an ophthalmoscopic view of the optic disc denoting where line scans were obtained (*upper middle*), a cross-sectional view through the optic disc at the selected line scan (*upper right*), circular scans around the optic disc (*lower right*), cross-sectional views of the retina (*lower middle*), and color-coded thickness mapping of the optic disc or retina (*lower right*). (*Courtesy of* Carol Rasmussen, MS, University of Wisconsin-Madison, Madison, WI.)

resulting data are analyzed by a spectrometer using a Fourier transformation. This allows for very fast scanning (20,000 A-scans per second) and for multiple related A-scans to create a B-scan or cross-sectional images of the optic nerve head, RNFL, and macula with a higher resolution (4–5 μm) than time-domain technology. Nevertheless, it is still essential that the eye be perfectly still for several seconds to capture useful images, and this is difficult to achieve in dogs without sedation. The high scanning speed reduces motion artifacts, and because multiple B-scans can be rapidly acquired, these can be combined to create a 3-dimensional representation of the fundus. The acquired images also can be automatically measured and evaluated. With some units, it is possible to measure choroidal, pre–lamina cribrosa and laminar structures in a living patient.

TECHNIQUES THAT EVALUATE THE RETINAL NERVE FIBER LAYER
Retinal Nerve Fiber Layer Photography

Because the axons of the retinal ganglion cells are one of the earliest structures damaged in glaucoma, evaluation of the RNFL is a critical component of the diagnosis and management of glaucoma. Damage to the RNFL occurs before detectable changes in the optic disc, and significant RFNL loss can occur before functional loss can be demonstrated on perimetry.[41] The brightly reflective tapetum lucidum, however, makes this tissue difficult to consistently clinically identify in dogs. The healthy RFNL will appear as slightly opaque with visibly radiating striations emanating from the optic disc. Glaucomatous defects in the RFNL appear as slit-groove–shaped or wedge-shaped defects or diffuse generalized loss. Techniques for evaluating the RFNL layer are described in the following sections.

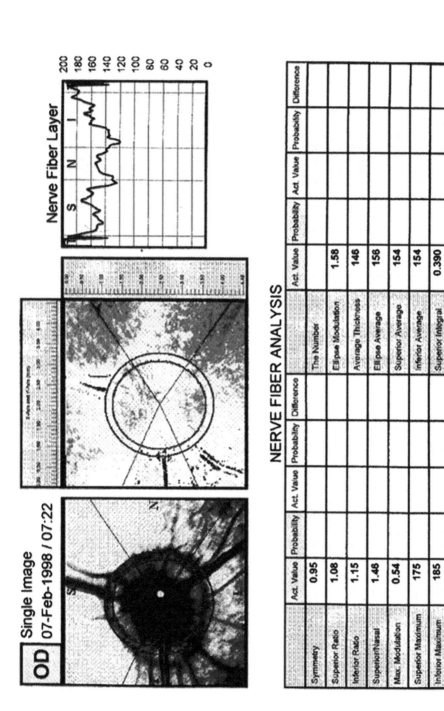

Fig. 19. Image from a normal eye with a scanning laser polarimeter (Gdx). Images include a fundus image from the scanned area and a color-coded thickness retardation map of the RNFL that shows thinner areas in blue and black and thicker areas in red, orange, and yellow. A variety of printouts are also presented. (*From* García-Sánchez GA, Gil-Carrasco F, Román JJ, et al. Measurement of the retinal nerve fiber layer thickness in normal and glaucomatous Cocker Spaniels by scanning laser polarimetry. Vet Ophthalmol 2007;10 Suppl 1:81; with permission.)

Ophthalmoscopy

A direct ophthalmoscope or a slit-lamp with a goniolens that has a central viewing lens for examination of the fundus is especially useful for evaluation of the RFNL. Examination is facilitated with the use of red-free (green) light (available on most direct and indirect ophthalmoscopes). This is because the RFNL is invisible to red light but more easily visualized with shorter-wavelength (green) light that does not penetrate the RFNL and is reflected by the superficial layers of the retina. Good visualization of the RFNL requires very clear media (often not a possible in dogs with PACG or some degree of cataract) and high contrast (which makes it difficult to observe in eyes with lightly pigmented fundi or a tapetum).

Red-Free Photography

This technique uses a fundus camera with a red-free filter and high-contrast black-and-white film or digitally acquired images that are converted to red-free and enhanced with various software packages to maximize contrast.

Confocal Scanning Laser Ophthalmoscopy and Optical Coherence Tomography

These previously discussed imaging techniques also are capable of evaluating the RFNL thickness and cross-sectional area values.

Scanning Laser Polarimetry

The RFNL is birefringent (like the cornea and to a lesser extent the lens).[51] The anterior-segment signals must be removed and the latest commercially available scanning laser polarimeter has a variable corneal compensator that allows for eye-specific compensation for anterior-segment birefringence and automated data analysis (**Fig. 19**). With this device, the images match the appearance of the RFNL in red-free fundus photographs, but its advantages over these techniques are its data analysis tools, especially its Nerve Fiber Layer Indicator (NFI), which provides a single number (range 1–100) that represents the overall integrity of the RFNL.

The diagnostic accuracy of the Gdx's (Laser Diagnostic Technologies, Inc, San Diego, CA, USA) NFI score in humans is very good, with a sensitivity of 91.7%, a specificity of 95%, and an overall accuracy of 93.2%.[52] The Heidelberg retinal tomograph (Heidelberg Engineering, Heidelberg, Germany) and OCT also have been shown to provide similar accuracies for discrimination between healthy and glaucomatous eyes.[53] In some studies, automated analysis of measurements with the Gdx and the HRT may better discriminate between healthy and glaucomatous eyes than general ophthalmologists who subjectively grade the appearance of the optic nerve head on stereoscopic optic disc photographs.[54] A study of glaucomatous cocker spaniels also demonstrated that scanning laser polarimetry was capable of detecting changes in RNFL thickness in early stages of the disease and that it may have value in detecting progressive changes in this tissue in dogs.[55]

REFERENCES

1. Spaeth GL, Waisbourd M. Definitions: what is glaucoma worldwide?. In: Shaarawy TM, Sherwood MB, Hitchings RA, et al, editors. Glaucoma: medical diagnosis & therapy. St Louis (MO): Elsevier Ltd; 2015. p. 311–24.
2. Foster PJ, Buhrmann R, Quigley HA, et al. The definition and classification of glaucoma in prevalence surveys. Br J Ophthalmol 2002;86:238–42.
3. Ahonen SJ, Pietilä E, Mellersh CS, et al. Genome-wide association study identifies a novel canine glaucoma locus. PLoS One 2013;8:e70903.

4. Kuchtey J, Kunkel J, Esson D, et al. Screening ADAMTS10 in dog populations supports Gly661Arg as the glaucoma-causing variant in beagles. Invest Ophthalmol Vis Sci 2013;54:1881–6.

5. Kuchtey J, Olson LM, Rinkoski T, et al. Mapping of the disease locus and identification of ADAMTS10 as a candidate gene in a canine model of primary open angle glaucoma. PLoS Genet 2011;7:e1001306.

6. Pearl R, Gould D, Spiess B. Progression of pectinate ligament dysplasia over time in two populations of flat-coated retrievers. Vet Ophthalmol 2015;18(1):6–12.

7. Miller PE. The glaucomas. In: Maggs DJ, Miller PE, Ofri R, editors. Slatter's fundamentals of veterinary ophthalmology. 5th edition. St Louis (MO): Elsevier; 2013. p. 247–71.

8. Gelatt KN. The canine glaucomas. In: Gelatt KN, Gilger BC, Kern TJ, editors. Veterinary ophthalmology. New Jersey: Wiley-Blackwell Hoboken; 2013. p. 1050–145.

9. Ahonen SJ, Kaukonen M, Nussdorfer FD, et al. A novel missense mutation in ADAMTS10 in Norwegian elkhound primary glaucoma. PLoS One 2014;9: e111941.

10. Ahram DF, Cook AC, Kecova H, et al. Identification of genetic loci associated with primary angle closure in the basset hound. Mol Vis 2014;20:497–510.

11. Dubin A, Bentley E, Miller PE. Evaluation and identification of risk factors for primary angle closure glaucoma in bouvier des Flandres dogs. In: Proceedings 45th Annual Meeting of the American College of Veterinary Ophthalmologists. Fort Worth, TX, October 8–11, 2014. p. 83.

12. Quigley HA, Friedmann DS, Congdon NG. Possible mechanisms of primary angle-closure and malignant glaucoma. J Glaucoma 2003;12:167–80.

13. Carreras FJ, Porcel D, González-Caballero F. Expanding forces in aqueous outflow pathways of a nonaccommodating mammal: an approach via comparative dynamic morphology. Comp Biochem Physiol 1997;117:197–209.

14. Ritch R, Stegman Z, Liebmann J. Mapstone's hypothesis confirmed. Br J Ophthalmol 1995;79:300.

15. Ruhl MB, Spiess BM. Goniodysplasie beim Bouvier des Flandres. Schweiz Arch Tierheilkd 1996;138:307–11.

16. Ekesten B, Narfström K. Correlation of morphologic features of the iridocorneal angle to intraocular pressure in samoyed dogs. Am J Vet Res 1991;52:1875–8.

17. Morrison JC, Van Buskirk EM. The canine eye: pectinate ligaments and aqueous outflow resistance. Invest Ophthalmol Vis Sci 1982;23:726–32.

18. Sihota R, Lakshmaiah NC, Walia KB, et al. The trabecular meshwork in acute and chronic angle closure glaucoma. Indian J Ophthalmol 2001;49:255–9.

19. Hamanaka T, Kasahara K, Takemura T. Histopathology of the trabecular meshwork and Schlemm's canal in primary angle-closure glaucoma. Invest Ophthalmol Vis Sci 2011;52:8849–61.

20. Reilly CM, Morris R, Dubielzig RR. Canine goniodysgenesis-related glaucoma: a morphologic review looking at inflammation and pigment dispersion. Vet Ophthalmol 2005;8:253–8.

21. Gelatt KN, MacKay EO. Prevalence of the breed-related glaucomas in pure-bred dogs in North America. Vet Ophthalmol 2004;7:97–111.

22. Tsai S, Bentley E, Miller PE, et al. Gender differences in iridocorneal angle morphology: a potential explanation for the female predisposition to primary angle closure glaucoma in dogs. Vet Ophthalmol 2012;15(Suppl 1):60–3.

23. Boillot T, Rosolen SG, Dulaurent T, et al. Determination of morphological, biometric and biochemical susceptibilities in healthy Eurasier dogs with suspected inherited glaucoma. PLoS One 2014;9:e111873.

24. Grozdanic SD, Matic M, Betts DM, et al. Recovery of canine retina and optic nerve function after acute elevation of intraocular pressure: implications for canine glaucoma treatment. Vet Ophthalmol 2007;10(Suppl 1):101–7.

25. Bentley E, Miller PE, Murphy CJ, et al. Combined cycloablation and gonioimplantation for treatment of glaucoma in dogs: 18 cases (1992–1998). J Am Vet Med Assoc 1999;215:1469–72.

26. Miller PE, Stanz KM, Dubielzig RR, et al. Mechanisms of acute intraocular pressure increases after phacoemulsification. Am J Vet Res 1997;58:1159–65.

27. Knollinger AM, La Croix NC, Barrett P, et al. An evaluation of a rebound tonometer for measuring intraocular pressure in dogs and horses. J Am Vet Med Assoc 2005;227:244–8.

28. Miller PE, Pickett JP, Majors LJ, et al. Clinical comparison of the Mackay-Marg and Tono-Pen applanation tonometers in the dog. Prog Vet Compar Ophthalmol 1991;1:171–6.

29. Waring GO, Bourne WM, Edelhauser HF, et al. The corneal endothelium: normal and pathologic structure and function. Ophthalmology 1982;89:531.

30. Kong X, Liu X, Huang X, et al. Damage to the blood-aqueous barrier in eyes with primary angle closure glaucoma. Mol Vis 2010;16:2026–32.

31. Miller PE, Schmidt GM, Vainisi SJ, et al. The efficacy of topical prophylactic anti-glaucoma therapy in primary closed angle glaucoma in dogs: a multicenter clinical trial. J Am Anim Hosp Assoc 2000;36:431–8.

32. Focht T, Bentley E, Miller PE. Can initial response to latanoprost therapy be used as a prognostic indicator in canine patients with primary closed angle glaucoma? In: Proceedings, 37th Annual Meeting of the American College of Veterinary Ophthalmologists. San Antonio, TX, November 1–4, 2006. p. 48.

33. Ekesten B, Torrång I. Age-related changes in ocular distances in normal eyes of samoyeds. Am J Vet Res 1995;56(1):127–33.

34. Yücel YH, Zhang Q, Weinreb RN, et al. Effects of retinal ganglion cell loss on magno-, parvo-, koniocellular pathways in the lateral geniculate nucleus and visual cortex in glaucoma. Prog Retin Eye Res 2003;22(4):465–81.

35. Gupta N, Ang LC, Noël de Tilly L, et al. Human glaucoma and neural degeneration in intracranial optic nerve, lateral geniculate nucleus and visual cortex. Br J Ophthalmol 2006;90:674–8.

36. Miller PE, Pickett JP. Comparison of the human and canine Schiotz tonometry conversion tables in clinically normal dogs. J Am Vet Med Assoc 1992;201:1021–5.

37. Park YW, Jeong MB, Kim TH, et al. Effect of central corneal thickness on intraocular pressure with the rebound tonometer and the applanation tonometer in normal dogs. Vet Ophthalmol 2011;14(3):169–73.

38. Pauli AM, Bentley E, Diehl KA, et al. Comparison of intraocular pressure with application of neck pressure via collar or a harness in dogs. J Am Anim Hosp Assoc 2006;42:207–11.

39. Broadwater JJ, Schoring JJ, Herring IP, et al. Effect of body position on intraocular pressure. Am J Vet Res 2008;69:527–30.

40. Nouri-Mahdavi K, Nassiri N, Giangiacomo A, et al. Detection of visual field progression in glaucoma with standard achromatic perimetry: a review and practical implications. Graefes Arch Clin Exp Ophthalmol 2011;249:1593–616.

41. Kerrigan-Baumrind LA, Quigley HA, Pease ME, et al. Number of ganglion cells in glaucoma eyes compared with threshold visual field tests in the same persons. Invest Ophthalmol Vis Sci 2000;41:741–8.

42. Sample PA. Short-wavelength automated perimetry: its role in the clinic and in understanding ganglion cell function. Prog Retin Eye Res 2000;19:369–83.

43. Graham SL, Fortune B. Electrophysiology in glaucoma assessment. In: Shaaraway TM, Sherwood MB, Hitchings RA, et al, editors. Glaucoma medical diagnosis and therapy. 2nd edition. Philadelphia: Elsevier Saunders; 2015. p. 149–68.

44. Grozdanic SD, Kecova H, Harper MM, et al. Functional and structural changes in a canine model of hereditary primary angle closure glaucoma. Invest Ophthalmol Vis Sci 2010;51:255–63.

45. Hamor RE, Gerding PA, Ramsey DT, et al. Evaluation of short-term increased intraocular pressure on flash- and pattern-generated electroretinograms of dogs. Am J Vet Res 2000;61:1087–91.

46. Strouthidis NG, Garway-Heath DF. New developments in Heidelberg retina tomograph for glaucoma. Curr Opin Ophthalmol 2008;19:141–8.

47. Rosolen SG, Saint-Macary G, Gautier V, et al. Ocular fundus images with confocal scanning laser ophthalmoscopy in the dog, monkey and minipig. Vet Ophthalmol 2001;4:41–5.

48. Grewal DA, Tanna AP. Diagnosis of glaucoma and detection of glaucoma progression using spectral domain optical coherence tomography. Curr Opin Ophthalmol 2013;24:150–61.

49. Anton A, Moreno-Montanes J, Blazquez E, et al. Usefulness of optical coherence tomography parameters of the optic disc and the retinal nerve fiber layer to differentiate glaucomatous, ocular hypertensive and normal eyes. J Glaucoma 2007; 16:1–8.

50. McLellan GJ, Rasmussen CA. Optical coherence tomography for the evaluation of retinal and optic nerve morphology in animal subjects: practical considerations. Vet Ophthalmol 2012;15(Suppl 2):13–28.

51. Da Pozzo S, Marchesan R, Ravalico G. Scanning laser polarimetry–a review. Clin Experiment Ophthalmol 2009;37:68–80.

52. Reus NJ, de Graaf M, Lemij HG. Accuracy of the GDx VCC, HRT 1 and clinical assessment of stereoscopic optic nerve head photographs for diagnosing glaucoma. Br J Ophthalmol 2007;91:313–8.

53. Medeiros FA, Zangwill LM, Bowd C, et al. Comparison of the GDx VCC scanning laser polarimeter, HRT II confocal scanning laser ophthalmoscope, and stratus OCT optical coherence tomograph for the detection of glaucoma. Arch Ophthalmol 2004;122:827–37.

54. Reus NJ, Lemij HG, Garway-Heath DF, et al. Clinical assessment of stereoscopic optic disc photographs for glaucoma: the European optic disc assessment trial. Ophthalmology 2010;117:717–23.

55. Garcia-Sánchez GA, Gil-Carrasco F, Román JJ, et al. Measurement of the retinal nerve fiber layer thickness in normal and glaucomatous cocker spaniels by scanning laser polarimetry. Vet Ophthalmol 2007;10(Suppl 1):78–87.

Microscopic Lesions in Canine Eyes with Primary Glaucoma

Gillian Beamer, VMD, PhD[a],*, Christopher M. Reilly, DVM, MAS[b],
Stefano Pizzirani, DVM, PhD[c]

KEYWORDS

- Glaucoma • Ocular pathology • Goniodysgenesis • Inner retinal degeneration
- Optic nerve cupping

KEY POINTS

- The glaucoma group of diseases produce similar ocular pathologic signs when evaluated in end-stage enucleated glaucomatous globes.
- The most common pathologic findings associated with glaucoma are collapsed cleft, inner retinal atrophy, and optic nerve cupping.
- Canine goniodysgenesis (GD) is a congenital iridocorneal angle (ICA) abnormality that predisposes to glaucoma—GD-associated glaucoma (GDAG) or primary angle closure glaucoma (PACG)—later in life.
- Tapetal (superior) retina undergoes less-severe degeneration when compared with nontapetal (inferior) retina.
- Progressive and irreversible retinal pathologic changes start early in the disease.

INTRODUCTION

Although the clinical classification of primary glaucoma in dogs is quite simple, the phenotypes of glaucoma in most of the species are indeed multiple. Ophthalmologists can often evaluate the dynamic changes of clinical signs at different times in the course of the disease, whereas pathologists are often presented with globes that have undergone abundant therapies and are at the end stage. These changes often overlap with different causes of disease. Therefore, an open collaboration between clinicians and pathologists can produce the most accurate interpretation in the

The authors have nothing to disclose.
[a] Department of Infectious Disease and Global Health, Tufts University, 200 Westboro Road, North Grafton, MA 01536, USA; [b] Microbiology & Immunology, School of Veterinary Medicine, University of California, 1 Shields Avenue, Davis, CA 95616, USA; [c] Ophthalmology, Department of Clinical Sciences, Cummings School of Veterinary Medicine, Tufts University, 200 Westboro Road, North Grafton, MA 01536, USA
* Corresponding author.
E-mail address: Gillian.Beamer@tufts.edu

pathology report and improve patient outcomes. The main pathogenesis of canine glaucoma involves processes that decrease aqueous outflow because of structural modifications of the outflow pathways through the angle, trabecular meshworks (TMs), and angular aqueous or scleral venous plexuses. The most distinctive microscopic lesions for primary glaucoma occur in the anterior portion of the eye. By light microscopy, the most recognizable structural abnormalities that occur are dysplastic changes of the ICA and the pectinate ligament (PL).

Regardless of the suspected or ultimate diagnoses, histopathology is often essential for accurate and complete diagnosis in enucleated (or eviscerated) globes. Although enucleation is considered by ophthalmologists to be the death of the eye, there typically remains a fellow visual eye, for which prognostication is crucial; this is particularly true for cases of unilateral GD and PACG, where the risk to the fellow eye after development of glaucoma in one eye is predictably high.[1] A variety of factors (end-stage disease, corneal opacity/edema, concurrent disease, atypical breed presentation, and/or lack of full ophthalmologic examination) may obscure the clinical diagnosis. Although histologic evaluation has limitations, it can reveal clinically unappreciable lesions, even with advanced diagnostic techniques. Ocular histopathologic interpretation benefits greatly from experience and training; most large veterinary diagnostic laboratories have pathologists with interest or expertise in ocular pathology, and there are several ocular-specific histopathology services. Increasingly, smaller veterinary histopathology and reference laboratories have access to ocular pathology expertise. It may be worth investigating these options with currently used laboratories (ie, directly requesting certain pathologists), specialized ocular pathology laboratories, or veterinary schools.

This article focuses on the histomorphologic elements that characterize and are important in canine primary glaucomas.

The anatomy of the normal canine outflow facilities is discussed by Pizzirani and Gong.[2]

GLAUCOMA-INDUCED CHANGES IN THE CANINE ANTERIOR SEGMENT
Goniodysgenesis: Background and Nomenclature

GD,[3,4] also known as pectinate ligament dysplasia (PLD),[3,5–12] or goniodysplasia[13,14] is a congenital ICA abnormality that, when extensive, may predispose to the development of glaucoma later in life.[3,10,15] A normal canine ICA (**Figs. 1** and **2**) and one with GD, but without glaucoma (**Fig. 3**), are shown for comparison. Histologically, GD is defined by an abnormally thick and imperforate PL (see **Fig. 3**).[3,4,10,15] The PL, however, can be segmentally imperforate, up to 25% of the angle, as a variation of normal, so segmental lesions should be interpreted with caution.[6,16] Other anatomic features have been associated with GD in several studies and unpublished observations (Reilly, 2015) but may be inconsistent or difficult to appreciate in histologic section. In particular, a frayed or arborized terminus of Descemet membrane (DM) may or may not be present (see **Fig. 3**; **Figs. 4–7**) in dogs with GD,[3] but this is not entirely sensitive or specific for GD.

Although the mechanisms of glaucoma development are incompletely understood, GD is considered a cause of primary glaucoma in the dog, referred to here as GDAG[3] or PACG[3,10,15,17–20]; it has been referred to as GD-related glaucoma in one study.[4] GDAG/PACG is also known as primary open-angle closed-cleft glaucoma,[3,10,21] primary closed-angle glaucoma, or simply primary glaucoma.[3] The last of these designations distinguishes GDAG/PACG from common secondary causes (eg, lens luxation, neovascular/inflammation associated, neoplasia associated) but may create

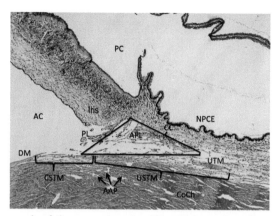

Fig. 1. Photomicrograph of the normal canine ICA. AH is produced by the nonpigmented ciliary epithelium (NPCE) and is pumped into the posterior chamber (PC). AH percolates through the pupil (not shown), into the anterior chamber (AC). The heavily perforated PL runs from the iris base to the terminus of DM. The PL is the anterior limit of the ciliary cleft (CC), spanned by accessory PL and uveal trabecular meshwork (UTM), into which all AH flows. From the CC, most AH exits the globe through the corneoscleral trabecular meshwork (CTSM) and uveoscleral trabecular meshwork (USTM) and into the angular aqueous plexus (AAP) and collector channels (CoCh) in to scleral venous circulation. This outflow system represents the conventional pathway. Some AH continues posteriorly, through the TM into the ciliary body and into the systemic circulation via the supraciliary and suprachoroidal spaces (not shown). The latter system represents nonconventional outflow. The cornea is to the right (original magnification ×4, hematoxylin-eosin).

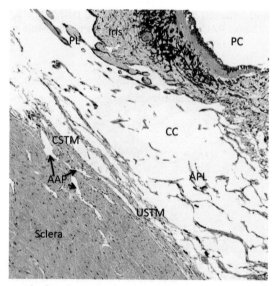

Fig. 2. Photomicrograph showing a higher magnification of the normal canine ICA. The anterior chamber, Descemet membrane, uveoscleral trabecular meshwork, and ciliary body are not shown in this image. AAP, angular aqueous plexus; APL, accessory pectinate ligaments or trabecular meshwork; CC, ciliary cleft; CSTM, corneoscleral trabecular meshwork; PC, posterior chamber; USTM, uveoscleral trabecular meshwork (original magnification ×10, hematoxylin-eosin).

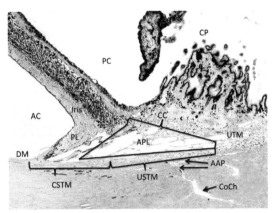

Fig. 3. Photomicrograph of the ICA with GD, but without elevated IOP/glaucoma. Note the thick PL extending from the iris base to the terminus of Descemet membrane (DM). DM is frayed, and overrides the insertion of the PL. The ciliary cleft (CC) is still open, and the other structures of the ICA are apparent. AAP, angular aqueous plexus; AC, anterior chamber; APL, accessory pectinate ligaments; CoCh, collector channels; CP, ciliary processes; CSTM, corneoscleral trabecular meshwork; PC, posterior chamber; USTM, uveoscleral trabecular meshwork (original magnification ×4, hematoxylin-eosin).

confusion with primary open-angle glaucoma (POAG), or other not yet recognized primary causes. POAG is very rare as a spontaneous cause of glaucoma in dogs, but it has been well characterized in a colony of beagle dogs and is a good model for human POAG.[3,10] Even without POAG, the confusing nomenclature of canine glaucoma is well documented,[3] and consensus is difficult to achieve, both among veterinary ophthalmologists and between ophthalmologists and pathologists. For the purposes of this review, GDAG and PACG are considered interchangeable and are referred to

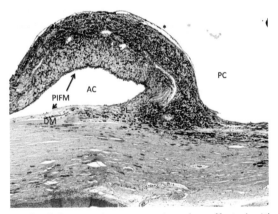

Fig. 4. Photomicrograph of the anterior segment in a dog affected with GDAG. A shorter, but thicker PL extends from the iris base to the end of DM, which is frayed. The corneoscleral and uveoscleral trabecular meshwork, angular aqueous plexus, ciliary cleft, and uveal meshwork are inapparent. A fibrovascular membrane is also present (PIFM) and extends on to the cornea, and perivascular basophilic stippling in the iris is lymphoplasmacytic infiltrate (uveitis). There is complete loss of the iris pigment epithelium (IPE), with a postiridal fibrous membrane (*asterisk*) and clusters of plump, heavily pigmented cells. AC, anterior chamber; PC, posterior chamber (original magnification ×4, hematoxylin-eosin).

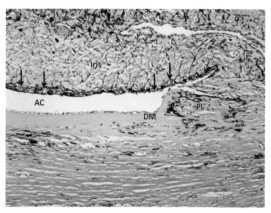

Fig. 5. Photomicrograph of the anterior segment in a dog affected with GDAG/PACG. A short, stout PL interdigitates with the frayed terminus of DM. Note the prominent vessels at the anterior face of the iris—this is a developing preiridal fibrovascular membrane (*arrows*). The corneoscleral trabecular meshwork is inapparent. AC, anterior chamber (original magnification ×10, hematoxylin-eosin).

together to reinforce this concept—GDAG/PACG; practically, they both reflect the most common cause of primary glaucoma as used in common veterinary parlance.

Breed predispositions are helpful in establishing an index of suspicion, although it is important to remember that breed predispositions should not dictate a diagnosis and that dogs of any or mixed breed may be affected. A more complete review of breed associations and breed-specific epidemiology is found elsewhere.[10,22]

Histopathologic Diagnosis and Challenges

In dogs, microscopic evaluation of the anterior segment often reveals morphologic lesions associated with impaired aqueous humor (AH) drainage, elevated intraocular

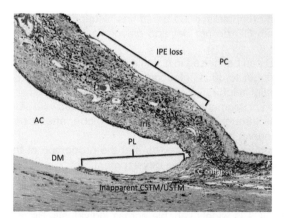

Fig. 6. Photomicrograph of the anterior segment in a dog affected with GDAG/PACG. A thin and long PL spans from the iris base to the end of DM. The ciliary cleft (CC) is collapsed, and the corneoscleral trabecular meshwork (CSTM)/uveoscleral trabecular meshwork (USTM) is inapparent. In addition, there is segmental loss of the iris pigment epithelium (IPE) and a thin fibrous postiridal membrane (*asterisk*). AC, anterior chamber; PC, posterior chamber (original magnification ×4, hematoxylin-eosin).

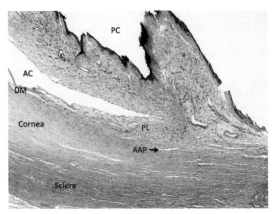

Fig. 7. Photomicrograph of the anterior segment in a subalbinotic (*blue-eyed*) dog with GDAG/PACG. Note the lack of pigment in the iris and PL stroma. The corneoscleral trabecular meshwork and ciliary cleft are inapparent. The angular aqueous plexus (AAP) is still appreciable. AC, anterior chamber; PC, posterior chamber (original magnification ×4, hematoxylin-eosin).

pressure (IOP), and resulting glaucoma. Distortion or obstruction of the ICA and/or the pupil is apparent at the light microscopic level in most spontaneous canine glaucoma cases.

- The posterior segment changes define glaucoma, whereas the changes seen in the anterior segment may provide morphologic information that can be helpful for identifying the cause
- Specific etiologic diagnoses, beyond primary or secondary, are critical for proper treatment and prognostication

In diagnosing GD microscopically, several factors must be taken into account. As with clinical presentation, breed predispositions are helpful, but can be misleading.

- Not every dog of a predisposed breed has histologic GD or GDAG/PACG
- Most dogs with GD do not develop glaucoma,[3,10,23] especially if segmentally affected
- Segmental GD can be missed in a single routine section of a globe, even if it may represent a trigger to cause glaucoma; additional sections of the ICA and cleft areas are usually helpful
  - Identification of segmental GD can be accomplished with several anteroposterior sections through the other half of the globe, after a parasagittal section (with optic nerve) is obtained
- It has been shown in several breeds that the proportion of the ICA affected is directly proportional to glaucoma development[7,16,24]

Several examples of the variations in ICA and PL morphology in GDAG/PACG are depicted in **Figs. 3–7** (reviewed later). It is important to reiterate that the specific morphology of the ICA is widely variable across individuals. Breed-related trends in histomorphology may be present but are not yet well described. Anecdotally, for example, basset hounds often have a distinctly inflammatory clinical and histopathologic constellation of lesions; the PL abnormality, however, remains the key to the microscopic diagnosis of GD. The abnormal PL may be short and stout, may be long and thin, and may vary between sections in a given eye. Close attention to concurrent lesions is important for furthering the broad understanding of glaucoma development in GDAG/PACG, as well as in postulating triggers in individual dogs.

Key histologic GD lesion: a sheet of irislike uveal tissue (ie, the abnormal PL) that extends from the iris base to the terminus of DM.

- The end of DM may be frayed or arborized (see **Figs. 3–5**), may interdigitate with the insertion of the PL (see **Figs. 4** and **5**), may overlie the PL (see **Fig. 3**), or may be overlain by the PL insertion (see **Fig. 6**)
- In some cases, the abnormal PL tapers in thickness toward DM (see **Fig. 7**, which also illustrates a subalbinotic [blue] iris)
- There is wide variation in the length and thickness of the abnormal PL in GD, ranging from short and stout (see **Figs. 3** and **5**) to long and thin (see **Figs. 4, 6**, and **7**)
- Chronic disease, inflammation, or other, potentially secondary changes may affect the morphology of the ICA/cleft and may confound or alter the interpretation of the original dysplastic morphology of PL; they may also contribute to disease progression (see Concurrent Lesions section)
- Confirmation of GD in eviscerated globes should not be expected, but in the authors' experience, rare cases will maintain suggestive morphology
- Submission of evisceration specimens is recommended to rule out other causes and the presence of undetected neoplasia or other lesions; in eviscerations, GDAG is a diagnosis of exclusion

Several breeds of GD-affected dogs are prone to subalbinism or heterochromia iridis (an entirely or a partially blue eye, respectively), which can make delineation of the ICA morphology more difficult. In the absence of stromal pigment or the anterior face of melanocytes along the iris face, there is little to distinguish an abnormal PL from preiridal fibrovascular tissue and peripheral anterior synechiae. An example GD in a subalbinotic (blue-eyed) globe is shown in **Fig. 7**.

A major limitation of histopathology for the diagnosis and study of GDAG/PACG pathogenesis is the typical late stage of disease at enucleation. However, histologic, immunohistochemical, and ultrastructural changes in the corneoscleral trabecular meshwork (CSTM)/uveoscleral trabecular meshwork (USTM) and the uveoscleral (US) pathway in canine GDAG/PACG have been described.[25] Smooth muscle actin expression in the CSTM/UTSM decreased with age, and more notably with glaucoma, both in POAG and GDAG/PACG.[26,27] The US pathway changed little with age, but exhibited loss of smooth muscle fibers, increased elastin-rich matrix, and increased pigment accumulation in both POAG and GDAG/PACG. This observation suggests that there may be overlap in the mechanisms of glaucoma in dogs predisposed to glaucoma, irrespective of the predisposing lesion, and that age-related changes may affect the progression in predisposed dogs.

Concurrent Lesions or Insights on Pathogenesis?

While the histomorphology of the PL is diagnostic for GD, concurrent histopathologic lesions can confound the diagnosis but may also offer clues into glaucoma pathogenesis. These factors, along with age-related changes, help to explain both the late onset of glaucoma in this fundamentally congenital malformation and the fact that most dogs with GD do not ever develop glaucoma. The following histopathologic features have been associated with, but not causally linked, with GD[3,4]:

1. Erosion of the iris pigment epithelium (IPE) from the posterior iris—generally adjacent to the pupil (see **Fig. 6**; **Figs. 8** and **9**)

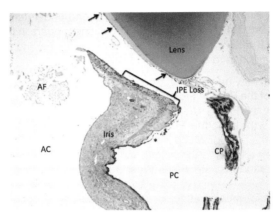

Fig. 8. Photomicrograph of the anterior segment in a dog affected with GDAG/PACG showing abnormal lens-iris contact and posterior synechiae in GDAG/PACG. The iris leaflet has a sigmoid contour, with segmental loss of the IPE (*bracket*) and a thin posterior synechiae (*arrows*), with pigmented and fibrovascular tissue lining the anterior lens. A thin fibrous membrane lines portions of the posterior iris (*asterisk*). This iris is also subalbinotic (*blue*), and there is protein exudate in the anterior chamber (aqueous flare, AF). CP, ciliary process; PC, posterior chamber (original magnification ×2, hematoxylin-eosin).

- This area may be analogous to the region of iris-lens contact and may be exacerbated by certain antiglaucoma therapies (ie, latanoprost)[28]
- This relationship can occasionally be inferred in histologic specimens (see **Fig. 8**)
- Postiridal membranes are common (see **Figs. 4, 6,** and **8**), and posterior synechiae (iris-lens) may become established (see **Fig. 8**)
- Intact IPE participates in ocular immune tolerance[29,30]
- Although not unique to GD—also reported in lens luxation[31]—it may contribute to both pigment dispersion and altered ocular immune function in GD

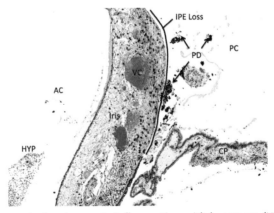

Fig. 9. Photomicrograph showing acute inflammation with hypopyon (HYP) in a dog with acute GDAG/PACG. There is also segmental loss of IPE (*with line*), pigment dispersion (PD) into the posterior chamber (PC), and generalized iridal edema (*clear space*) and vascular congestion (VC). AC, anterior chamber; CP, ciliary process (original magnification ×4, hematoxylin-eosin).

2. Dispersion of pigment cells (mainly IPE and melanomacrophages) or free pigment into the anterior chamber, posterior chamber, CSTM/USTM, and US region[8,9]– more so ventrally (see **Fig. 9**; **Fig. 10**)
    - Also described in primary lens luxation,[31] and is seen in aging dogs[32]
    - May be contributed to by lens-iris contact, iris epithelial cysts and their rupture, or disruption of the epithelium by inflammation or cellular/fibrovascular membranes
    - Dispersed melanin is phagocytosed by macrophages (melanomacrophages)— and rarely corneal endothelium (**Fig. 11**)
    - Melanin and associated collagen type 1 may act as a proinflammatory autoantigen[33–36]
3. Mild to moderate inflammation in the anterior uveal stroma, remnant ICA structures, ciliary cleft (CC), and/or anterior chamber[8,9,36]
    - Neutrophils, with or without hypopyon in acute cases, that is, less than 7 days of clinical signs, likely recruited by recently occurred spontaneous tissue damage (see **Fig. 9**)
    - Lymphocytes, plasma cells in most cases (see **Fig. 6**; **Fig. 12**)
    - Macrophages present, but may be indistinct or laden with melanin
    - Significant increases in levels of tumor necrosis factor α[37] and transforming growth factor $\beta2$ (S.P., G.B., unpublished data [2015]) have been demonstrated in the AH of dogs with PACG, compared with normal controls
    - Increased COX-2 expression has been demonstrated in the ICA structures of glaucomatous dogs, particularly the CSTM/USTM and angular aqueous plexus[38,39]

Recently preiridal membranes—both cellular[40,41] and fibrovascular[36,42]—have been described or observed in most GDAG/PCAG cases (see **Figs. 4, 5,** and **12**).

- Generally induced by inflammation, neoplasia, or retinal hypoxia (eg, retinal separation)
- In GDAG/PACG, it may be secondary to glaucomatous lesions, mild inflammation, retinal hypoxia, and so on

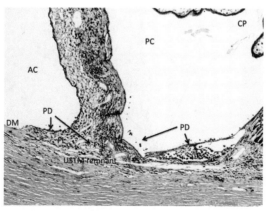

Fig. 10. Photomicrograph of the anterior segment in a dog affected with GDAG/PACG. Pigment dispersion (PD) into the inferior anterior chamber (AC) and posterior chamber (PC) and remnant USTM/uveal stroma. CP, ciliary process (original magnification ×4, hematoxylin-eosin).

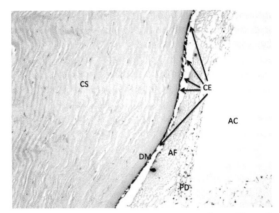

Fig. 11. Photomicrograph of the anterior segment in a dog affected with GDAG/PACG. Corneal endothelial (CE) cells show included pigment as a result of pigment dispersion. There is also pigment dispersed (PD) into the anterior chamber (AC), along with proteinaceous exudate (aqueous flare, AF). CS, corneal stroma (original magnification ×20, hematoxylin-eosin).

- Could contribute to the occlusion of flow holes, and to the adhesion of the PL and accessory pectinate ligaments to other CC structures, promoting permanent closure[3,10]
- Entropion uveae (or posterior curling of the pupillary iris), which indicates periiridal membrane formation and contraction, identified as an early indicator of PACG in humans[43]

The concurrence of fibrovascular membranes, particularly when peripheral, can severely confound accurate diagnosis. An ICA profile with GD and a preiridal fibrovascular membrane (PIFM) that reflects onto the peripheral cornea—as in a peripheral anterior synechiae—is shown in **Fig. 4**. The presence of vascular endothelial growth factor (VEGF) in the AH, as well as VEGF receptors 1 and 2 in PIFMs, has been

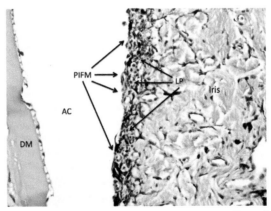

Fig. 12. Photomicrograph of the anterior segment in a dog affected with GDAG/PACG showing signs of chronic uveitis and thin preiridal fibrovascular membrane (PIFM). AC, anterior chamber; LP, lymphocytes and plasma cells (original magnification ×20, hematoxylin-eosin).

documented in canine PACG,[42,44] and likely plays a role in canine PIFM formation. In addition, macrophages may directly participate in the process of fibrovascular tissue proliferation, either through cell-cell signaling to fibroblasts and/or through macrophage differentiation into fibroblasts under appropriate conditions.[40,45,46] As outlined above, cellular and fibrovascular membranes often also involve the posterior iris (see **Figs. 4**, **6**, and **8**), where they may replace damaged IPE and contribute to posterior synechiae and further elevate the IOP.

While these associated lesions are not necessarily unique to GDAG/PCAG, and may confound the accurate histologic diagnosis, they also suggest potential pathogenic mechanisms. Comparison of the ICA from normotensive globes with GD (see **Fig. 3**) and those with GDAG/PACG (see **Figs. 4–7** and **12**) confirms that there is eventual collapse and remodeling of the CC and CTSM/USTM. Many of the associated lesions could contribute to progressive, and eventually sustained, collapse of the ICA/CC— IPE loss and pigment dispersion, inflammation, cellular or fibrovascular membrane proliferation—in eyes that are predisposed via GD or other anatomic factors. Furthermore, as the lens thickens and hardens with age and lens-iris contact is putatively increased, periods of temporary pupil block may increase, in turn increasing periods of CC collapse and plausibly increasing the likelihood that this collapse becomes permanent. Disruption of the IPE may also alter immune privilege in the anterior segment, promoting inflammation and its consequences. Further studies into the interplay of the anatomic features of GD and associated lesions are key for understanding pathogenesis and management of this blinding canine disease.

Goniodysgenesis: Static or Progressive?

Published reports of GD being a progressive condition[8,12,15] are at least somewhat at odds with the initial pathogenesis, that is, a failure of tissue to regress, rather than abnormal proliferation of tissue. It is clear, however, that changes to the anterior segment in GDAG/PCAG are progressive. Given the constellation of inflammatory, pigmentary, and fibrovascular lesions that often accompany GDAG/PACG, it is not surprising that the clinical or gonioscopic appearance of the ICA in affected dogs may change over time, and that histomorphology of the anterior segment may change with the stage of disease. However, it remains to be proven that the key histologic lesion of GD—an abnormally thick and imperforate PL—is truly progressive. A recent report describes temporal progression of GD (called PLD in that study) in flat-coated retrievers and clearly demonstrates progressive changes in the clinical features of the anterior segment with time. As histopathology was not a component of that study, the histologic correlates of clinically apparent progression are not known and it is plausible that pigment dispersion, loss of TM endothelial cells, and cross-linking of the exposed beam-collagen with progressive ICA/CC collapse and, potentially, proliferation of preiridal membranes could mimic true progression of the underlying PL abnormality. Although the decrease of the ICA/CC is clearly a progressive phenomenon, the fine mechanisms leading to the morphologic changes of this region in primary glaucoma have not yet been described and/or differentiated from a normal age-matched population.

GLAUCOMA-INDUCED CHANGES IN THE CANINE POSTERIOR SEGMENT

The posterior segment of the eye includes vitreous body, retina, choroid, and optic nerve. Of these structures, the retina and optic nerve undergo the most substantial degenerative and atrophic structural changes secondary to elevated IOP and/or changes in the lamina cribrosa. Changes in the choroid and vitreous also occur in association with glaucoma, but are less well documented. All ocular lesions are best captured in surgical specimens that have been immediately placed in fixative. Post-mortem examination is less reliable because retinal tissue is extremely sensitive to lack of fixation and autolyzes rapidly resulting in artifacts that may obscure lesions.

General Microscopic Features of Primary Glaucoma in the Posterior Segment

There are no pathognomonic features of primary glaucoma in the posterior segment of the eye, and microscopic lesions are identical in primary and secondary forms of glaucoma. The main changes include retinal degeneration and atrophy, stereotypically progressing from inner layer to eventually extend to complete atrophy, and optic nerve cupping. In particular, microscopic examination of the posterior segment is quite helpful to document the extent and severity of disease and to examine structures that are not visible by clinical examination.

Microscopic Lesions of Early Primary Glaucoma: Atrophy of the Inner Retina

Early lesions of glaucoma occur in the inner retina (nerve fiber layer, ganglion cells, inner plexiform layer, and inner nuclear layer), although the outer plexiform layer seems to undergo early collapse as well. Specifically, the inner limiting membrane and Muller cells become prominent with atrophy and loss of the nerve fiber layer. Increased IOP also results in retinal ganglion cell (RGC) degeneration, apoptosis, and loss, resulting in a thin or nearly absent inner nuclear layer. Anecdotal observations suggest that canine RGCs are more sensitive to increased IOP than equine or feline ganglion cells, but confirmation and identification of underlying mechanisms are still needed. Typical for any cells undergoing degenerative or death-related changes, degenerating, necrotic, and apoptotic ganglion cells show a range of morphologies including cytoplasmic lytic or shrunken nuclei and hypereosinophilic (pink) cytoplasm (**Fig. 13**). The number of visible RGCs is not a precise indicator to assess their degeneration because different sectors of the retina have widely variable numbers of RGCs normally.

Evidence of RGC apoptosis occurs very early after the clinical onset of the disease and is believed to be irreversible.[47,48] The molecular mechanisms that contribute to

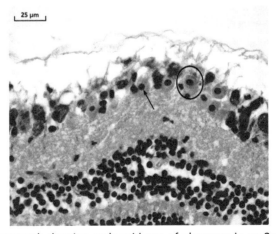

Fig. 13. Photomicrograph showing early evidence of glaucoma in an 8-year-old castrated male cocker shown by RGC necrosis. Multiple RCGs in this field of inner retina are undergoing necrosis. The black circle highlights one affected cell identified by hypereosinophilic (*pink*) cytoplasm and a shrunken, dark nucleus. The arrow identifies another example of an RCG with a shrunken nucleus. These changes are observed in primary and secondary glaucoma (original magnification ×40, hematoxylin-eosin).

the ganglion cell structural changes are multiple, complex, and not fully elucidated. However, much can be extrapolated from in vitro and in vivo studies, which show that impeded release of brain-derived neurotrophic factors, oxidative stress, imbalanced proapoptotic and antiapoptotic signals (involving caspases and heat shock proteins), activation of glial cells, abnormal accumulations of excitatory neurotransmitters, decreased vascular perfusion, autoimmunity or immune-functioning cytokines, and genetic predispositions can all contribute to the complex pathogenesis of ganglion cell degeneration and loss.[39,49–54]

Microscopic Lesions of Chronic Primary Glaucoma: Panretinal Atrophy, Optic Nerve Cupping, and Choroidal and Scleral Thinning

With chronically elevated IOP, the entire globe enlarges and the CC and lamina cribrosa undergo important structural changes. It is thought that mechanical and vascular mechanisms contribute to the degenerative and atrophic changes seen in the posterior segment. However, the physical alterations that affect the globe as a whole may also contribute to generalized thinning of the retina, choroid, and sclera either directly or indirectly.

As glaucoma progresses, the inner retinal layers undergo degeneration and atrophy first. The structural changes include thinning of the inner nuclear layer and both plexiform layers, which manifests as a reduction in nuclei and collapse of the inner and most of the outer plexiform layer (**Fig. 15**B). Eventually, the outer retinal layer also undergoes degeneration and atrophy with loss of the outer nuclear layer and outer plexiform layer and thinning/loss of the rod and cone photoreceptor segments. When all layers of the retina are affected, the term panretinal atrophy is applied, normal retinal structures are practically absent.

Structural and cellular alterations that are secondary to panretinal degeneration/atrophy become prominent such as gliosis, which is increased cellularity due to microglia (the macrophage cells of neural and neuroectodermal tissues) and/or other sustentacular cells such as astrocytelike Muller cells, or fibroblasts/fibrocytes. As a result, the retina is replaced by a fibrocellular membrane, which is essentially retinal scarring. As in all other tissues, scarring is a manifestation of wound healing, but within the eye, scarring is completely deficient in preserving or restoring function. In some instances, the glial and fibrotic response may actually accelerate retinal degeneration and atrophy, in particular if autoimmunity or proinflammatory cytokines are present. The latter has been suggested in experimental models of glaucoma and correlation studies examining potential biomarkers.[50,55]

As retinal cells undergo degeneration and apoptosis, the interneuronal connections that are crucial for transmitting and translating light signals to electrochemical reactions conducted through the optic nerve to the visual cortex are irremediably lost. The loss of this signal integration network ultimately impairs function and structure of the optic nerve, resulting in irreversible functional optic neuropathy, axonal degenerative changes (dilated axon sheaths and cylinders, axonophagia, axon loss, and cupping of the optic nerve head [**Fig. 14**]). Cupping of the optic nerve head is the final end-stage hallmark of increased IOP, and it is not unique to primary glaucoma.

A current obstacle to more effective treatment of glaucoma is the fact that the neurosensory retina has very limited capacity for regeneration. Abundant research is now being conducted to identify and improve regenerative responses and to identify and sustain compensatory mechanisms that could protect the retina exposed to elevated IOP.[56–58] These insights have not yet translated into routine clinical veterinary practice, but results in experimental settings have been encouraging.

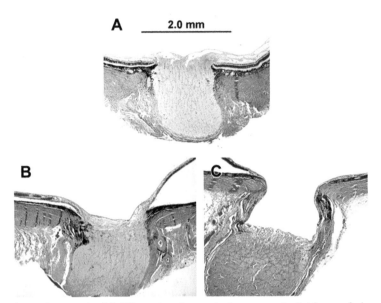

Fig. 14. Photomicrograph of 3 different canine posterior segments. Evidence of glaucoma in canine eyes shown by mild and marked cupping of the optic nerve head. Normal canine optic nerve head is shown (*A*) for comparison, where the optic nerve head aligns with the retina. Mild cupping of the optic nerve head is shown (*B*) where the optic nerve is slightly depressed from its normal position. Marked cupping of the optic nerve head is shown in (*C*) where the depression and tissue loss due to increased IOP is dramatic. These changes are observed in primary and secondary glaucoma (Bar = 2 mm, original magnification ×2, hematoxylin-eosin).

Changes in the Choroid and Tapetum with Primary Glaucoma

There are no lesions of the choroid that are pathognomonic for primary glaucoma, and no published studies have rigorously addressed the topic in veterinary medicine. In human studies, the choroid becomes thinner with elevated IOP,[59,60] and presumably the same is true for veterinary species.

Photic Retinopathy or the So-Called Tapetal Sparing

In glaucomatous (primary and secondary) dogs, a different distribution of the severity of the retinal changes between dorsal and ventral sensory retina has been observed for a long time.[3,30,48,61,62] The sensory retina corresponding to the tapetal area shows less-severe signs of atrophy when compared with the ventral, nontapetal retina (**Fig. 15**), with atrophic signs in the early stages of the disease characteristically and expectedly distributed primarily to the inner layers of the sensory retina. Parry[61] was the first to report a sparing effect in the dorsal retina in dogs with glaucoma. Other investigators have coined the term tapetal sparing because of the observed better preservation of the retina in the corresponding dorsal area and as if the tapetum could provide a sort of protection to the retina.[3]

Interestingly, the ventral retina shows 2 distinct patterns of atrophy and degeneration, which suggests 2 different underlying mechanisms. The characteristic histopathologic signs of glaucoma in the inner retina are associated with focal, multifocal, or segmental areas of outer retinal atrophy involving the photoreceptor and outer nuclear layers. Often, the severity of the outer lesions is more advanced when compared with

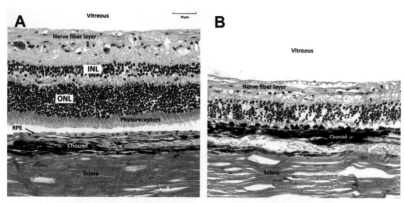

Fig. 15. Retinal photomicrographs from the enucleated left eye of a 10-year-old, spayed female Shih-Tzu affected with primary glaucoma. (*A*) Dorsal retina. (*B*) Ventral retina. The difference in retinal thickness between the 2 sections is evident. Although the nerve fiber layers are comparable, the atrophy affecting the outer layers is greater in the ventral retina. The retinal pigmented epithelium represents a monolayer of nonpigmented epithelial cells in (*A*), whereas in (*B*) it is hypertrophic. Photoreceptors are still recognizable in (*A*), whereas they are severely atrophied in (*B*) (Bar = 50 μm, original magnification ×20, hematoxylin-eosin). INL, inner nuclear layer; ONL, outer nuclear layer.

the inner changes (**Fig. 16**). The neuroretina corresponding to the outer changes in the sensory retina is also involved, and actually, the changes in the outer sensory retina may likely represent kiss lesions caused by primary modifications affecting the retinal pigmented epithelium (RPE).[63] RPE cells appear initially to be enlarged and proliferate. Different amounts of melanin-laden, large round phagocytic cells (melanophages) can be often seen in the subretinal space (**Fig. 17**). Melanophage migration from the subretinal space into the outer and inner layers is often noted.

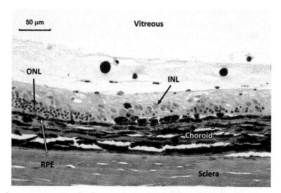

Fig. 16. Retinal photomicrograph from the enucleated right eye of a 7-year-old, spayed female American cocker affected with primary glaucoma. In the central area of the image, corresponding to the proliferation of retinal pigmented epithelium (RPE) cells and melanophages accumulation, the outer retina is completely atrophic, whereas nuclei belonging to the inner nuclear layer are still recognizable. In the left side of the image, where the pigmented RPE is normal, the nuclei of the outer nuclear layer are present, although the layer is decreased in thickness. Melanophages are present at the vitreoretinal interface (Bar = 50 μm, original magnification ×20, hematoxylin-eosin). INL, inner nuclear layer; ONL, outer nuclear layer.

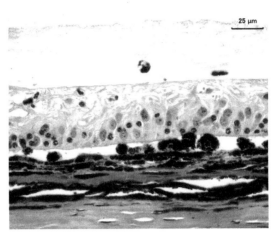

Fig. 17. Retinal photomicrograph from the same patient in **Fig. 16**. There is a clear accumulation of large round melanin-laden macrophages in the subretinal space and mild clumping of the melanin of the RPE and choroidal melanocytes. The outer retina is affected by severe atrophy, and few residual outer nuclei have migrated among the inner nuclei. The atrophy of the outer retina is more severe than that of the inner retina (Bar = 25 μm, original magnification ×40, hematoxylin-eosin).

Choroidal infarction with subsequent retinal ischemia or decreased number and caliper of the short posterior ciliary arteries have been proposed as the possible pathogenic mechanisms for the outer retinal atrophy seen in the nontapetal area.[48,54] The vascular hypotheses, however, do not suit with the vertical sectorial distribution of the choroidal vascularization.[64,65]

It is the authors' opinion that the differences observed between the dorsal and ventral retina could be ascribable to photic damage to the ventral retina. Indeed, identical histologic features have been described in photic retinopathy in dogs and other primate and nonprimate mammals.[66–70]

The nontapetal RPE is pigmented, whereas the tapetal RPE is not. The pathogenesis may involve melanin's capacity to absorb photic energy and subsequently release that energy to photoreceptors.[71–73] The authors speculate that dogs with glaucoma with mydriasis and deteriorating vision may stare at light sources more frequently or for longer duration, so exposing their retinas to higher amounts of photic energy, mostly in the longer wavelengths.

Interestingly, subalbinotic dogs without a tapetal region, still show the disparity in the severity of the retinal changes observed in the dorsal and ventral retina,[3] questioning the real sparing effect of the tapetum. RPE originates from the neuroectoderm, so it is not affected by the lack of pigment originating in the neurocrest. As a matter of fact, ventral RPE is pigmented in dogs with blue iris (like the posterior epithelium of the iris is).

Changes in the Lens with Primary Glaucoma

There are no lens lesions that are specific to primary glaucoma.

Changes in the Vitreous with Primary Glaucoma

There are no changes in the vitreous that are pathognomonic for primary glaucoma. The presence of mucinous material within the optic nerve may be entrapped vitreous and is often seen in canine patients with glaucoma and could suggest an association (**Fig. 18**). However, caution in this interpretation is recommended because this

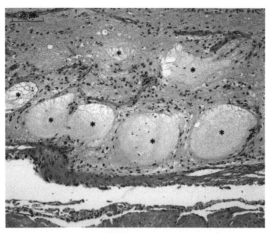

Fig. 18. Optic nerve photomicrograph showing mucinous material (*asterisks*) within the optic nerve in a dog affected with primary glaucoma. The light blue to gray material is accumulation of mucinous material in the optic nerve head, which may be entrapped vitreous. This finding is observed in canine chronic glaucoma and has also been reported in other conditions (Bar = 100 μm, original magnification ×10, hematoxylin-eosin).

particular disease manifestation may reflect the temporal pattern (rapid and severe spikes in IOP that tend to occur with primary glaucoma), rather than a single underlying cause. This change is known as Schnabel cavernous degeneration or Schnabel cavernous optic atrophy, and it has also been described as an age-associated and vasculopathy-associated change in humans.[74,75]

Changes in the Sclera with Primary Glaucoma

With chronically elevated IOP, the entire globe enlarges. This change is not unique to primary glaucoma. As a result, the sclera, which is primarily composed of collagen, becomes stretched and thin. The change is easily recognized as an enlarged, buphthalmic eye clinically, but challenging to appreciate by microscopy, except in the most extreme cases. Relying on microscopy alone to identify scleral thinning is not advised because multiple facets contribute to erroneous interpretation including tissue shrinkage due to fixation and processing, sampling and orientation artifacts, folding of eye sections when they are captured on glass slides, and size/breed variations from normal. To the authors' knowledge, no controlled studies have correlated in vivo scleral measurements with or without glaucoma to light microscopy measurements using age-, sex-, and breed-matched controls. Thus although scleral thinning is a well-recognized consequence of chronically elevated IOP that is quite recognizable clinically, reliance on it as a single diagnostic criterion for glaucoma is not encouraged.

SUMMARY

GDAG/PACG is a common and devastating disease in the dog, and its accurate and timely diagnosis is essential for prolonging vision, particularly following enucleation of one eye. The key histologic feature in affected eyes is a thick, imperforate PL (although the mechanisms that lead to angle closure and aqueous outflow impairment are incompletely understood), associated with the retinal changes that are characteristic for glaucoma (inner retinal degeneration with RGC apoptosis and optic nerve cupping). Lens-iris contact, disruption of the iris pigment epithelial barrier, pigment dispersion, uveitis, and preiridal and postiridal fibrovascular membrane proliferation are often concurrent and may contribute to the pathogenesis. GD is known to be heritable in many breeds, and genetic investigations are beginning to identify candidate gene mutations that may shed light on pathogenesis. Histopathologic examination by pathologists with experience in the diagnosis and concurrent lesions is highly recommended, even in end-stage eyes, particularly if clinical examination is limited.

REFERENCES

1. Miller PE, Schmidt GM, Vainisi SJ, et al. The efficacy of topical prophylactic antiglaucoma therapy in primary closed angle glaucoma in dogs: a multicenter clinical trial. J Am Anim Hosp Assoc 2000;36(5):431–8.
2. Pizzirani S, Gong H. Functional anatomy of the outflow facilities. Vet Clin Small Anim, in press.
3. Dubielzig RR, Ketring KL, McLellan GJ, et al. The glaucomas. In: Dubielzig RR, Ketring KL, McLellan GJ, et al, editors. Veterinary ocular pathology. A comparative review. Edinburgh (United Kingdom): Saunders Elsevier; 2010. p. 418–48.
4. Reilly CM, Morris R, Dubielzig RR. Canine goniodysgenesis-related glaucoma: a morphologic review of 100 cases looking at inflammation and pigment dispersion. Vet Ophthalmol 2005;8(4):253–8.
5. van der Linde-Sipman JS. Dysplasia of the pectinate ligament and primary glaucoma in the Bouvier des Flandres dog. Vet Pathol 1987;24(3):201–6.
6. Read RA, Wood JL, Lakhani KH. Pectinate ligament dysplasia (PLD) and glaucoma in flat coated retrievers. I. Objectives, technique and results of a PLD survey. Vet Ophthalmol 1998;1(2–3):85–90.
7. Wood JL, Lakhani KH, Read RA. Pectinate ligament dysplasia and glaucoma in flat coated retrievers. II. Assessment of prevalence and heritability. Vet Ophthalmol 1998;1(2–3):91–9.
8. Bjerkas E, Ekesten B, Farstad W. Pectinate ligament dysplasia and narrowing of the iridocorneal angle associated with glaucoma in the English Springer Spaniel. Vet Ophthalmol 2002;5(1):49–54.
9. Kato K, Sasaki N, Matsunaga S, et al. Possible association of glaucoma with pectinate ligament dysplasia and narrowing of the iridocorneal angle in Shiba Inu dogs in Japan. Vet Ophthalmol 2006;9(2):71–5.
10. Plummer CE, Regnier A, Gelatt KN. The canine glaucomas. In: Gelatt KN, Gilger BC, Kern TJ, editors. Veterinary Ophthalmology, vol. 2, 5th edition. Ames (IA): John Wiley & Sons, Inc; 2013. p. 1050–145.
11. Spiess, Bolliger, Borer G, et al. Prevalence of pectinate ligament dysplasia in golden retrievers in Switzerland. Schweiz Arch Tierheilkd 2014;156(6):279–84 [in German].
12. Pearl R, Gould D, Spiess B. Progression of pectinate ligament dysplasia over time in two populations of flat-coated retrievers. Vet Ophthalmol 2015;18(1):6–12.
13. Ruhli MB, Spiess BM. Goniodysplasia in the Bouvier des Flandres. Schweiz Arch Tierheilkd 1996;138(6):307–11 [in German].
14. Kato K, Sasaki N, Matsunaga S, et al. Incidence of canine glaucoma with goniodysplasia in Japan: a retrospective study. J Vet Med Sci 2006;68(8):853–8.
15. Grozdanic SD, Kecova H, Harper MM, et al. Functional and structural changes in a canine model of hereditary primary angle-closure glaucoma. Invest Ophthalmol Vis Sci 2010;51(1):255–63.
16. Ekesten B, Narfstrom K. Correlation of morphologic features of the iridocorneal angle to intraocular pressure in Samoyeds. Am J Vet Res 1991;52(11):1875–8.

17. Tsai S, Bentley E, Miller PE, et al. Gender differences in iridocorneal angle morphology: a potential explanation for the female predisposition to primary angle closure glaucoma in dogs. Vet Ophthalmol 2012;15(Suppl 1):60–3.

18. Dees DD, Fritz KJ, Maclaren NE, et al. Efficacy of prophylactic antiglaucoma and anti-inflammatory medications in canine primary angle-closure glaucoma: a multicenter retrospective study (2004-2012). Vet Ophthalmol 2014;17(3): 195–200.

19. Ahram DF, Cook AC, Kecova H, et al. Identification of genetic loci associated with primary angle-closure glaucoma in the basset hound. Mol Vis 2014;20:497–510.

20. Ahram DF, Grozdanic SD, Kecova H, et al. Variants in nebulin (NEB) are linked to the development of familial primary angle closure glaucoma in basset hounds. PLoS One 2015;10(5):e0126660.

21. Oshima Y, Bjerkas E, Peiffer RL Jr. Ocular histopathologic observations in Norwegian Elkhounds with primary open-angle, closed-cleft glaucoma. Vet Ophthalmol 2004; 7(3):185–8.

22. Gelatt KN, MacKay EO. Prevalence of the breed-related glaucomas in pure-bred dogs in North America. Vet Ophthalmol 2004;7(2):97–111.

23. Ekesten B, Torrang I. Heritability of the depth of the opening of the ciliary cleft in Samoyeds. Am J Vet Res 1995;56(9):1138–43.

24. Wood JL, Lakhani KH, Mason IK, et al. Relationship of the degree of goniodysgenesis and other ocular measurements to glaucoma in Great Danes. Am J Vet Res 2001;62(9):1493–9.

25. Samuelson D, Streit A. Microanatomy of the anterior uveoscleral outflow pathway in normal and primary open-angle glaucomatous dogs. Vet Ophthalmol 2012; 15(Suppl 1):47–53.

26. Ryland TR, Lewis PA, Chisholm M, et al. Localization of smooth muscle actin in the iridocorneal angle of normal and spontaneous glaucomatous beagle dogs. Vet Ophthalmol 2003;6(3):205–9.

27. Hassel B, Samuelson DA, Lewis PA, et al. Immunocytochemical localization of smooth muscle actin-containing cells in the trabecular meshwork of glaucomatous and nonglaucomatous dogs. Vet Ophthalmol 2007;10(Suppl 1):38–45.

28. Tsai S, Almazan A, Lee SS, et al. The effect of topical latanoprost on anterior segment anatomic relationships in normal dogs. Vet Ophthalmol 2013;16(5):370–6.

29. Mochizuki M. Regional immunity of the eye. Acta Ophthalmol 2010;88(3):292–9.

30. Sugita S, Horie S, Yamada Y, et al. Suppression of bystander T helper 1 cells by iris pigment epithelium-inducing regulatory T cells via negative costimulatory signals. Invest Ophthalmol Vis Sci 2010;51(5):2529–36.

31. Alario AF, Pizzirani S, Pirie CG. Histopathologic evaluation of the anterior segment of eyes enucleated due to glaucoma secondary to primary lens displacement in 13 canine globes. Vet Ophthalmol 2013;16(Suppl 1):34–41.

32. Pizzirani S, Desai SJ, Pirie CG, et al. Age related changes in the anterior segment of the eye in normal dogs. Vet Ophthalmol 2010;13(6):421.

33. Kim MC, Kabeer NH, Tandhasetti MT, et al. Immunohistochemical studies on melanin associated antigen (MAA) induced experimental autoimmune anterior uveitis (EAAU). Curr Eye Res 1995;14(8):703–10.

34. Bora NS, Kim MC, Kabeer NH, et al. Experimental autoimmune anterior uveitis. Induction with melanin-associated antigen from the iris and ciliary body. Invest Ophthalmol Vis Sci 1995;36(6):1056–66.

35. Jha P, Manickam B, Matta B, et al. Proteolytic cleavage of type I collagen generates an autoantigen in autoimmune uveitis. J Biol Chem 2009;284(45): 31401–11.

36. Pizzirani S, Carroll V, Pirie CG, et al. Pathologic factors involved with the late onset of canine glaucoma associated with goniodysgenesis. Preliminary study. Paper presented at: ACVO 39th Annual Conference. Boston, October 15–18, 2008.

37. Durieux P, Etchepareborde S, Fritz D, et al. Tumor necrosis factor-alpha concentration in the aqueous humor of healthy and diseased dogs: a preliminary pilot study. J Fr Ophtalmol 2015;38(4):288–94.

38. Marshall JL, Stanfield KM, Silverman L, et al. Enhanced expression of cyclooxygenase-2 in glaucomatous dog eyes. Vet Ophthalmol 2004;7(1):59–62.

39. Tatton WG, Chalmers-Redman RM, Tatton NA. Apoptosis and anti-apoptosis signalling in glaucomatous retinopathy. Eur J Ophthalmol 2001;11(Suppl 2): S12–22.

40. Gornik KR, Pizzirani S, Brown FS, et al. Use of immunohistochemical markers to determine the cellular origin of pre-iridal fibrovascular membranes in enucleated canine globes with ocular inflammation. Paper presented at: 45th Annual Meeting of the American College of Veterinary Ophthalmologists. Fort Worth, October 8–11, 2014.

41. Bauer BS, Sandmeyer LS, Hall RB, et al. Immunohistochemical evaluation of fibrovascular and cellular pre-iridal membranes in dogs. Vet Ophthalmol 2012; 15(Suppl 1):54–9.

42. Binder DR, Herring IP, Zimmerman KL, et al. Expression of vascular endothelial growth factor receptor-1 and -2 in normal and diseased canine eyes. Vet Ophthalmol 2012;15(4):223–30.

43. Sihota R, Saxena R, Agarwal HC. Entropion uveae: early sphincter atrophy, signposting primary angle closure glaucoma? Eur J Ophthalmol 2004;14(4): 290–7.

44. Sandberg CA, Herring IP, Huckle WR, et al. Aqueous humor vascular endothelial growth factor in dogs: association with intraocular disease and the development of pre-iridal fibrovascular membrane. Vet Ophthalmol 2012;15(Suppl 1):21–30.

45. Mantovani A. Macrophage diversity and polarization: in vivo veritas. Blood 2006; 108(2):408–9.

46. Seta N, Kuwana M. Derivation of multipotent progenitors from human circulating CD141 monocytes. Exp Hematol 2010;38(7):557–63.

47. Smedes SL, Dubielzig RR. Early degenerative changes associated with spontaneous glaucoma in dogs. J Vet Diagn Invest 1994;6(2):259–63.

48. Whiteman AL, Klauss G, Miller PE, et al. Morphologic features of degeneration and cell death in the neurosensory retina in dogs with primary angle-closure glaucoma. Am J Vet Res 2002;63(2):257–61.

49. Dreyer EB, Grosskreutz CL. Excitatory mechanisms in retinal ganglion cell death in primary open angle glaucoma (POAG). Clin Neurosci 1997;4(5):270–3.

50. Agarwal R, Agarwal P. Glaucomatous neurodegeneration: an eye on tumor necrosis factor-alpha. Indian J Ophthalmol 2012;60(4):255–61.

51. Almasieh M, Wilson AM, Morquette B, et al. The molecular basis of retinal ganglion cell death in glaucoma. Prog Retin Eye Res 2012;31(2):152–81.

52. Krizaj D, Ryskamp DA, Tian N, et al. From mechanosensitivity to inflammatory responses: new players in the pathology of glaucoma. Curr Eye Res 2014; 39(2):105–19.

53. Wert KJ, Lin JH, Tsang SH. General pathophysiology in retinal degeneration. Dev Ophthalmol 2014;53:33–43.

54. Fick CM, Dubielzig RR. Short posterior ciliary artery anatomy in normal and acutely glaucomatous dogs. Vet Ophthalmol 2015. [Epub ahead of print].

55. Pinazo-Duran MD, Zanon-Moreno V, Garcia-Medina JJ, et al. Evaluation of presumptive biomarkers of oxidative stress, immune response and apoptosis in primary open-angle glaucoma. Curr Opin Pharmacol 2013;13(1):98–107.
56. Wen R, Tao W, Li Y, et al. CNTF and retina. Prog Retin Eye Res 2012;31(2):136–51.
57. Cui Q, Ren C, Sollars PJ, et al. The injury resistant ability of melanopsin-expressing intrinsically photosensitive retinal ganglion cells. Neuroscience 2015;284:845–53.
58. Wang Y, Xie T. Extracellular, stem cells and regenerative ophthalmology. J Glaucoma 2014;23(8 Suppl 1):S30–3.
59. Kubota T, Jonas JB, Naumann GO. Decreased choroidal thickness in eyes with secondary angle closure glaucoma. An aetiological factor for deep retinal changes in glaucoma? Br J Ophthalmol 1993;77(7):430–2.
60. Banitt M. The choroid in glaucoma. Curr Opin Ophthalmol 2013;24(2):125–9.
61. Parry HB. Degenerations of the dog retina. III. Retinopathy secondary to glaucoma. Br J Ophthalmol 1953;37(11):670–9.
62. Scott EM, Boursiquot N, Beltran WA, et al. Early histopathologic changes in the retina and optic nerve in canine primary angle-closure glaucoma. Vet Ophthalmol 2013;16(Suppl 1):79–86.
63. Grierson I, Hiscott P, Hogg P, et al. Development, repair and regeneration of the retinal pigment epithelium. Eye 1994;8(Pt 2):255–62.
64. Hayreh SS. Segmental nature of the choroidal vasculature. Br J Ophthalmol 1975;59(11):631–48.
65. Olver JM. Functional anatomy of the choroidal circulation: methyl methacrylate casting of human choroid. Eye 1990;4(Pt 2):262–72.
66. Pizzirani S, Davidson MG, Gilger BC. Transpupillary diode laser retinopexy in dogs: ophthalmoscopic, fluorescein angiographic and histopathologic study. Vet Ophthalmol 2003;6(3):227–35.
67. Buyukmihci N. Photic retinopathy in the dog. Exp Eye Res 1981;33(1):95–109.
68. Wallow IH, Sponsel WE, Stevens TS. Clinicopathologic correlation of diode laser burns in monkeys. Arch Ophthalmol 1991;109(5):648–53.
69. Smiddy WE, Hernandez E. Histopathologic results of retinal diode laser photocoagulation in rabbit eyes. Arch Ophthalmol 1992;110(5):693–8.
70. Green WR, Robertson DM. Pathologic findings of photic retinopathy in the human eye. Am J Ophthalmol 1991;112(5):520–7.
71. Algvere PV, Torstensson PA, Tengroth BM. Light transmittance of ocular media in living rabbit eyes. Invest Ophthalmol Vis Sci 1993;34(2):349–54.
72. Boettner EA, Wolter JR. Transmission of the ocular media. Invest Ophthalmol 1962;1(6):776–83.
73. Mainster MA. Ophthalmic applications of infrared lasers – thermal considerations. Invest Ophthalmol Vis Sci 1979;18(4):414–20.
74. Giarelli L, Falconieri G, Cameron JD, et al. Schnabel cavernous degeneration: a vascular change of the aging eye. Arch Pathol Lab Med 2003;127(10):1314–9.
75. Rummelt V, Lang GK, Yanoff M, et al. A 32-year follow-up of the rigid Schreck anterior chamber lens. A clinicopathological correlation. Arch Ophthalmol 1990;108(3):401–4.

Medical Treatment of Primary Canine Glaucoma

Anthony F. Alario, DVM[a],*, Travis D. Strong, DVM, MS[b], Stefano Pizzirani, DVM, PhD[c]

KEYWORDS

- Glaucoma • Medical therapy • Carbonic anhydrase inhibitors
- Prostaglandin analogues • Novel therapies • Delivery systems

KEY POINTS

- Glaucoma is a painful and blinding group of diseases with no cure; currently, treatment is aimed at chronically managing the condition, with an ultimate goal of a comfortable and preferably visual eye.
- Medical therapy remains the predominant method for managing glaucoma in veterinary patients. It may be used alone or in combination with surgical techniques to control intraocular pressure (IOP).
- The veterinary practitioner is faced with a large array of hypotensive agents, most of which have shown promise in managing IOP if the diagnosis is made early; however, there is no one drug that has been shown to universally treat this condition.
- Because angle-closure glaucoma is the most common canine glaucoma, medications acting to improve trabecular outflow are used rarely.
- Glaucoma is a progressive disease and medical therapy, if effective, needs to be continued for the lifetime of affected patients.

INTRODUCTION

The field of ocular therapeutics is rapidly evolving, with new information published on a regular basis. With such a substantial amount of research available and a plethora of medical options for the clinician to choose from, the simple question, "What is the best way to medically treat canine glaucoma?" becomes far more complex than expected. Before diving into the subject matter at hand, there are several concepts that merit further discussion to assist the reader in interpreting the information provided in this article.

The authors have nothing to disclose.
[a] VCA Capital Area Veterinary Emergency and Specialty, 1 Intervale Road, Concord, NH 03301, USA; [b] Lloyd Veterinary Medical Center, Iowa State University College of Veterinary Medicine, 1600 16th Street, Ames, IA 50011, USA; [c] Department of Clinical Sciences, Cummings School of Veterinary Medicine, Tufts University, 200 Westboro Road, North Grafton, MA 01536, USA
* Corresponding author.
E-mail address: aalario@gmail.com

Vet Clin Small Anim 45 (2015) 1235–1259
http://dx.doi.org/10.1016/j.cvsm.2015.06.004
0195-5616/15/$ – see front matter © 2015 Elsevier Inc. All rights reserved.

vetsmall.theclinics.com

With the data presented regarding the efficacy of each of the glaucoma drugs, the research model used in the study is discussed. For research purposes, most study populations are either genetically similar colony beagles affected with primary open-angle glaucoma (POAG) or normotensive research beagles. The availability and uniformity of the populations allow for high-quality, controlled studies to be performed and objective evaluation of a drug's efficacy at reducing IOP. These populations, however, do not represent the typical population encountered by the veterinary clinician in practice. In contrast to the research models, the vast majority of clinical idiopathic canine glaucoma is of the primary narrow-angle type, which behaves differently from POAG. As such, it is difficult to justify the use of medications that increase trabecular outflow when, in the most common phenotype of canine glaucoma, the anatomic anterior conventional outflow pathways are irrevocably collapsed. Additionally, it is well documented that the IOP-lowering effect of many drugs is greater in glaucomatous eyes than normotensive control eyes. Therefore, it is expected that the efficacy of drugs used in the clinical setting will vary to a much larger degree than the results of the controlled studies performed in a laboratory setting.

Another evolving concept regarding the medical management of glaucoma is the notion of nonresponders to specific medical therapy. For any given drug, there is a subset of individuals whose response to a specific antiglaucoma medication is substantially less than the rest of the population studied. The exact cause of poor response is not entirely clear, although there is strong support of a genetic basis that determines the efficacy of any particular drug in an individual patient. In humans, single-nucleotide polymorphisms have been identified in patients who responded well to timolol (>20% IOP reduction, high responders) and in individuals who demonstrated a poor response to latanoprost (nonresponders).[1,2] Although not specifically studied in dogs, clinical experience dictates that this principle holds true for clinical glaucoma patients as well. This may help explain the often conflicting results of various studies evaluating the efficacy of glaucoma drugs in canine patients. Therefore, prudence and judgment must be exercised when evaluating the extensive research on the topic of canine glaucoma, and developing overgeneralized conclusions about the efficacy of each drug for the entire canine population should be refrained from.

The last concept that merits discussion is that the definition of glaucoma has changed over the past several decades. At least in the veterinary literature, glaucoma has historically been nearly synonymous with elevated IOP. Current research has shed light on ocular damage occurring even at IOP levels previously thought safe in canine patients. This, along with variability in signalment, patient history, and clinical course of the various forms of glaucoma, has led veterinary ophthalmologists to re-evaluate their description of the disease. Glaucoma is no longer a singular entity but a single common endpoint for a variety of ocular conditions that result in retinal ganglion cell (RGC) death and optic nerve degeneration. Unfortunately the inciting cause for many forms of glaucoma, especially primary canine glaucoma, remains an enigma. Currently, the mainstay of medical therapy for glaucoma remains aimed at reducing IOP, because it is the main known risk factor. In the future, this generic approach to medical management of glaucoma patients is likely to change, hopefully replaced with tailored therapies that target the underlying cause of the glaucoma and prevent or delay optic nerve degeneration.

TOPICAL OCULAR HYPOTENSIVE DRUGS

Topical hypotensive drugs have become the predominant method for treating canine glaucoma. They have largely replaced systemic forms of therapy due to their high efficacy and lower side-effect profiles. Despite being applied directly to the eye, significant amounts of the medication can still be systemically absorbed and cause unwanted side effects. This is especially true of topical adrenergic type drugs, such as β-blockers and α_2-agonists. Therefore, clinicians must exercise caution when prescribing topical hypotensive drugs, especially in smaller patients and those with cardiac or respiratory issues. Commonly used ocular hypotensive drugs are discussed later. Each drug is segregated by class and mechanism of action.

CHOLINERGIC AGONISTS (MIOTICS)
Mechanism of Action

Cholinergic agonists directly or indirectly stimulate the parasympathetic nervous system in the eye via acetylcholine receptors. Direct-acting agents (pilocarpine and carbachol) directly activate acetylcholine receptors, whereas indirect-acting cholinergic agents (demecarium bromide) inhibit acetylcholinesterase activity, thereby increasing the concentration and exposure time of acetylcholine at its receptor site. Activation of these receptors leads to miosis, ciliary muscle contraction, reduction in IOP, and transient disruption of the blood-aqueous barrier. The mechanism of IOP reduction is well documented in humans and nonhuman primates. In these species, cholinergic activation leads to contraction of the longitudinal fibers of the ciliary muscle, which are anchored anteriorly to an anatomic structure called the scleral spur. It is this anatomic relationship between the longitudinal fibers of the ciliary muscle and the scleral spur that result in widening of the conventional outflow pathway with the application of cholinergic agents.[3] Small animals, including canines, lack a true scleral spur and have a poorly developed ciliary muscle. Although the exact mechanism by which IOP is lowered in these animals is unknown, the attachment of the ciliary muscle tendons to the posterior scleral lamellae of the scleral sulcus may justify their action.[4] Studies have confirmed that in addition to lowering IOP, topical and intracameral cholinergic agonists have been shown to increase conventional outflow facility in both normotensive and POAG beagles.[5,6] This supports the hypothesis that despite differing anatomy and lack of a scleral spur, the IOP-lowering effects in small animals is likely achieved via increased flow through the conventional outflow pathway.

Pilocarpine

Pilocarpine is a direct-acting, nonspecific parasympathomimetic drug that is commercially available in concentrations ranging from 0.5% to 8% in methylcellulose or polyvinyl alcohol vehicles. The pH of commercial formulations of this drug are acidic (4.5–5.5) and can be irritating to the ocular surface, leading to clinical signs of blepharospasm, epiphora, conjunctival hyperemia, and nictitating membrane elevation in some patients. Formulations with a buffered tip may alleviate some of these adverse reactions with no loss of efficacy.[3] Studies examining the use of various concentrations of pilocarpine in glaucomatous (POAG) and normotensive beagles demonstrate a 30% to 40% decrease in IOP with an associated increase in the coefficient of tonographic outflow facility.[3,7] The IOP-lowering effect lasts for at least 6 hours and is greater in glaucomatous than in normotensive beagles.[7] A recent study examined the effects of pilocarpine in combination with latanoprost, a topical prostaglandin analogue, at reducing IOP in normotensive mixed breed dogs. Although pilocarpine and latanoprost each significantly reduced IOP from baseline in the dogs examined, there was no significant additive effect from the combination therapy.[8]

Clinical use

The use of pilocarpine should only be considered when early stages of POAG are encountered. In reality the improved efficacy of newer hypotensive medications has rendered pilocarpine obsolete for the clinical treatment of canine glaucoma. Furthermore, in advanced cases of canine glaucoma when the trabecular pathways are irreversibly compromised, pilocarpine has no rational use.[3] The low pH of commercial formulations and the correlated ocular irritation that some patients may experience is another reason to avoid the topical use of this medication.

Contraindications

Although pilocarpine produces increased flare, it does not affect the integrity of the blood-aqueous barrier.[9,10] Its use with concomitant uveitis, however, should be well pondered because the associated miosis may lead to posterior synechia formation and subsequent iris bombé. Pilocarpine should also be avoided in cases of anterior lens luxation, because pupillary block may result.

Carbachol

Carbachol is a direct-acting parasympathomimetic with extremely poor lipid solubility, limiting its clinical use in veterinary ophthalmology to intracameral injection at the end of cataract surgery to reduce the risk of postoperative ocular hypertension (POH).[3,11,12] Because of conflicting results, the use of carbachol at the end of phacoemulsification therapy remains debated among veterinary ophthalmologists and is ultimately used at the discretion of the surgeon.[3,11,12]

Demecarium Bromide

Demecarium bromide is an indirect-acting parasympathomimetic drug that reversibly binds to and inhibits acetylcholinesterase. Although no longer commercially available, this medication can be compounded in 0.125% and 0.25% preparations for ophthalmic use. The IOP-lowering effect of demecarium bromide is similar to that of pilocarpine in both normotensive and glaucomatous beagles; however, the duration of action is significantly longer (up to 55 hours for the 0.25% solution).[5] The same is true of the miotic effect of the drug, which can persist for up to 77 hours.[5]

Clinical use

Historically, demecarium bromide was used as a topical therapy in chronic primary canine glaucoma. Despite its long duration of action, twice-daily therapy has been recommended in dogs to prevent IOP fluctuations that often accompany the disease.[5] A prospective, multicenter clinical trial confirmed that prophylactic use of demecarium bromide, 0.25%, in combination with a topical steroid significantly delayed the onset of glaucoma in the second eye of dogs with unilateral closed-angle glaucoma. The median time until treatment failure was 31 months in the demecarium bromide/steroid group compared with 8 months in the control group.[13] A more recent retrospective study evaluating the prophylactic use of various antiglaucoma medications found drastically shorter median times to treatment failure for all drugs used, including demecarium bromide. The results for demecarium bromide were concentration dependent, with a median time to treatment failure of 330 days and 143 days for the 0.125% and 0.25% solutions, respectively. Despite this striking difference, the results were not statistically significant.[14]

Contraindications

Similar to other parasympathomimetic drugs, demecarium bromide should be avoided in cases of glaucoma secondary to uveitis, due to its ability to temporarily disrupt the blood-aqueous barrier.[3] It should also be avoided in cases of anterior lens luxation, because pupil block glaucoma may result. Despite this, successful medical therapy using demecarium bromide in cases of posterior and subluxation of the crystalline lens has been reported in dogs.[15] Given the nonspecific nature of the drug, systemic signs of toxicity may occur with the use of this drug. These include salivation, vomiting, diarrhea, and abdominal cramps. To minimize the risk of toxicity, demecarium bromide should be avoided in patients treated with flea preparations containing organophosphates.[5]

DRUGS ACTING ON ADRENOCEPTORS
Epinephrine and Dipivefrin

Epinephrine and dipivefrin, its more lipophilic prodrug, are nonspecific adrenergic agonists that lower IOP in humans and canine patients. The mechanism by which these drugs reduce IOP in humans is still unclear. It is hypothesized that they both decrease aqueous humor (AH) production and increase conventional outflow.[16–19] The effect of epinephrine on AH dynamics in humans has been debated, because multiple studies provide conflicting data regarding the drug's true effect on AH production.[16–18] The most recent study by Wang and colleagues[16] suggests the reduction in AH production observed in humans is due to decreased blood flow to the ciliary body. The increased conventional outflow facility is mediated through β-receptors found in the trabecular meshwork.[16,19] The IOP-lowering effects of epinephrine and dipivefrin have been reported in both normotensive and glaucomatous beagles. The effect tended to be greater in the latter group, lowering IOP by 5 to 6 mm Hg with minimal ocular irritation and tearing.[20]

Clinical use
Despite the promising experimental results in normotensive and glaucomatous beagles, topical epinephrine and dipivefrin are seldom used clinically to control IOP in idiopathic canine glaucoma. The main indication for these drugs is medical control of POAG, which is not the type of glaucoma typically encountered in clinical veterinary practice.[3] Additionally, the mydriatic effect of these drugs may raise concerns in patients with primary narrow-angle glaucoma because further crowding of the angle may occur. Because corneal esterases convert dipivefrin to phenylephrine, the combined use of indirect-acting parasympathomimetic drugs, such as demecarium bromide, with dipivefrin is not advised.[3]

α_2-Adrenergic Agonists

Mechanism of action
α_2-Adrenergic agonists decrease IOP in human eyes via reduction of AH production and increased uveoscleral outflow facility.[3,21] Activation of presynaptic α_2-receptors inhibits norepinephrine release, thereby blocking the tonic stimulatory effect of the sympathetic nervous system on AH production at the level of the ciliary epithelium. Further reductions in AH secretion are attributed to postsynaptic ciliary epithelial α_2-receptor stimulation, an effect mediated by reduced intracellular cyclic adenosine monophosphate (cAMP) levels.[3,21] α_2-Agonists have also been shown to modulate the expression and enzymatic activity of matrix metalloproteinases (MMPs) and tissue inhibitors of MMPs in the outflow pathways, resulting in the degradation of extracellular matrix material. This leads to decreased resistance to uveoscleral outflow and thus assists in reducing the IOP within the eye.[21]

Apraclonidine
Apraclonidine is only mildly α_2-selective and is currently available in a 0.5% ophthalmic preparation. The efficacy of this drug in glaucomatous beagles has been

evaluated. Administration of a single drop of the 0.5% solution resulted in a significant IOP reduction of 16% (3.0 mm Hg) 8 hours after treatment. Apraclonidine also resulted in a significant mydriasis of 29% (2.2 mm) in treated eyes, lasting for up to 8 hours after administration of the drug.[22] Side effects of apraclonidine in dogs are typically mild and include reduction in heart rate and blanching of the conjunctiva after topical application.[22] This is in stark contrast to cats, where apraclonidine has been shown to cause undesirable side effects, such as bradycardia, gastrointestinal upset, salivation, and vomiting.[23] Because of the limited efficacy of apraclonidine, it is not recommended as a first-line antiglaucoma drug in dogs and should generally be avoided in feline patients.[22,23]

Brimonidine

Brimonidine tartrate is a highly selective α_2-agonist labeled to reduce IOP in human patients with glaucoma.[3] Despite its effectiveness and low side-effect profile in humans, brimonidine does not seem as efficacious in canine patients. After single- and multiple-drop applications of brimonidine in beagles affected with POAG, a trend of insignificant IOP reduction was observed. Side effects were mild and included reduced heart rate and miosis.[24] Based on these results, brimonidine is not recommended as a sole agent to manage canine glaucoma.

β-Adrenergic Antagonists (β-Blockers)

Mechanism of action

β-blockers decrease IOP primarily via reduced AH production.[25] Although the exact mechanism by which this effect is mediated is unclear, 3 theories have been proposed to explain the effect of this class of drug. The first attributes IOP reduction to blockade of β_2-receptors on the ciliary epithelium. This inhibits the tonic stimulatory influence of norepinephrine on intracellular cAMP production and thus reduces AH production. The second mechanism by which β-blockers may reduce IOP is via blockade of sodium potassium ATPase, which reduces active transport and ultrafiltration in the ciliary epithelium. Lastly, β-blockers are believed to reduce IOP via a vasoactive mechanism, modulating blood flow to the ciliary body and iris root.[3,26] To date, β-blockers have not been shown to modulate AH outflow.[3,25]

Timolol

Timolol maleate is a nonselective β-blocker available as 0.25% and 0.50% ophthalmic preparations.[27–29] Given its success at controlling glaucoma in humans, timolol has received a significant amount of attention in the past decades as a possible first-line medication for glaucoma therapy in dogs. There is a considerable amount of clinical and laboratory research evaluating this drug in both normotensive and glaucomatous dogs of various breeds.[25,27–33] Unfortunately, the data from these studies often provide conflicting results regarding the efficacy of the drug, leaving clinicians to wonder whether to include it in the their treatment of clinical patients with glaucoma. The matter is further confounded by a distinct lack of prospective, controlled clinical studies evaluating the efficacy of this drug in a clinical setting. A summary of pertinent research regarding the efficacy of timolol is provided in **Tables 1** and **2**.

Clinical use Despite conflicting reports of its efficacy at lowering IOP in dogs, timolol has been a mainstay of glaucoma therapy for the past few decades. Topical application of timolol maleate, 0.25%, is recommended in dogs weighing less than 9 kg, whereas the 0.5% solution is advisable in larger dogs. The frequency of administration should be every 8 to 12 hours in larger dogs and every 12 hours in small dogs to minimize systemic side effects. With the development of newer antiglaucoma drugs,

Table 1
Summary of pertinent studies evaluating intraocular pressure reducing effect of timolol in normotensive dogs

Study	Wilkie et al, 1991	Maehara et al, 2004	Takiyama et al, 2006	Gum et al, 1991	Gelatt et al, 1995	Smith et al, 2010
Population	Normotensive dogs[12]	Normotensive mongrel dogs[13]	Normotensive beagles[7]	Normotensive beagles[5]	Normotensive beagles[5]	Normotensive dogs of various breed[18]
Dosing	Timolol, 0.5%, single drop	Timolol, 0.5%, q12 h over 28 d	Timolol, 0.5%, gel-forming solution q24 h over 7 d	Timolol, 0.25%–8%, q24 h	Timolol, 4% or 6%, ± pilocarpine, 2%, q12 h over 5 d	Timolol, 0.5%, ± latanoprost, 0.005%, q12 h, over 4 d
IOP reduction, treated eye	Mean: 16.1% (2.5 mm Hg)	Net reduction: 26% (4.1 mm Hg) Max: 27% (day 7)	Mean: 33.1% (5.3 mm Hg) At t_{24h}: 21.8% (3.5 mm Hg)	No significant decrease in IOP, trend toward IOP reduction for 2% and 4%	Timolol: none Significant reduction with pilocarpine	Timolol: none Significant reduction with latanoprost ± timolol
IOP reduction, fellow eye	Mean: 9.0% (1.4 mm Hg)	Nonsignificant trend toward IOP reduction	Nonsignificant trend toward IOP reduction (1.8 mm Hg)	No significant decrease in IOP, trend toward IOP reduction for 2% and 4%	Timolol: none	Timolol: none Significant reduction with latanoprost ± timolol
Side effects	Miosis (OU) Bradycardia	Bradycardia Reduction in MAP	Miosis (nonsignificant) No change in BP	Miosis Bradycardia	Bradycardia	Timolol ± latanoprost: Bradycardia Miosis

Abbreviations: BP, blood pressure; MAP, mean arterial pressure; max, maximum IOP reduction; OU, both eyes; t24, 24 hours post drop.

Table 2
Summary of pertinent studies evaluating intraocular pressure reducing effects of timolol in glaucomatous dogs

Study	Gum et al, 1991	Gelatt et al, 1995	Plummer et al, 2006	Peng et al, 2012
Population	POAG beagles[33]	POAG beagles[9]	POAG beagles[13]	POAG beagles[13]
Dosing	Timolol, 0.25%–8%, q24 h or single drop	Timolol, 4% or 6%, ± pilocarpine, 2%, q12 h over 5 d	Timolol, 0.5%, q12 h Dorzolamide, 2%, q8 h Timolol, 0.5%, + dorzolamide, 2%, q12 h	Timolol, 0.5%, q24 h over 5 d Timolol-soaked contact lenses
IOP reduction, treated eye	0.25% And 0.5%: 16% (4–5 mm Hg) 2%–8%: 26%–46% (8–14 mm Hg) dose-dependent reduction	Timolol alone: 23.5%–33.8% mm Hg (8–11.5 mm Hg) dose dependent IOP reduction enhanced by pilocarpine	Timolol: 2.83–3.75 mm Hg (max day 4) Dorzolamide: 6.47–7.5 mm Hg (max day 4) Combo: 6.56–8.42 mm Hg (max day 4) Significant greater reduction than either drug alone	Timolol: 4.64 mm Hg Contact lens delivery: decrease in IOP but not significantly different from timolol drop
IOP reduction, fellow eye	Trend toward IOP reduction, but change not significant	No significant effect	Timolol alone: no effect Combo: 3.67–7 mm Hg (max day 4)	Timolol: 3.17 mm Hg Contact lens delivery: none
Side effects	Bradycardia	Bradycardia	Miosis Bradycardia	Miosis Bradycardia

Abbreviations: Combo, combination of timolol and dorzolamide; max, maximum IOP reduction.

timolol no longer seems a decisive first-line drug in the fight against glaucoma. In the authors' clinical experience, it is typically used as an auxiliary medication, when carbonic anhydrase inhibitors (CAIs) and prostaglandins fail to adequately control the IOP.

Contraindication and side effects The most common ocular side effect of timolol is local intolerance, which results from a stinging or burning sensation on instillation. Other possible ocular side effects include photophobia, ptosis, blepharoconjunctivitis, reduced tear film break-up time, and superficial punctate keratitis.[34,35] Miosis after timolol administration is also well documented in both the treated and nontreated eye of canine patients receiving the drug.[27,28,30,32,34,36] The bilateral miosis and IOP reduction are often attributed to systemic absorption of the drug through the mucosa of the nasolacrimal duct, which recent studies confirm is significant.[37] Systemic absorption of topical β-blockers is also responsible for the frequently encountered cardiovascular and pulmonary adverse effects of the drug. These include bradycardia, systemic hypotension, cardiac arrhythmias, syncope, bronchospasm, and dyspnea.[3,34,37] Topical β-blockers are specifically contraindicated in patients with significant cardiac or pulmonary diseases.[38]

Other topical β-blockers
In addition to timolol, several other topical β-blockers are labeled as ocular hypotensive agents for humans. These include betaxolol, levobunolol, metipranolol, and carteolol. All but betaxolol are nonselective β-blockers. Betaxolol is selective for β_1-receptors, with less effect toward β_2-receptors.[39] Of the β-blockers, betaxolol possesses the greatest neuroprotective profile due to its stronger affinity for both sodium and calcium ion channels.[39] Although there are no studies specifically evaluating the IOP-lowering effect of this drug in the canine population, betaxolol (0.5%), was found as effective as a combination of demecarium bromide and topical steroid at delaying the onset of glaucoma in the fellow eye of clinical patients with primary narrow-angle glaucoma.[13] The effects of levobunolol have also been evaluated in normotensive mixed breed dogs. Levobunolol was found to significantly reduce IOP alone and to a greater extent in combination with dorzolamide. Compared with a timolol/dorzolamide combination drop, levobunolol alone was not as effective at lowering IOP. When used in combination with dorzolamide, levobunolol was significantly more effective than the timolol/dorzolamide combination.[40,41]

CARBONIC ANHYDRASE INHIBITORS
Mechanism of Action

AH formation is partially dependent on the production of bicarbonate by the enzyme carbonic anhydrase (CA). This enzyme is found in high levels in the nonpigmented epithelium of the ciliary body and is responsible for the hydration of carbon dioxide to carbonic acid. Carbonic acid dissociates spontaneously to bicarbonate and a free hydrogen ion.[42] The free intracellular bicarbonate molecules are transferred to the intercellular spaces and ultimately the posterior chamber of the eye where they associate with sodium and other cations. This generates an osmotic gradient allowing water to be drawn from the reservoir of the ciliary body stroma into the posterior chamber, resulting in the formation of aqueous humor.[3,42,43] There are 7 isoenzymes of CA but only CA II seems clinically relevant with regards to AH formation. For CAIs to reduce AH production, 98% to 100% of the CA II in the ciliary epithelium must be inhibited.[3,42,44] Ultimately, suppression of this enzyme can decrease AH production by up to 40%, accounting for the IOP reduction seen clinically.[3]

Systemic Carbonic Anhydrase Inhibitors

Of the systemic CAIs, methazolamide is most commonly used in the clinical setting to reduce IOP. Methazolamide is supplied in 25- and 50-mg tablets. The recommended dose of methazolamide in dogs is 5 to 10 mg/kg orally every 8 to 12 hours. Ideally, the lowest dose possible should be used to achieve the desired effect and reduce systemic side effects. Methazolamide has been shown to reduce IOP in normal dogs by 18% to 21%. This was associated with a 28% reduction in the AH formation.[45] In glaucomatous beagles, oral methazolamide, at a dose of 5 mg/kg twice daily, significantly reduced IOP by up to 12 mm Hg; however, there was no additive effect when used in combination with dorzolamide, a topical CAI.[44]

Topical Carbonic Anhydrase Inhibitors

Dorzolamide and brinzolamide are the 2 most frequently prescribed topical CAIs in veterinary ophthalmology. Both are potent inhibitors of CA II, with substantially less activity against CA IV.[46] Additionally, when given via the topical route they are able to produce local drug concentrations similar to those achieved with systemically administered CAIs but with plasma concentrations approximately 100 times less. These 2 attributes allow topical CAIs to achieve similar reductions in IOP and AH production with practically zero systemic side effects.[46] As a result, topical CAIs have largely replaced systemic CAIs as a preferred treatment of nearly all forms of canine glaucoma.

Dorzolamide is available as a topical 2% ophthalmic preparation and has been evaluated in normotensive and glaucomatous dogs. In normal beagles, dorzolamide (2%) was found to reduce IOP by 18% (3.1 mm Hg) from 30 minutes to 6 hours after treatment. The maximum effect of a single drop occurred at 6 hours postdosing, resulting in an IOP reduction of 22.5% (3.8 mm Hg).[47] When given every 8 hours in a multidose trial, the maximum IOP reduction of 24% (4.1 mm Hg) was achieved 3 hours post–drug application. AH flow rate was concurrently reduced by 43% in treated eyes over the same time period.[47] When given to beagles with various stages of POAG, dorzolamide (2%) also significantly reduced IOP by 6.47 mm Hg with a single-dose application and 7.5 mm Hg when applied topically every 8 hours. This accounts for an IOP decrease between 30% and 40%.[29]

The IOP-lowering effect of brinzolamide has also been evaluated in normotensive beagle dogs. When applied topically every 12 hours, brinzolamide (1%) significantly reduced IOP in treated eyes by 3.5 mm Hg, with a maximum effect between 5 and 6 hours after treatment. IOP returned to baseline levels by 10 to 11 hours after dosing, suggesting administration every 8 hours would provide superior pharmacologic effect compared with administration every 12 hours.[48] To date, there are no published controlled studies describing the efficacy of brinzolamide in glaucomatous dogs; however, it is the opinion of the authors that it seems as effective as dorzolamide at reducing IOP. The main advantage of this drug over dorzolamide is less ocular irritation after topical application. This is largely due to the pH of the brinzolamide (7.5) being far closer to physiologic pH (7.4) than dorzolamide (5.6).[3]

Clinical Use

CAIs are indicated in all forms of canine glaucoma, including secondary glaucoma.[3] As discussed previously, topical CAIs have largely replaced their systemically administered counterparts as one of the first-line drugs in the fight against glaucoma. This is largely due to their minimal side-effect profile and similar efficacy. Because there is no clear additive effect of using topical and systemic CAIs concurrently,[44,48] the authors do not recommend routine use of systemic CAIs in the clinical setting. Topical

CAIs are typically used at a twice-daily frequency when used as a prophylactic treatment of preventing/delaying the onset of glaucoma in the fellow nonaffected eye or when used in combination with a β-blocker, such as timolol. When used alone to treat glaucoma, a minimum frequency of every 8 hours is recommended. In severe or refractory cases of glaucoma, therapy every 4 to 6 hours may be warranted.

Contraindication and Side Effects

Because CA is a ubiquitous enzyme found in numerous locations in the body, side effects of systemically administered CAIs are common. These include gastrointestinal disturbances (anorexia, vomiting, and diarrhea), diuresis, malaise, and increased respiratory rate as a mechanism to compensate for metabolic acidosis.[3] Hypokalemia has also been reported with both short- and long-term use of systemic CAIs; however, normal food intake is typically enough to prevent significant potassium depletion. Close monitoring is indicated when prescribing systemic CAIs to anorexic patients or patients with preexisting hypokalemia, because clinically relevant potassium depletion may occur.[3,49] There have been no systemic side effects reported with the use of topical CAIs in canine patients. The most common side effect of topical CAIs is local irritation and squinting after application. As discussed previously, this is more common with dorzolamide than brinzolamide due to its relatively low pH.[3] Dorzolamide has also been reported to produce blepharitis in some dogs. This typically resolves when therapy is discontinued.[49]

PROSTAGLANDIN ANALOGUES
Mechanism of Action

All commercially available prostaglandin analogues are synthetic derivatives of prostaglandin $F_{2\alpha}$. They have been modified from their naturally occurring parent compound to improve corneal permeability but maintain a high affinity for prostanoid FP receptors, which mediate their IOP-lowering effects.[3,50] Prostaglandin analogues primarily reduce IOP via increased uveoscleral outflow. Recent reports also suggest some increase in conventional outflow facility may occur as well.[3,50–52] The exact mechanisms by which prostaglandin analogues increase uveoscleral outflow is under investigation. Substantial evidence from current studies suggest that up-regulation in endogenous MMPs plays a significant role in reducing the density of collagen fibers in the extracellular matrix of the ciliary muscle, thus increasing the facility of uveoscleral outflow.[3,53,54] Other mechanisms by which this class of drugs may reduce IOP include the release of endogenous prostaglandins and increased scleral permeability.[52,55,56] Recent investigations in both humans and dogs confirm that concurrent use of topical anti-inflammatory medications (both nonsteroidal anti-inflammatory drugs and steroids) with latanoprost decreases the IOP-lowering effect of this drug, presumably via reduction in endogenous prostaglandin activation.[56,57]

Latanoprost

Latanoprost is one of the most commonly used topical medications for canine glaucoma and is available as a 0.005% topical solution. The recent development of generic formulations of this drug has made it more accessible to the veterinary community. There have been extensive studies examining the IOP-lowering effects of latanoprost in both normotensive and glaucomatous dogs.[58,59] When administered once daily to normotensive dogs of various breeds, latanoprost significantly reduced IOP in the treated eye by approximately 22% to 40%, depending on the study.[8,31,56,58,60] The maximum hypotensive effect was noted on the fifth day of therapy, and the greatest reduction in IOP was noted 6 hours after application.[58,60] In laboratory beagles with POAG, latanoprost also significantly reduced IOP by approximately 50% (19.1–26.6 mm Hg) when administered at both a once- and twice-daily dosing frequency. Latanoprost also significantly dampened the diurnal fluctuation of IOP, an effect that was most dramatic when given twice daily or once daily at night. For this reason twice-daily treatment is recommended to treat canine glaucoma.[59]

Other Prostaglandin Analogues

Other commonly prescribed prostaglandin analogues that have been evaluated in canine patients include bimatoprost and travoprost ophthalmic preparations. These drugs possess the same mechanism of action as latanoprost, bind to the same FP receptors, and have been shown to have similar efficacy to latanoprost in both normotensive and glaucomatous dogs.[59–63] The most significant difference between these drugs and latanoprost is the cost because generic formulations are not currently available for these medications. Use of these drugs is usually cost prohibitive in many cases.

Clinical Use

In dogs, prostaglandin analogues are indicated for all forms of idiopathic canine glaucoma and may help in some forms of secondary glaucoma.[31,59–61] In the authors' practice, it has largely replaced mannitol as an emergency treatment of canine glaucoma, because the IOP-lowering effects of these drugs often take place within 1 hour of initiating treatment. Prostaglandin analogues may be used as monotherapy or in conjunction with other topical hypotensive agents to treat canine glaucoma.[31] They may also be used as prophylactic therapy in the fellow eye of patients affected with idiopathic glaucoma.[14] Recommended dosage schemes include both once- and twice-daily dosing. If once-daily dosing is elected, application is recommended at night to mitigate some of the detrimental effects of the associated miosis. In persistent or advanced cases of glaucoma, twice-daily application is preferred and has been shown experimentally to dampen daily IOP fluctuations better than once-daily application.[59,61,62] Latanoprost may be indicated after phacoemulsification to mitigate POH, but a recent study found no significant beneficial effect with regard to the frequency or severity of POH when applying this medication topically at the end of surgery.[11]

Contraindication and Side Effects

Adverse effects of topically applied prostaglandin analogues are rare, with conjunctival hyperemia reported most frequently.[58,59] A consistent side effect of this class of drug is a profound miosis, which typically begins within the first hour after topical application. This effect persists for less than 24 hours, at which time a rebound mydriasis often is seen.[56,58,59] Because of this profound miosis, topical prostaglandins are contraindicated when treating glaucoma secondary to anteriorly luxated lenses because it may lead to pupillary block and exacerbate existing ocular hypertension.[49] Despite this, they have been used successfully to medically treat posterior and subluxation of the crystalline lens in canine patients.[15,64] Due to their propensity to disrupt the blood-aqueous barrier, topical prostaglandin analogues should be used with caution in cases of glaucoma secondary to uveitis.[49,65] Recent reports in the human literature are challenging this relative contraindication.[66,67]

OSMOTIC AGENTS

Osmotic agents are typically used as an emergency treatment of acute congestive glaucoma but are not indicated for ongoing IOP control.[3] All osmotic agents are administered orally or intravenously and increase the osmolarity of plasma. Because the main ocular fluids (aqueous and vitreous) are separated from the plasma by semi-permeable membranes (blood-aqueous and blood-vitreous barriers), this increase in plasma osmolarity creates an osmotic gradient favoring the diffusion of water out of the intraocular tissues. This fluid shift helps reduce IOP in 2 ways. First, it inhibits the ultrafiltration process in the ciliary body, thereby reducing AH production. Second, it recalls fluid from the vitreous body, leading to shrinkage of the vitreous and posterior displacement of the iris-lens diaphragm.[49] Because the efficacy of osmotic agents relies solely on their ability to create an osmotic gradient between plasma and intraocular fluids, an intact blood-ocular barrier is essential. The effects of osmotic agents may be severely diminished with concurrent uveitis and blood-ocular barrier disruption.[3,49] The most commonly used osmotic agents in veterinary ophthalmology include mannitol, hypertonic hydroxyethyl starch (HES), and glycerin.

Mannitol

Mannitol is a 6-carbon sugar that is not metabolized to any significant extent by the body and must be excreted by the kidneys. Given its poor oral absorption it must be administered intravenously. The recommended dose for lowering IOP in dogs is 1 to 2 g/kg of body weight, administered slowly over 20 to 30 minutes. The authors occasionally use lower doses (0.5 g/kg) with good results. Mannitol concentrations vary between 10% and 25%. Concentrations above 15% tend to crystallize at lower temperature. The bottles or vials should be kept warmed and administered at body temperature, ideally through a filtering catheter. The first fifth of the dose may be administered over the first 2 to 5 minutes for maximum effect. The IOP-lowering effects are typically evident within the first 30 to 60 minutes and may last up to 6 to 10 hours.[3,49] In normotensive dogs, mannitol, administered at a dose of 1 g/kg, significantly reduced IOP by 24%.[68] Because mannitol expands the extracellular fluid volume, it has the potential to overload the cardiovascular system. This may lead to pulmonary edema in patients with cardiac disease or anesthetized patients.[3,49] Water consumption should be restricted for at least 2 hours after the injection. The systemic status of patients receiving mannitol should be monitored closely, however, because it is a diuretic and dehydration may occur in compromised patients. Mannitol is also contraindicated in patients with renal disease.[49]

Hydroxyethyl Starch

Hypertonic HES is a hyperosmotic agent used in to treat hemorrhagic shock and elevated intracranial pressure in human and veterinary patients. The IOP-lowering effects of HES have recently been evaluated in both normotensive and acutely glaucomatous dogs.[68] Hypertonic HES (7.5%/6%), administered at a dose of 4 mL/kg over 15 minutes, demonstrated IOP reduction comparable to 20% mannitol, administered at a 1 g/kg dose over the same time period, although the duration of action is slightly shorter. Additionally, HES was found to reduce IOP by up to 24% in 6 of 7 clinical cases of acute congestive primary glaucoma.[68] The major side effects of HES include hypernatremia and hypokalemia, especially in patients with preexisting dehydration.[3]

Glycerin

Glycerin, or glycerol, is a trihydric alcohol that is rapidly absorbed after oral administration and is ultimately metabolized by the body to glucose. Glycerol is administered orally at dose of 1 to 2 g/kg/d, typically with a meal. When administered to healthy dogs at a dose of 1.44 g/kg, a significant reduction in IOP was detected between 1 and 10 hours after administration.[69] In a more recent study, oral glycerol, at a dose of 1.5 g/kg, administered to healthy canines reduced IOP by 17% from baseline values; however, this decrease in IOP was not significant compared with the control group.[70] Major side effects of glycerin include nausea or vomiting, an effect that seems to be dose dependent. Weight gain may occur with chronic use. This drug is specifically contraindicated in patients with diabetes mellitus because it is eventually converted to glucose.[70]

PROPHYLACTIC TREATMENT OF PRIMARY CANINE GLAUCOMA

Prophylactic therapy in the fellow eye of patients diagnosed with primary or idiopathic canine glaucoma is common practice among veterinary ophthalmologists. Despite this, there is a paucity of research clearly evaluating the benefit of such therapy in at-risk patients. In a prospective, multicenter clinical trial, both betaxolol, 0.5% (1 drop topically every 12 hours), and demecarium bromide, 0.25%, with a topical steroid (1 drop of each every 24 hours) significantly delayed the onset of glaucoma in the fellow eye compared with untreated control eyes. The median times until the development of glaucoma was 30 months with the betaxolol (0.5%), 31 months with the demecarium bromide (0.25%)/steroid combination, and 8 months with no therapy. There was no significant difference found between the 2 forms of prophylactic therapy; rather, they both seemed equally effective in delaying the onset of glaucoma in the fellow eye.[13]

In a more recent study by Dees and colleagues,[14] 4 different prophylactic therapies were evaluated in the fellow eye of dogs with primary narrow-angle glaucoma both with and without adjunctive anti-inflammatory therapy. Although mathematical differences in the median time until the onset of glaucoma existed, these values were not statically significant form each other. Median time to medical failure after treatment with demecarium bromide (0.125%), latanoprost (0.005%), dorzolamide (2%), and demecarium bromide (0.25%) were 330.0, 284.0, 272.5, and 143 days, respectively. Dogs treated concurrently with topical anti-inflammatory agents (prednisolone acetate, neomycin/polymyxin/dexamethasone, or diclofenac) tended to have longer disease-free intervals than those treated only with a topical hypotensive agent (median time 324 days vs 195 days). These results were not statistically significant. The major limitation of this study is the lack of an untreated control group, but, given the clinical nature of the study, it was deemed inappropriate to withhold treatment from the patients.

Despite the seemingly large range in efficacy between studies and the relative paucity of information on the subject, prophylactic therapy in the treatment of idiopathic canine glaucoma is generally recommended in the clinical setting. From the data it seems that the choice of prophylactic antihypertensive agent may not be as important as the inclusion of a topical anti-inflammatory drop.[14] The authors typically recommend the use of dorzolamide (2%) every 12 hours and topical prednisolone acetate (1%) or neomycin/polymyxin/dexamethasone drops every 24 to 48 hours for the prophylactic treatment of confirmed or suspected idiopathic canine glaucoma. Immune-mediated mechanisms are commonly reported in medical literature and the association of an anti-inflammatory for the treatment/prevention of canine glaucoma is surely justified, especially considering the role that intraocular mononuclear cells may assume in the species.[71,72]

NEUROPROTECTIVE THERAPY IN PRIMARY CANINE GLAUCOMA

Because glaucoma is primarily a progressive, irreversible degenerative disease of the optic nerve, the ideal therapy should address the several mechanisms that lead to

RGC death and nerve degeneration.[73] Currently, however, lowering IOP is the only established medical therapy that may delay the onset and slow the progression of blindness.

Recent studies have focused attention on preventing RGC death by addressing the issue of excitotoxicity. Early studies examining the selective N-methyl-D-aspartate receptor antagonist memantine showed promise at preventing RGC loss in the face of glaucoma; however, recent stage III clinical trials in humans have produced disappointing results. At this time, this drug seems of little clinical use in the fight against RGC death and glaucoma.[74]

The most promising research examining neuroprotection in the face of ocular hypertension focuses on supplementation of neurotrophic factors that are normally obtained by RGCs via retrograde transport, a process that is interrupted with elevated IOP. Specifically, treatment with brain-derived neurotrophic factor and ciliary neurotrophic factor has shown in animal models of glaucoma to prevent RGC death in the face of optic nerve injuries.[74] Despite these promising results, no clinically relevant therapies are available as of the date of publication.

In addition to their IOP-lowering effects, many of the drugs commonly used to clinically treat glaucoma also have neuroprotective effects that warrant discussion. α_2-Agonists directly inhibit proapoptotic pathways and reduce excitotoxicity by inhibiting glutamate release. In addition to their inhibitory effects at the β-receptors, β-blockers act to reduce Na^+ and Ca^{++} influx into RGCs, protecting them from neuronal damage and apoptosis. Prostaglandin analogues, such as latanoprost, have been shown to impede glutamate release and hypoxia induced apoptosis. Topical CAIs, such as dorzolamide and brinzolamide, have been shown to increase blood flow to both the optic nerve and choroid, which may serve a protective role during ocular hypertension.[74]

Ultimately the role of neuroprotective agents is likely to grow as further research into the pathophysiology of this multifactorial disease provides new therapeutic targets. Currently, the authors do not routinely recommend medications specifically aimed at neuroprotection but rely on conventional ocular hypotensive therapy to alleviate the major risk factor associated with optic nerve damage, elevated IOP. Fortunately, most of these medications also provide some neuroprotective properties.

EMERGING TREATMENTS FOR GLAUCOMA

In an endeavor to increase the pharmacologic armamentaria to treat glaucoma, researchers are pursuing a growing list of molecular targets, including Rho kinases (ROCK1 and ROCK2), nitric oxide (NO) and other gaseous transmitters, endothelin-1, cannabinoids, and adenosine receptor agonists, among several others.[75–77] A few of the promising medical treatment approaches currently being studied that may have potential translational use in veterinary medicine are introduced. These include nitric oxide donors, Rho kinase inhibitors, and a brief survey of novel drug-delivery strategies.

Nitric Oxide and Other Gaseous Transmitters (Gasotransmitters)

With the discovery in 1987 that endogenously produced NO is a physiologically active molecule with far-reaching effects, the study of gaseous signaling compounds (gasotransmitters) has flourished, spurring an expansive field of research.[78] Besides their numerous effects on different body tissues,[79,80] these compounds have several compelling intraocular effects in various animal models and humans. The ocular production of these gases seems to influence many aspects of ocular physiology, including regional blood flow, inflammation, and AH dynamics, notably lowering IOP by enhancement of AH egress through the main drainage route of the eye (conventional pathway).[81–83]

NO is a freely diffusible, diatomic gas having a half-life of a mere few seconds.[84] This simple gas is produced endogenously by a closely related group of enzymes named NO synthases (NOSs) through the conversion of L-arginine to NO and L-citrulline. Three isoforms have been identified. Endothelial NOS (eNOS) and neuronal NOS (nNOS) are expressed constitutively in a variety of tissues, produce picomolar to low nanomolar levels of NO under physiologic conditions, and are tightly regulated in their expression and activity.[82,85] Alternatively, inducible NOS is expressed during tissue insult, is involved in inflammatory cascades, produces dramatically elevated micromolar to millimolar levels of NO, and directs more prolonged elevations of NO than either eNOS or nNOS.[86] The pathways involved in NO production, regulation, and signaling have been thoroughly explored, with additional discoveries made routinely.[82] Recently, the first NO-donating compound for ocular hypertension and glaucoma therapy, latanoprostene bunod, met a primary endpoint in a phase 3 trial with positive results (Bausch + Lomb [Rochester, NY, USA] and Nicox S.A. [Fort Worth, TX, USA]). Growing evidence gleaned from various animal models (including normal and early glaucomatous dogs) and human studies reveals a multitude of roles for NO in regulating the intraocular mileu.[84,87,88] Of particular importance, NO has been shown integral in the regulation of AH outflow through the conventional pathway in several animal and human studies.[89–92]

Treatment with topical NO donors has been shown to relax and shrink trabecular meshwork cells as well as meaningfully lower IOP through decreasing resistance to outflow.[87,90,93,94]

Because the preponderance of current antiglaucoma medications target AH production and uveoscleral outflow, there remains an enormous therapeutic potential for compounds, such as NO, that exert direct effects on the conventional pathway. Furthermore, numerous additional studies hint at the profound effects NO may have on regulating intraocular inflammation,[95] chorioretinal and optic nerve head blood flow,[96,97] AH formation,[98,99] and episcleral vascular resistance[100] as well as limiting RGC degeneration in models of glaucoma and ischemia.[101–103]

Although eNOS and nNOS expression have been noted in human trabecular meshwork tissue,[104–106] there are no studies to the authors' knowledge that demonstrate ocular expression and localization under normal physiologic conditions of the NOS isoforms in domestic animal species (eg, dogs, cats, and horses).

Rho Kinase Inhibitors

Rho kinases (ROCK1 and ROCK2) are ubiquitously expressed serine/threonine kinases that on activation by Rho family GTPases affect a wide range of cellular activities.[107] Notable among these effects is the enhancement of smooth muscle contraction through increasing myosin light chain phosphorylation and stabilizing filamentous actin.[108] ROCKs are ubiquitously involved in systemic physiology, and their aberrant regulation may promote disease states associated with cytoskeletal and contractile derangements, including systemic hypertension and tumor metastasis.[109,110] As such, ROCK inhibitors are avidly researched for their therapeutic potential against numerous systemic diseases. As a subset of their systemic expression, ROCKs are expressed in various ocular structures in humans and several laboratory animals, including trabecular meshwork, retina, ciliary body, and cornea, among others.[111–114] Given that these proteins are highly conserved across animal taxa, similar ocular expression is confirmed or expected in common veterinary species.[115]

Some of the cells present in the trabecular meshwork share similarities with smooth muscle cells in having contractile properties, and several studies have demonstrated that ROCKs are involved in contractile signaling in the trabecular meshwork.[116,117] In turn, the dynamic nature of the trabecular meshwork cells influences AH outflow and IOP, with decreased outflow associated with ROCK activation and contraction of trabecular meshwork cells.[111,118]

Administering ROCK inhibitors has resulted in the lowering of IOP in animal studies.[111,118] In human patients, ROCK inhibitors represent a promising emerging treatment option for glaucoma.[111] Several ROCK inhibitors have demonstrated encouraging initial results, with 3 ongoing phase II trials as of May 2015. Furthermore, ripasudil is a topical ROCK inhibitor already approved for clinical use in Japan.[119] As a topical, twice-daily medication, this ROCK inhibitor acts directly on the trabecular meshwork to reduce IOP by decreasing the stiffness and increasing the expansion of the juxtacanalicular connective tissue and the cells of the inner wall of Schlemm canal.[119,120]

Beyond their capacity to decrease outflow resistance through the conventional pathway, ROCK inhibitors may enhance retinal blood flow through their relaxing effects on vascular smooth muscle cells, which may in turn protect RGCs from degeneration associated with glaucoma.[121] Additionally, Rho kinase inhibitors have demonstrated the added benefit of potentially decreasing scarring after glaucoma filtering surgery through the inhibition of myofibroblast formation.[122] Because postoperative scarring can progressively impede the flow of AH across the bypass and lead to elevated IOP, inhibiting the postoperative scarring process would have a significant impact on the success of glaucoma surgery.

These compounds provide the greatest benefit in patients affected with POAG, and their limitation resides in their unknown efficacy when the ciliary cleft and the conventional outflow pathways are seriously compromised, as in primary angle-closure glaucoma, the most common form of glaucoma clinically seen in dogs.

Emerging Drug-Delivery Platforms

A vast majority of veterinary ophthalmic drugs are administered to the ocular surface, owing to its ease of access for caretakers. Topical instillation, however, is inefficient for several reasons, including rapid tear turnover and absorption through the conjunctiva.[123] Furthermore, a large amount of the medication drains through the nasolacrimal duct, leading to gastrointestinal tract absorption.[124] Because of the short residence time on the ocular surface, there is a resultant low corneal bioavailability (approximately 1%–5%), which in turn often necessitates frequent instillation.[125] In addition, compliance with respect to topical treatment in human patients affected with glaucoma can be as poor as 50%[126]; although compliance for veterinary patients is poorly studied, anecdotal evidence indicates it is often suboptimal. Common ophthalmic preservatives may also adversely affect the corneal surface, as well as potentially exacerbating glaucoma.[127]

The limitations and drawbacks to topical medications have spurred basic and clinical research into improved drug delivery strategies. Innovations to topical medications for enhancing bioavailability include modification of solution viscosity and/or corneal penetration by gels, polymers, liposomes, nanoparticles, and microemulsions, among many others.[127] Contact lenses provide many potential benefits as prospective drug delivery devices, notably a continuous and steady delivery of medication to the corneal surface. Consistent with their potential, a surge of recent publications has touted their utility and promise for treating glaucoma through the continuous, long-term release of desired compounds.[128,129] Other researchers have published encouraging reports of sustained control of IOP for a 4-week period with single sub-conjunctival injections of brimonidine-loaded microspheres.[130] Coated nanoparticles have also been used to deliver medications directly to the intraocular milieu, an approach analogous to the administration of vascular endothelial growth factor inhibitors for the treatment of age-related macular degeneration in humans.[131,132] Moreover, researchers in the burgeoning fields of gene and stem cell therapies are reporting encouraging results for ameliorating the effects of glaucoma, with these modalities likely yielding novel therapeutic options in the upcoming years.[133–135]

SUMMARY

Glaucoma is a painful and blinding group of diseases with no cure. Currently, treatment is aimed at chronically managing the condition, with an ultimate goal of a comfortable and preferably visual eye. Medical therapy remains the predominant method for managing glaucoma in veterinary patients. It may be used alone or in combination with surgical techniques to control IOP. The veterinary practitioner is faced with a large array of hypotensive agents, most of which have shown promise in managing most forms of canine glaucoma. There is no one drug, however, that has been shown to universally treat this condition. Therefore, a polypharmacy approach is typically required and practitioners must be well versed in several medical treatment options to treat the diverse presentations of this devastating disease.

REFERENCES

1. McCarty CA, Burmester JK, Mukesh BN, et al. Intraocular pressure response to topical beta-blockers associated with an ADRB2 single-nucleotide polymorphism. Arch Ophthalmol 2008;126(7):959–63.
2. Sakurai M, Higashide T, Ohkubo S, et al. Association between genetic polymorphisms of the prostaglandin F2alpha receptor gene, and response to latanoprost in patients with glaucoma and ocular hypertension. Br J Ophthalmol 2014;98(4):469–73.
3. Plummer CE, Regnier A, Gelatt KN. The canine glaucomas. In: Gelatt KN, Gilger BC, Kern T, editors. Veterinary Ophthalmology. 5th edition. Ames (IA): John Wiley and Sons, Inc; 2013. p. 1050–145.
4. Pizzirani S, Gong H. Functional anatomy of the outflow facilities. Vet Clin North Am Small Anim Pract 2015, in press.
5. Gum GG, Gelatt KN, Gelatt JK, et al. Effect of topically applied demecarium bromide and echothiophate iodide on intraocular pressure and pupil size in beagles with normotensive eyes and beagles with inherited glaucoma. Am J Vet Res 1993;54(2):287–93.
6. Chiou CY, Trzeciakowski J, Gelatt KN. Reduction of intraocular pressure in glaucomatous dogs by a new cholinergic drug. Invest Ophthalmol Vis Sci 1980; 19(10):1198–203.
7. Gwin RM, Gelatt KN, Gum GG, et al. The effect of topical pilocarpine on intraocular pressure and pupil size in the normotensive and glaucomatous beagle. Invest Ophthalmol Vis Sci 1977;16(12):1143–8.
8. Sarchahi AA, Abbasi N, Gholipour MA. Effects of an unfixed combination of latanoprost and pilocarpine on the intraocular pressure and pupil size of normal dogs. Vet Ophthalmol 2012;15(Suppl 1):64–70.
9. Freddo TF, Neville N, Gong H. Pilocarpine-induced flare is physiological rather than pathological. Exp Eye Res 2013;107:37–43.

10. Freddo TF, Patz S, Arshanskiy Y. Pilocarpine's effects on the blood-aqueous barrier of the human eye as assessed by high-resolution, contrast magnetic resonance imaging. Exp Eye Res 2006;82(3):458–64.
11. Crasta M, Clode AB, McMullen RJ Jr, et al. Effect of three treatment protocols on acute ocular hypertension after phacoemulsification and aspiration of cataracts in dogs. Vet Ophthalmol 2010;13(1):14–9.
12. Stuhr CM, Miller PE, Murphy CJ, et al. Effect of intracameral administration of carbachol on the postoperative increase in intraocular pressure in dogs undergoing cataract extraction. J Am Vet Med Assoc 1998;212(12):1885–8.
13. Miller PE, Schmidt GM, Vainisi SJ, et al. The efficacy of topical prophylactic antiglaucoma therapy in primary closed angle glaucoma in dogs: a multicenter clinical trial. J Am Anim Hosp Assoc 2000;36(5):431–8.
14. Dees DD, Fritz KJ, Maclaren NE, et al. Efficacy of prophylactic antiglaucoma and anti-inflammatory medications in canine primary angle-closure glaucoma: a multicenter retrospective study (2004-2012). Vet Ophthalmol 2014;17(3):195–200.
15. Binder DR, Herring IP, Gerhard T. Outcomes of nonsurgical management and efficacy of demecarium bromide treatment for primary lens instability in dogs: 34 cases (1990–2004). J Am Vet Med Assoc 2007;231(1):89–93.
16. Wang YL, Hayashi M, Yablonski ME, et al. Effects of multiple dosing of epinephrine on aqueous humor dynamics in human eyes. J Ocul Pharmacol Ther 2002; 18(1):53–63.
17. Townsend DJ, Brubaker RF. Immediate effect of epinephrine on aqueous formation in the normal human eye as measured by fluorophotometry. Invest Ophthalmol Vis Sci 1980;19(3):256–66.
18. Schneider TL, Brubaker RF. Effect of chronic epinephrine on aqueous humor flow during the day and during sleep in normal healthy subjects. Invest Ophthalmol Vis Sci 1991;32(9):2507–10.
19. Wang YL, Toris CB, Zhan G, et al. Effects of topical epinephrine on aqueous humor dynamics in the cat. Exp Eye Res 1999;68(4):439–45.
20. Gwin RM, Gelatt KN, Gum GG, et al. Effects of topical 1-epinephrine and dipivalyl epinephrine on intraocular pressure and pupil size in the normotensive and glaucomatous Beagle. Am J Vet Res 1978;39(1):83–6.
21. Arthur S, Cantor LB. Update on the role of alpha-agonists in glaucoma management. Exp Eye Res 2011;93(3):271–83.
22. Miller PE, Nelson MJ, Rhaesa SL. Effects of topical administration of 0.5% apraclonidine on intraocular pressure, pupil size, and heart rate in clinically normal dogs. Am J Vet Res 1996;57(1):79–82.
23. Miller PE, Rhaesa SL. Effects of topical administration of 0.5% apraclonidine on intraocular pressure, pupil size, and heart rate in clinically normal cats. Am J Vet Res 1996;57(1):83–6.
24. Gelatt KN, MacKay EO. Effect of single and multiple doses of 0.2% brimonidine tartrate in the glaucomatous Beagle. Vet Ophthalmol 2002;5(4):253–62.
25. Maehara S, Ono K, Ito N, et al. Effects of topical nipradilol and timolol maleate on intraocular pressure, facility of outflow, arterial blood pressure and pulse rate in dogs. Vet Ophthalmol 2004;7(3):147–50.
26. Frishman WH, Fuksbrumer MS, Tannenbaum M. Topical ophthalmic beta-adrenergic blockade for the treatment of glaucoma and ocular hypertension. J Clin Pharmacol 1994;34(8):795–803.
27. Gelatt KN, Larocca RD, Gelatt JK, et al. Evaluation of multiple doses of 4 and 6% timolol, and timolol combined with 2% pilocarpine in clinically normal beagles and beagles with glaucoma. Am J Vet Res 1995;56(10):1325–31.

28. Gum G, Larocca RD, Gelatt KN, et al. The effect of topical timolol maleate on intraocular pressure in normal beagles and beagles with inherited glaucoma. Progress in Veterinary and Comparative Ophthalmology 1991;1:141–50.

29. Plummer CE, MacKay EO, Gelatt KN. Comparison of the effects of topical administration of a fixed combination of dorzolamide-timolol to monotherapy with timolol or dorzolamide on IOP, pupil size, and heart rate in glaucomatous dogs. Vet Ophthalmol 2006;9(4):245–9.

30. Peng CC, Ben-Shlomo A, Mackay EO, et al. Drug delivery by contact lens in spontaneously glaucomatous dogs. Curr Eye Res 2012;37(3):204–11.

31. Smith LN, Miller PE, Felchle LM. Effects of topical administration of latanoprost, timolol, or a combination of latanoprost and timolol on intraocular pressure, pupil size, and heart rate in clinically normal dogs. Am J Vet Res 2010;71(9): 1055–61.

32. Takiyama N, Shoji S, Habata I, et al. The effects of a timolol maleate gel-forming solution on normotensive beagle dogs. J Vet Med Sci 2006;68(6):631–3.

33. Wilkie DA, Latimer CA. Effects of topical administration of timolol maleate on intraocular pressure and pupil size in dogs. Am J Vet Res 1991;52(3):432–5.

34. Svec AL, Strosberg AM. Therapeutic and systemic side effects of ocular beta-adrenergic antagonists in anesthetized dogs. Invest Ophthalmol Vis Sci 1986; 27(3):401–5.

35. Zimmerman TJ, Boger WP 3rd. The beta-adrenergic blocking agents and the treatment of glaucoma. Surv Ophthalmol 1979;23(6):347–62.

36. Wilkie DA, Latimer CA. Effects of topical administration of timolol maleate on intraocular pressure and pupil size in cats. Am J Vet Res 1991;52(3):436–40.

37. Volotinen M, Hakkola J, Pelkonen O, et al. Metabolism of ophthalmic timolol: new aspects of an old drug. Basic Clin Pharmacol Toxicol 2011;108(5):297–303.

38. Willis AM, Diehl KA, Robbin TE. Advances in topical glaucoma therapy. Vet Ophthalmol 2002;5(1):9–17.

39. Zimmerman TJ. Topical ophthalmic beta blockers: a comparative review. J Ocul Pharmacol Ther 1993;9(4):373–84.

40. Pugliese M, Scardillo A, Niutta PP, et al. Comparison of effects of topical levobunolol to a combination of timolol-dorzolamide on intraocular pressure and pulse rate of healthy dogs. Vet Res Commun 2009;33(Suppl 1):205–7.

41. Scardillo A, Pugliese M, De Majo M, et al. Effects of topical 0.5% levobunolol alone or in association with 2% dorzolamide compared with a fixed combination of 0.5% timolol and 2% dorzolamide on intraocular pressure and heart rate in dogs without glaucoma. Vet Ther 2010;11(3):E1–6.

42. Jampel HD, Chen X, Chue C, et al. Expression of carbonic anhydrase isozyme III in the ciliary processes and lens. Invest Ophthalmol Vis Sci 1997;38(2): 539–43.

43. Sugrue MF. Pharmacological and ocular hypotensive properties of topical carbonic anhydrase inhibitors. Prog Retin Eye Res 2000;19(1):87–112.

44. Gelatt KN, MacKay EO. Changes in intraocular pressure associated with topical dorzolamide and oral methazolamide in glaucomatous dogs. Vet Ophthalmol 2001;4(1):61–7.

45. Skorobohach BJ, Ward DA, Hendrix DV. Effects of oral administration of methazolamide on intraocular pressure and aqueous humor flow rate in clinically normal dogs. Am J Vet Res 2003;64(2):183–7.

46. Maren TH, Conroy CW, Wynns GC, et al. Ocular absorption, blood levels, and excretion of dorzolamide, a topically active carbonic anhydrase inhibitor. J Ocul Pharmacol Ther 1997;13(1):23–30.

47. Cawrse MA, Ward DA, Hendrix DV. Effects of topical application of a 2% solution of dorzolamide on intraocular pressure and aqueous humor flow rate in clinically normal dogs. Am J Vet Res 2001;62(6):859–63.

48. Whelan NC, Welch P, Pace A, et al. A comparison of the efficacy of topical brinzolamide and dorzolamide alone and in combination with oral methazolamide in decreasing normal canine intraocular pressure. 30th Annual Meeting of the Americal College of Veterinary Ophthalmologists. Chicago (IL), October 1999.

49. Willis AM. Ocular hypotensive drugs. Vet Clin North Am Small Anim Pract 2004; 34(3):755–76.

50. Sambhara D, Aref AA. Glaucoma management: relative value and place in therapy of available drug treatments. Ther Adv Chronic Dis 2014;5(1):30–43.

51. Richter M, Krauss AH, Woodward DF, et al. Morphological changes in the anterior eye segment after long-term treatment with different receptor selective prostaglandin agonists and a prostamide. Invest Ophthalmol Vis Sci 2003;44(10): 4419–26.

52. Toris CB, Gabelt BT, Kaufman PL. Update on the mechanism of action of topical prostaglandins for intraocular pressure reduction. Surv Ophthalmol 2008; 53(Suppl1):S107–20.

53. Gaton DD, Sagara T, Lindsey JD, et al. Increased matrix metalloproteinases 1, 2, and 3 in the monkey uveoscleral outflow pathway after topical prostaglandin F(2 alpha)-isopropyl ester treatment. Arch Ophthalmol 2001;119(8):1165–70.

54. Ooi YH, Oh DJ, Rhee DJ. Effect of bimatoprost, latanoprost, and unoprostone on matrix metalloproteinases and their inhibitors in human ciliary body smooth muscle cells. Invest Ophthalmol Vis Sci 2009;50(11):5259–65.

55. Aihara M, Lindsey JD, Weinreb RN. Enhanced FGF-2 movement through human sclera after exposure to latanoprost. Invest Ophthalmol Vis Sci 2001;42(11): 2554–9.

56. Pirie CG, Maranda LS, Pizzirani S. Effect of topical 0.03% flurbiprofen and 0.005% latanoprost, alone and in combination, on normal canine eyes. Vet Ophthalmol 2011;14(2):71–9.

57. Chiba T, Kashiwagi K, Chiba N, et al. Effect of non-steroidal anti-inflammatory ophthalmic solution on intraocular pressure reduction by latanoprost in patients with primary open angle glaucoma or ocular hypertension. Br J Ophthalmol 2006;90(3):314–7.

58. Studer ME, Martin CL, Stiles J. Effects of 0.005% latanoprost solution on intraocular pressure in healthy dogs and cats. Am J Vet Res 2000;61(10): 1220–4.

59. Gelatt KN, MacKay EO. Effect of different dose schedules of latanoprost on intraocular pressure and pupil size in the glaucomatous Beagle. Vet Ophthalmol 2001;4(4):283–8.

60. Carvalho AB, Laus JL, Costa VP, et al. Effects of travoprost 0.004% compared with latanoprost 0.005% on the intraocular pressure of normal dogs. Vet Ophthalmol 2006;9(2):121–5.

61. Gelatt KN, Mackay EO. Effect of different dose schedules of bimatoprost on intraocular pressure and pupil size in the glaucomatous Beagle. J Ocul Pharmacol Ther 2002;18(6):525–34.

62. Gelatt KN, MacKay EO. Effect of different dose schedules of travoprost on intraocular pressure and pupil size in the glaucomatous Beagle. Vet Ophthalmol 2004;7(1):53–7.

63. Mackay EO, McLaughlin M, Plummer CE, et al. Dose response for travoprost(R) in the glaucomatous beagle. Vet Ophthalmol 2012;15(Suppl 1):31–5.

64. Montgomery KW, Labelle AL, Gemensky-Metzler AJ. Trans-corneal reduction of anterior lens luxation in dogs with lens instability: a retrospective study of 19 dogs (2010-2013). Vet Ophthalmol 2014;17(4):275–9.

65. Johnstone McLean NS, Ward DA, Hendrix DV. The effect of a single dose of topical 0.005% latanoprost and 2% dorzolamide/0.5% timolol combination on the blood-aqueous barrier in dogs: a pilot study. Vet Ophthalmol 2008;11(3): 158–61.

66. Goldberg I, Li XY, Selaru P, et al. A 5-year, randomized, open-label safety study of latanoprost and usual care in patients with open-angle glaucoma or ocular hypertension. Eur J Ophthalmol 2008;18(3):408–16.

67. Markomichelakis NN, Kostakou A, Halkiadakis I, et al. Efficacy and safety of latanoprost in eyes with uveitic glaucoma. Graefes Arch Clin Exp Ophthalmol 2009;247(6):775–80.

68. Volopich S, Mosing M, Auer U, et al. Comparison of the effect of hypertonic hydroxyethyl starch and mannitol on the intraocular pressure in healthy normotensive dogs and the effect of hypertonic hydroxyethyl starch on the intraocular pressure in dogs with primary glaucoma. Vet Ophthalmol 2006;9(4):239–44.

69. Lorimer DW, Hakanson NE, Pion PD, et al. The effect of intravenous mannitol or oral glycerol on intraocular pressure in dogs. Cornell Vet 1989;79(3):249–58.

70. Wasserman NT, Kennard G, Cochrane ZN, et al. Effects of oral isosorbide and glycerol on intraocular pressure, serum osmolality, and blood glucose in normal dogs. Vet Ophthalmol 2013;16(1):20–4.

71. Pizzirani S, Carroll V, Pirie CG, et al. Pathological factors involved with the late onset of canine glaucoma associated with goniodysgenesis: preliminary study. Presented at the 39th Annual Meeting of the American College of Veterinary Ophthalmologists. Boston (MA), October 2008.

72. Reilly CM, Morris R, Dubielzig RR. Canine goniodysgenesis-related glaucoma: a morphologic review of 100 cases looking at inflammation and pigment dispersion. Vet Ophthalmol 2005;8(4):253–8.

73. Pizzirani S. Definition, classification, and pathophysiology of canine glaucoma. Vet Clin North Am Small Anim Pract 2015, in press.

74. Vasudevan SK, Gupta V, Crowston JG. Neuroprotection in glaucoma. Indian J Ophthalmol 2011;59(Suppl):S102–13.

75. Agarwal R, Agarwal P. Newer targets for modulation of intraocular pressure: focus on adenosine receptor signaling pathways. Expert Opin Ther Targets 2014;18(5):527–39.

76. Lee AJ, Goldberg I. Emerging drugs for ocular hypertension. Expert Opin Emerg Drugs 2011;16(1):137–61.

77. Shoshani YZ, Harris A, Shoja MM, et al. Endothelin and its suspected role in the pathogenesis and possible treatment of glaucoma. Curr Eye Res 2012;37(1): 1–11.

78. Palmer RM, Ferrige AG, Moncada S. Nitric oxide release accounts for the biological activity of endothelium-derived relaxing factor. Nature 1987;327(6122): 524–6.

79. Wu L, Wang R. Carbon monoxide: endogenous production, physiological functions, and pharmacological applications. Pharmacol Rev 2005;57(4):585–630.

80. Farrugia G, Szurszewski JH. Carbon monoxide, hydrogen sulfide, and nitric oxide as signaling molecules in the gastrointestinal tract. Gastroenterology 2014; 147(2):303–13.

81. Bucolo C, Drago F. Carbon monoxide and the eye: Implications for glaucoma therapy. Pharmacol Ther 2011;130(2):191–201.

82. Cavet ME, Vittitow JL, Impagnatiello F, et al. Nitric oxide (NO): an emerging target for the treatment of glaucoma. Invest Ophthalmol Vis Sci 2014;55(8): 5005–15.

83. Zhao J, Tan S, Liu F, et al. Heme oxygenase and ocular disease: a review of the literature. Curr Eye Res 2012;37(11):955–60.

84. Thomas DD, Liu X, Kantrow SP, et al. The biological lifetime of nitric oxide: implications for the perivascular dynamics of NO and O2. Proc Natl Acad Sci U S A 2001;98(1):355–60.

85. Murad F. Nitric oxide signaling: would you believe that a simple free radical could be a second messenger, autacoid, paracrine substance, neurotransmitter, and hormone? Recent Prog Horm Res 1998;53:43–59 [discussion: 59–60].

86. Becquet F, Courtois Y, Goureau O. Nitric oxide in the eye: multifaceted roles and diverse outcomes. Surv Ophthalmol 1997;42(1):71–82.

87. Borghi V, Bastia E, Guzzetta M, et al. A novel nitric oxide releasing prostaglandin analog, NCX 125, reduces intraocular pressure in rabbit, dog, and primate models of glaucoma. J Ocul Pharmacol Ther 2010;26(2):125–32.

88. Impagnatiello F, Borghi V, Gale DC, et al. A dual acting compound with latanoprost amide and nitric oxide releasing properties, shows ocular hypotensive effects in rabbits and dogs. Exp Eye Res 2011;93(3):243–9.

89. Ellis DZ. Guanylate cyclase activators, cell volume changes and IOP reduction. Cell Physiol Biochem 2011;28(6):1145–54.

90. Behar-Cohen FF, Goureau O, D'Hermies F, et al. Decreased intraocular pressure induced by nitric oxide donors is correlated to nitrite production in the rabbit eye. Invest Ophthalmol Vis Sci 1996;37(8):1711–5.

91. Schuman JS, Erickson K, Nathanson JA. Nitrovasodilator effects on intraocular pressure and outflow facility in monkeys. Exp Eye Res 1994;58(1):99–105.

92. Stamer WD, Lei Y, Boussommier-Calleja A, et al. eNOS, a pressure-dependent regulator of intraocular pressure. Invest Ophthalmol Vis Sci 2011;52(13): 9438–44.

93. Nathanson JA. Nitrovasodilators as a new class of ocular hypotensive agents. J Pharmacol Exp Ther 1992;260(3):956–65.

94. Kotikoski H, Alajuuma P, Moilanen E, et al. Comparison of nitric oxide donors in lowering intraocular pressure in rabbits: role of cyclic GMP. J Ocul Pharmacol Ther 2002;18(1):11–23.

95. Koriyama Y, Kamiya M, Arai K, et al. Nipradilol promotes axon regeneration through S-nitrosylation of PTEN in retinal ganglion cells. Adv Exp Med Biol 2014;801:751–7.

96. Delaey C, Van de Voorde J. The effect of NO donors on bovine retinal small arteries and posterior ciliary arteries. Invest Ophthalmol Vis Sci 1998;39(9):1642–6.

97. Okamura T, Kitamura Y, Uchiyama M, et al. Canine retinal arterial and arteriolar dilatation induced by nipradilol, a possible glaucoma therapeutic. Pharmacology 1996;53(5):302–10.

98. Millar JC, Shahidullah M, Wilson WS. Intraocular pressure and vascular effects of sodium azide in bovine perfused eye. J Ocul Pharmacol Ther 2001;17(3): 225–34.

99. Shahidullah M, Yap M, To CH. Cyclic GMP, sodium nitroprusside and sodium azide reduce aqueous humour formation in the isolated arterially perfused pig eye. Br J Pharmacol 2005;145(1):84–92.

100. Funk RH, Gehr J, Rohen JW. Short-term hemodynamic changes in episcleral arteriovenous anastomoses correlate with venous pressure and IOP changes in the albino rabbit. Curr Eye Res 1996;15(1):87–93.

101. Karim MZ, Sawada A, Mizuno K, et al. Neuroprotective effect of nipradilol [3,4-dihydro-8-(2-hydroxy-3-isopropylamino)-propoxy-3-nitroxy-2H-1-benzopyran] in a rat model of optic nerve degeneration. J Glaucoma 2009;18(1):26–31.

102. Mizuno K, Koide T, Yoshimura M, et al. Neuroprotective effect and intraocular penetration of nipradilol, a beta-blocker with nitric oxide donative action. Invest Ophthalmol Vis Sci 2001;42(3):688–94.

103. Watanabe M, Tokita Y, Yata T. Axonal regeneration of cat retinal ganglion cells is promoted by nipradilol, an anti-glaucoma drug. Neuroscience 2006;140(2):517–28.

104. Nathanson JA, McKee M. Identification of an extensive system of nitric oxide-producing cells in the ciliary muscle and outflow pathway of the human eye. Invest Ophthalmol Vis Sci 1995;36(9):1765–73.

105. Boissel JP, Schwarz PM, Forstermann U. Neuronal-type NO synthase: transcript diversity and expressional regulation. Nitric Oxide 1998;2(5):337–49.

106. Selbach JM, Gottanka J, Wittmann M, et al. Efferent and afferent innervation of primate trabecular meshwork and scleral spur. Invest Ophthalmol Vis Sci 2000;41(8):2184–91.

107. Riento K, Ridley AJ. Rocks: multifunctional kinases in cell behaviour. Nat Rev Mol Cell Biol 2003;4(6):446–56.

108. Schofield AV, Bernard O. Rho-associated coiled-coil kinase (ROCK) signaling and disease. Crit Rev Biochem Mol Biol 2013;48(4):301–16.

109. Huveneers S, Daemen MJ, Hordijk PL. Between Rho(k) and a hard place: the relation between vessel wall stiffness, endothelial contractility, and cardiovascular disease. Circ Res 2015;116(5):895–908.

110. Rath N, Olson MF. Rho-associated kinases in tumorigenesis: re-considering ROCK inhibition for cancer therapy. EMBO Rep 2012;13(10):900–8.

111. Inoue T, Tanihara H. Rho-associated kinase inhibitors: a novel glaucoma therapy. Prog Retin Eye Res 2013;37:1–12.

112. Isobe T, Mizuno K, Kaneko Y, et al. Effects of K-115, a rho-kinase inhibitor, on aqueous humor dynamics in rabbits. Curr Eye Res 2014;39(8):813–22.

113. Koizumi N, Okumura N, Ueno M, et al. New therapeutic modality for corneal endothelial disease using Rho-associated kinase inhibitor eye drops. Cornea 2014;33(Suppl 11):S25–31.

114. Van de Velde S, Van Bergen T, Sijnave D, et al. AMA0076, a novel, locally acting Rho kinase inhibitor, potently lowers intraocular pressure in New Zealand white rabbits with minimal hyperemia. Invest Ophthalmol Vis Sci 2014;55(2):1006–16.

115. Stankova V, Tsikolia N, Viebahn C. Rho kinase activity controls directional cell movements during primitive streak formation in the rabbit embryo. Development 2015;142(1):92–8.

116. Rao PV, Deng PF, Kumar J, et al. Modulation of aqueous humor outflow facility by the Rho kinase-specific inhibitor Y-27632. Invest Ophthalmol Vis Sci 2001;42(5):1029–37.

117. Ko MK, Tan JC. Contractile markers distinguish structures of the mouse aqueous drainage tract. Mol Vis 2013;19:2561–70.

118. Gong H, Yang CY. Morphological and hydrodynamic correlations with increasing outflow facility by rho-kinase inhibitor Y-27632. J Ocul Pharmacol Ther 2014;30(2–3):143–53.

119. Garnock-Jones KP. Ripasudil: first global approval. Drugs 2014;74(18):2211–5.

120. Yang CY, Liu Y, Lu Z, et al. Effects of Y27632 on aqueous humor outflow facility with changes in hydrodynamic pattern and morphology in human eyes. Invest Ophthalmol Vis Sci 2013;54(8):5859–70.

121. Sugiyama T, Shibata M, Kajiura S, et al. Effects of fasudil, a Rho-associated protein kinase inhibitor, on optic nerve head blood flow in rabbits. Invest Ophthalmol Vis Sci 2011;52(1):64–9.
122. Honjo M, Tanihara H, Kameda T, et al. Potential role of Rho-associated protein kinase inhibitor Y-27632 in glaucoma filtration surgery. Invest Ophthalmol Vis Sci 2007;48(12):5549–57.
123. Velpandian T. Intraocular penetration of antimicrobial agents in ophthalmic infections and drug delivery strategies. Expert Opin Drug Deliv 2009;6(3):255–70.
124. Kompella UB, Kadam RS, Lee VH. Recent advances in ophthalmic drug delivery. Ther Deliv 2010;1(3):435–56.
125. Kearns VR, Williams RL. Drug delivery systems for the eye. Expert Rev Med Devices 2009;6(3):277–90.
126. Rotchford AP, Murphy KM. Compliance with timolol treatment in glaucoma. Eye 1998;12(Pt 2):234–6.
127. Rasmussen CA, Kaufman PL. Exciting directions in glaucoma. Canadian journal of ophthalmology. Can J Ophthalmol 2014;49(6):534–43.
128. Carvalho IM, Marques CS, Oliveira RS, et al. Sustained drug release by contact lenses for glaucoma treatment-a review. J Control Release 2015;202:76–82.
129. Peng CC, Burke MT, Carbia BE, et al. Extended drug delivery by contact lenses for glaucoma therapy. J Control Release 2012;162(1):152–8.
130. Fedorchak MV, Conner IP, Medina CA, et al. 28-day intraocular pressure reduction with a single dose of brimonidine tartrate-loaded microspheres. Exp Eye Res 2014;125:210–6.
131. Kim NJ, Harris A, Gerber A, et al. Nanotechnology and glaucoma: a review of the potential implications of glaucoma nanomedicine. Br J Ophthalmol 2014;98(4):427–31.
132. Lambert WS, Carlson BJ, van der Ende AE, et al. Nanosponge-mediated drug delivery lowers intraocular pressure. Transl Vis Sci Technol 2015;4(1):1.
133. Ding QJ, Zhu W, Cook AC, et al. Induction of trabecular meshwork cells from induced pluripotent stem cells. Invest Ophthalmol Vis Sci 2014;55(11):7065–72.
134. Flachsbarth K, Kruszewski K, Jung G, et al. Neural stem cell-based intraocular administration of ciliary neurotrophic factor attenuates the loss of axotomized ganglion cells in adult mice. Invest Ophthalmol Vis Sci 2014;55(11):7029–39.
135. Solinis MA, Del Pozo-Rodriguez A, Apaolaza PS, et al. Treatment of ocular disorders by gene therapy. Eur J Pharm Biopharm 2014. [Epub ahead of print].

Surgical Treatment of Canine Glaucoma

Filtering and End-Stage Glaucoma Procedures

Federica Maggio, DVM[a],*, Dineli Bras, DVM, MS[b]

KEYWORDS

- Canine • Dog • Glaucoma • Gonioimplants • Glaucoma drainage devices
- Enucleation • Evisceration • Chemical ablation of ciliary bodies

KEY POINTS

- Surgical strategies for glaucoma are aimed at controlling intraocular pressure through procedures that either decrease aqueous humor production, increase its outflow, or through a combination of both.
- Gonioimplants or glaucoma drainage devices are used alone or in combination with cyclodestructive procedures to decrease intraocular pressure by diverting aqueous humor from the anterior chamber to the subconjunctival or frontal sinus spaces.
- Medical treatment, by means of topical anti-inflammatory and glaucoma medications, is still required long-term in the postoperative management of filtering procedures.
- Bleb fibrosis, caused by severe inflammatory response in the subconjunctival tissues, represents a common complication of filtration surgery in dogs, eventually leading to implant failure.
- Modulation of wound healing is the key to a successful management of postoperative filtering devices, through proper surgery timing and control of inflammation.

INTRODUCTION

Glaucoma is a group of diseases that commonly leads to vision loss in cats and dogs. Although the definition of the disease has evolved over the years to indicate a neurodegenerative disorder of retinal ganglion cells and their axons, an increase in intraocular pressure (IOP) represents a constant risk factor in dogs and the only available therapeutic target. The goal of glaucoma therapy is to prevent further optic nerve damage and preserve vision. Because of the rapidly progressive course of canine primary

The authors have nothing to disclose.
[a] Ophthalmology Department, Tufts Veterinary Emergency Treatment and Specialties (Tufts VETS), 525 South Street, Walpole, MA 02081, USA; [b] Ophthalmology Department, Veterinary Specialists Center of Puerto Rico, Km 0.1 Carr. 873, San Juan, PR 00969, USA
* Corresponding author.
E-mail address: Federica.Maggio@tufts.edu

glaucoma, early surgical intervention has been suggested to improve the surgical outcome.[1]

Surgical treatment of glaucoma is aimed at decreasing IOP in the affected eyes. This is attained through techniques that modulate the inflow/outflow of aqueous humor (AH), by decreasing its production and/or increasing its drainage (**Fig. 1**). Several different criteria affect the choice for the proper surgical treatment, with vision preservation or its potential recovery being decisive.

Cyclodestructive procedures (addressed elsewhere in this issue) and filtering techniques are used to control IOP in visual patients. The use of gonioimplants allows AH to be diverted from the anterior chamber to different venues, such as the subconjunctival, frontal sinus, or suprachoroidal and intrascleral spaces.

For blind glaucomatous globes, the main goal shifts toward pain and corneal complications management and quality of life for the patient. The primary aim of end-stage procedures is to control or prevent ocular discomfort (**Fig. 2**). Globe removal is obviously recommended when glaucoma is secondary to intraocular tumors, or to chronic inflammatory and traumatic conditions associated with blindness.

This article focuses on the description of the available filtering procedures in visual eyes, and of the salvage procedures in nonvisual patients.

FILTERING PROCEDURES

Several surgical filtering procedures have been described in glaucomatous dogs including iridencleisis, cyclodialysis, corneoscleral trephination, and posterior sclerectomy.[2] They are unfortunately met with uniform failure and are only mentioned for historical purposes. The current technique in filtering procedures for canine glaucomas involves the use of anterior chamber shunts or glaucoma drainage devices (GDDs).

Trabeculectomy has long been considered the gold standard of filtering glaucoma surgery in people.[3] However, in recent years, studies aimed at comparing the long-term outcomes of trabeculectomy and GDDs implantation have drawn comparable results between procedures,[4,5] with the increased advantage of a more consistent aqueous outflow and decreased complications from hypotony in GDDs techniques.[3] Recent surveys have shown a significant increase in the use of GDDs over trabeculectomy in human patients with prior ocular surgery or with neovascular or uveitic glaucoma.[6]

Various different devices have been studied in canine patients over the years, from the Krupin-Denver model to the Joseph, Baerveldt, T-shaped nonvalved, and Ahmed

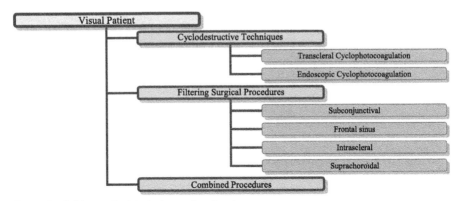

Fig. 1. Available surgical techniques for visual eyes.

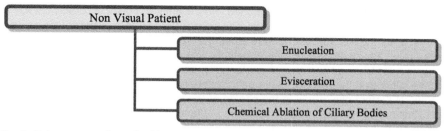

Fig. 2. Salvage procedures for blind eyes.

implants (**Fig. 3**).[7–15] The subconjunctival space is the most common site for AH diversion, but experimental studies have investigated other possible outlets, such as the jugular vein via the facial vein, the subcutaneous space, and the parotid duct, with limited to no success.[16,17] The Cullen shunt to the frontal sinus has also been described.[18,19]

GENERAL CONSIDERATIONS IN CURRENT GONIOIMPLANT DESIGN

The earliest benchmark glaucoma device, envisioning a tube and plate design, was created and subsequent modified by Molteno in the early 1970s. Since then, several other models and modifications have been available on the market; however, the predominant general design is similar across devices and generally consists of a silicone tube connected to a plate, also made of silicone, polypropylene or, lately,

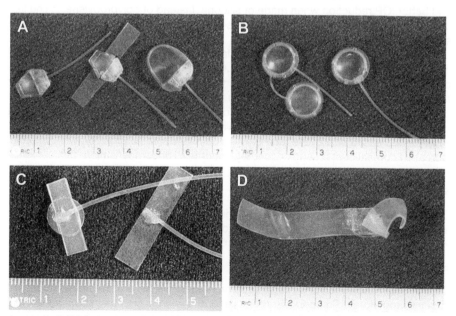

Fig. 3. Commercial and self-constructed anterior shunts. (*A*) Ahmed (small, large, and attached to a 10 × 30 mm silicone band). (*B*) Molteno (single and double plate). (*C*) Self-constructed T shunt (with and without a valve). (*D*) Joseph. (*From* Gelatt KN, Gelatt JP. Surgical procedures for the glaucomas. In: Gelatt KN, Gelatt JP, editors. Veterinary ophthalmic surgery. Saunders Ltd; 2011. p. 284; with permission.)

polyethylene. The tubular portion, inserted into the anterior chamber, drains the AH to the platform, located subconjunctivally. The AH is thus diverted from the anterior chamber into a filtering bleb that surrounds the plate, and from there it is absorbed by the local vasculature. Less common models substitute the plate for an encircling silicone band, such as in the Shocket and Joseph implants. These implants have been investigated in canine patients in the past, but have been progressively abandoned.[8]

Several factors play a role in the choice of the gonioimplant. Both valved (Ahmed and Krupin) and nonvalved (Baerveldt and Molteno) devices are commonly available (**Table 1**). The presence of a valve provides a unidirectional flow, preventing postsurgical hypotony, secondary uveitis, and potential retinal detachment. The valve usually "vents" in response to IOPs higher than 8 to 12 mm Hg, but bleb fibrosis can elicit failure. The main advantage of nonvalved devices is long-term IOP control caused by less severe capsular fibrosis.[20] In nonvalved devices, a back pressure eventually develops secondary to the development of a mature filtration bleb, but IOP inconsistency with hypotension or hypertension is often experienced in the early postoperative period.

Size and material of the implant may also affect the surgical outcome. Although it is well established that the size of the plate and subsequently of the bleb is directly correlated to the degree of IOP reduction,[21] there seems to be an upper limit to plate size beyond which there is no appreciable improvement of pressure control.[22,23] According to Laplace's law, the larger the radius of the bleb (determined by the size of the implant), the more tension is exerted on the capsule surface, with increased stimulation of collagen deposition and fibrosis.[24] The optimal plate size for dogs has not been determined; however, the plate size of the most common currently available devices ranges from 96 to 184.00 mm^2.

Ahmed implants in human patients seem to show a decreased rate of complications and better IOP reduction when made of silicone, instead of polypropylene.[25] The last generation of Ahmed implants currently used in dogs is also composed of silicone and seems to be well tolerated.

In most commercially available gonioimplants the silicone tubing has an inside diameter of 0.3 mm and an outside diameter of 0.6 mm. Such diameter allows an AH outflow of 3 to 6 μL/min, which accounts for the normal AH outflow in dogs and cats.[26] Larger tubings, such as the one used in the Cullen valved frontal sinus shunt (0.64 mm inside diameter and 12 mm outside diameter) could potentially decrease the incidence of tube occlusion by fibrin and inflammatory cells, which is a known complication in dogs. However, the increased size of the tube may be detrimental to its pliability, with potential increased corneal contact and secondary endothelial decompensation.[18,19]

SUBCONJUNCTIVAL IMPLANTS

Currently, the most commonly used GDDs in filtering canine glaucoma surgery are the silicone Ahmed valves VFP7 and VFP8, and polypropylene Ahmed valves S2 and S3, with a surface area of 184 mm^2 and 96 mm^2, respectively (**Fig. 4**).

Preparation

Careful patient selection and preparation are imperative for a successful outcome of implant procedures. Preoperative topical and/or systemic steroidal and nonsteroidal medications and topical antibiotics are administered 2 to 7 days before surgery. IOP must be lowered to near-normal values, ideally between 10 and 20 mm Hg. AH paracentesis may be required preoperatively (**Fig. 5**). Use of osmotic agents, such as intravenous mannitol, may also be recommended to reduce the volume of the vitreous body.

Table 1
Available anterior chamber shunts in small animals

Implant[a]	AC Tubing	Scleral Explant
Nonvalved		
Baerveldt	Silicone ID 0.3 mm OD 0.6 mm No valve	Oval-to-half-circle base, radiopaque Three sizes: 400, 700, and 1000 mm^2
Molteno et al	Silicone ID 0.3 mm OD 0.63 mm No valve	Polypropylene base single/double plates: 320 mm^2 single plate 640 mm^2 double plate
Schocket et al	Silastic ID 0.3 mm OD 0.64 mm No valve	No. 20 silicone band; 360° Variable, 900 mm^2
T-implant	Silicone ID 0.3 mm OD 0.6 mm No valve	Silicone, 7 × 30 mm 420 mm^2
White	Silicone ID 0.3 mm OD 0.64 mm Unidirectional No valve	Silicone compressible reservoir and base with tubing (1.04 mm ID and 1.42 mm OD)
Valved		
Ahmed Modified by Gelatt	Silicone ID 0.3 mm OD 0.6 mm Valve opens at 8–10 mm Hg	Five-sided polypropylene body Three different sizes Silicone strap (12 × 30 mm) added
Hitchings	Silicone ID 0.3 mm OD 0.64 mm Valve, slit (side): opens at 4–20 mm Hg	1 × 9 mm silicone strap 180°–360°
Joseph	Silicone ID 0.3 mm OD 0.64 mm Valve, slit (side): opens at 4–20 mm Hg	Silicone strap 1 × 9 mm 8.5 cm long <1600 mm^2 Bedford, used as nonvalve in dogs
Krupin et al	Silastic ID 0.3 mm OD 0.64 mm Valve, slit opens at 11 mm Hg; closes at 9 mm Hg	Later No. 220 episcleral explant, 180°–360° in length

Abbreviations: AC, anterior chamber; ID, inner diameter; OD, outer diameter.
[a] Implant dimensions are calculated for the entire surface areas of each implant.
From Gelatt KN, Gelatt JP. Surgical procedures for the glaucomas. In: Gelatt KN, Gelatt JP, editors. Veterinary ophthalmic surgery. Saunders Ltd; 2011. p. 285; with permission.

Technique

- The patient is placed in dorsal recumbency and the surgical area is routinely aseptically prepared. Neuromuscular block by atracurium or cisatracurium, in addition to stay sutures placed at the limbus, aids in optimal globe rotation

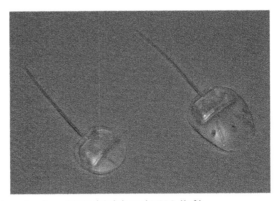

Fig. 4. Silicone Ahmed valves, VFP7 (*right*) and VFP8 (*left*).

and exposure. The stay sutures must avoid the intended surgical site. The superotemporal quadrant is the most common location for placement because of ease of exposure (**Fig. 6**A), followed by the superonasal, inferotemporal and inferonasal quadrants. In case of failure of the implant, it is recommended to avoid placing a second implant in the same location: additional implants, if needed, follow the previously reported sequence.

- A linear conjunctival incision, 8 to 10 mm wide, is performed 10 to 12 mm from the limbus using blunt and sharp dissection with tenotomy scissors (see **Fig. 6**B). Wet-field cautery is used to minimize hemorrhage. The dissection is extended caudally in the sub-Tenon space to create a pocket to accommodate the implant plate.
- Antimitotic agents can be used to reduce conjunctival capsule fibrosis. One or two sterile surgical cellulose sponges are inserted in the pocket and soaked with mitomycin-C (MMC; 0.3 mL of 0.25–0.5 mg/mL) or 5-fluorouracil (5-FU; 0.1–0.2 mL of 50 mg/mL). Care is taken to avoid contact with the conjunctival wound edges and surrounding tissues. After 5 minutes, the sponges are removed and the site is irrigated with 30 mL of balanced saline solution.

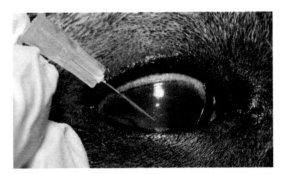

Fig. 5. Aqueous humor paracentesis in a dog with chronic glaucoma. The needle is inserted at the limbus and progressed into the anterior chamber, avoiding any contact with the intraocular tissues. According to the severity of IOP increase, the needle is withdrawn as soon as the fluid fills the hub, or one drop is allowed to fall. A Haab stria is visible along the dorsomedial corneal quadrant.

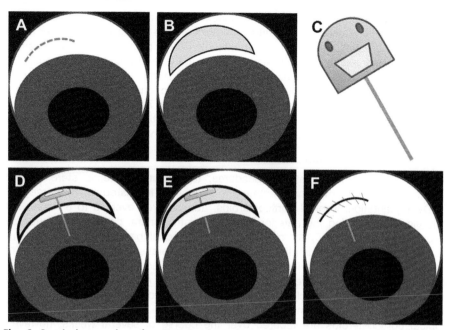

Fig. 6. Surgical procedure for GDD implantation. (*A*) The superotemporal quadrant is exposed and the globe is stabilized by stay sutures or mosquitoes. (*B*) A linear deep fornix-based incision, 8–10 mm in length, is performed on the conjunctiva with Westcott scissors, using a combination of sharp and blunt dissection. (*C*) A drawing of the implant is represented here; the implant is primed by injecting balanced saline solution into the tubular portion with a 25 to 27G cannula. (*D*) The implant is inserted into the surgical pocket. The rostral margin of the plate is positioned about 10–12 mm from the limbus and secured by two half-thickness scleral 8-0 nylon sutures. (*E*) The implant tube is trimmed with a wide upward-facing bevel. After creation of a scleral track by a 22G needle at the limbus, the tube is inserted in the anterior chamber. (*F*) The conjunctiva and Tenon capsule are closed with 8-0 absorbable suture in a simple continuous pattern.

- To ensure effective device function, the implant (see **Fig. 6**C) is primed by inject-ing balanced saline solution into the tubular portion with a 25 to 27G cannula, forcing it through the valve and out of the plate.
- The implant is gently grasped and inserted into the surgical pocket. The rostral margin of the plate is positioned about 10 to 12 mm from the limbus and secured by two half-thickness scleral 8-0 nylon sutures (see **Fig. 6**D). Care must be taken to avoid deep scleral penetration of the suture needle and subsequent scleral hemorrhages. The knots are cut short and then rotated and buried into the plate suture holes, to avoid irritation. The tube is irrigated with tissue plasminogen acti-vator (TPA) to prevent fibrin occlusion.
- If performing combined procedures (extracapsular lens phacoemulsification, endoscopic cyclophotocoagulation [ECP]), the tube is tucked under the conjunc-tival pocket and intraocular surgery is then performed. The GDD procedure is resumed once the intraocular surgery is completed.
- The tube should cross the limbal area at a 90° angle. The length of the tube is care-fully estimated before it is trimmed. Ideally, it should protrude in the anterior cham-ber for 3 to 4 mm. Westcott tenotomy scissors are used to create a wide, anteriorly and upward-facing bevel, to ease insertion and to prevent fibrin occlusion[27] and

corneal endothelial contact. The conjunctival flap is then carefully elevated and a 22G needle attached to a syringe is advanced into the anterior chamber at the limbus, creating a scleral track. The needle is kept parallel to the iris, removed, and rapidly exchanged with the beveled tube (see **Fig. 6**E). Anterior chamber deflation should be avoided. Some surgeons use viscoelastic substances to preserve the created scleral track and prevent anterior chamber collapse.

- The conjunctiva and Tenon capsule are closed with 7-0 or 8-0 absorbable suture in a simple continuous pattern (see **Fig. 6**F). Additional intracameral TPA may then be injected at the surgeon's discretion. The final result is shown in **Fig. 7**.

Postoperative Management

As with cyclophotocoagulation procedures, topical and systemic steroidal and nonsteroidal anti-inflammatory treatment is paramount in postoperative therapy for GDDs implantation. Topical corticosteroids, administered every 6 to 8 hours, not only aid in addressing the anterior uveitis postintracameral penetration,[1] but may help in suppressing the cyclooxygenase pathway and inhibiting fibroblasts proliferation, both responsible for implant fibrosis.[14,28,29] Several studies support the use of systemic corticosteroids to limit capsular fibrosis and achieve better IOP control in the human field[30–32]; however, a report of the American Academy of Ophthalmology has recently disproved the claim.[33] Despite this current debate, systemic corticosteroids are currently recommended, when possible, in veterinary ophthalmology.[1] Topical corticosteroids are tapered over the course of several weeks; however, long-term treatment with topical prednisolone acetate 1% every 24 to 48 hours is warranted.[14] Topical and systemic antibiotics are administered for 2 weeks postoperatively. Topical antiglaucoma medications are typically maintained long-term.

Expected IOP values in the immediate postoperative period range from 5 mm Hg with nonvalved devices to 8 to 12 mm Hg with valved devices. Eventually capsule fibrosis develops, usually within 3 to 6 weeks, prompting bleb revision and/or the injection of 5-FU to address implant failure. In bleb revision the overlying conjunctiva is incised and a portion of the fibrotic capsule over the implant site is removed. This provides immediate but short-term relief, because capsular fibrosis relapses within a variable amount of time. A bleb diversion device into the orbital space has been recently evaluated in five dogs with previous failed Ahmed implant, but IOP control failed in three of the five eyes within 5 months.[34]

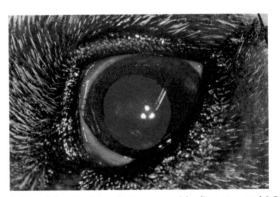

Fig. 7. The standard size of shunt tubing (0.6 mm outside diameter and 0.3 mm inside diameter) within the anterior chamber in a dog with primary glaucoma. (*From* Gelatt KN, Gelatt JP. Surgical procedures for the glaucomas. In: Gelatt KN, Gelatt JP, editors. Veterinary ophthalmic surgery. Saunders Ltd; 2011. p. 286; with permission.)

Success Rate

Because of changes in patient selection, criteria for IOP target values, surgical goals, and variations in implants over the last 30 years, comparisons among studies are challenging. Krupin, modified Joseph, Ahmed, and modified Ahmed devices have all been investigated in the late 1980s and 1990s with variable results.[7,8,11] A high incidence of complications, from implant failure to implant extrusion, uncontrolled IOP, additional surgery required for IOP control, and vision loss, have also been reported with the use of Baerveldt implants.[9,10]

The success rate has improved in more recent studies. Westermeyer and colleagues[14] reported a staggering success in a nine-case series of Ahmed implantation in glaucomatous dogs, with eight of nine eyes visual at 1-year follow-up. Temporalis muscle fascia or porcine intestinal submucosa grafts were used to protect the tube portion under the conjunctiva, and all cases were treated with MMC intraoperatively and chronic topical steroidal treatment postsurgery. Surgical bleb revision was necessary in four eyes, whereas conjunctival necrosis, likely secondary to MMC use, occurred in four eyes.

Combined Procedures

With the introduction of cyclodestructive techniques, recent studies have investigated the combination of gonioimplantation and ablation of the ciliary bodies in glaucomatous dogs. In two separate studies, glaucomatous eyes underwent both gonioimplantation with Ahmed devices and either cyclocryoablation or transscleral cyclophotocoagulation (TSCP). Bentley and colleagues[13] reported IOP control in 73% and vision preservation in 58% of treated eyes 1 year postoperatively. Similar results were reported by Sapienza and van der Woerdt,[12] with IOP control in 76% and vision preservation in 41% of patients at 1 year. Progressive failure of the gonioimplant device was observed starting 6 months postoperatively.

A few studies have suggested that the combination of cyclodestructive and filtering procedures performed at the same time may result in a lower success rate, when compared with the techniques performed separately. The rationale behind this is that cyclodestruction causes massive release of intraocular inflammatory mediators and postoperative increases in IOP, with increased amount of cytokine-laden AH outflow through the implant, likely leading to its premature fibrosis.[14,35] For this reason, several studies have suggested a staggered two-stage technique, with early Ahmed gonioimplantation followed by later TSCP or ECP.[35–37]

ECP allows direct visualization and optimal laser energy delivery, resulting in decreased intraocular inflammation when compared with TSCP.[38] Combination treatment involving the use of ECP and GDDs may improve long-term success rate, while minimizing the complication of IOP spikes in the postoperative period.

FRONTAL SINUS SHUNTS

A less popular drainage implant, aimed at diverting AH to the frontal sinus in dogs, has been investigated and reported by Grahn and Cullen.[18,19] The aim of this type of shunting procedure is to prevent bleb fibrosis and implant failure by diverting the AH to an epithelium-lined, air-filled space, such as the frontal sinus.

The Cullen canine valved frontal sinus glaucoma shunt consists of two portions: a silicone tube that is inserted in the anterior chamber and a frontal sinus portion, provided with a valved plug tip and an anchoring bulb (**Fig. 8**). A skin incision is performed dorsomedial to the globe, above the rostral compartment of the frontal sinus. The frontal sinus then is entered with a 3/32-in Steinman pin and Jacob chuck and the valved portion of the device is inserted into the surgical hole and secured to the periosteum by fluorocarbon

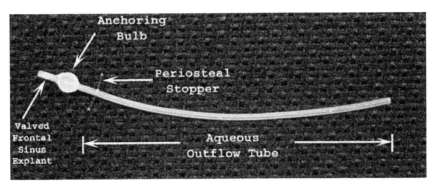

Fig. 8. Cullen frontal sinus glaucoma shunt. (*From* Cullen CL. Cullen frontal sinus glaucoma shunt: preliminary findings in dogs with primary glaucoma. Vet Ophthalmol 2004;7(5):312, with permission.)

suture material. A subcutaneous tunnel is created by blunt dissection with mosquito forceps; the tunnel connects the frontal sinus site and a 12-o'clock incision previously performed over the dorsal bulbar conjunctiva of the surgery eye. The tip of the silicone tubing is then pulled through the tunnel to exit the dorsal conjunctiva. The tubing is properly trimmed and beveled as previously described, and inserted into the limbal track created by a 16G needle at 12 o'clock. A modified Chinese finger-trap suture pattern is used to secure the shunt to the sclera, and the overlying conjunctiva is closed with 7-0 polyglactin in a simple interrupted pattern.[18] Reported complications of the Cullen shunt relate to the thick and more rigid intracameral tube, including corneal decompensation from endothelium contact; anterior uveitis with fibrin formation; and tube displacement from the anterior chamber.[18,19,39] Despite the risks of possible retrograde bacterial contamination from the dorsal sinus, only one case of endophthalmitis has been reported.[40]

SUPRACHOROIDAL SHUNTS

The suprachoroidal space has been considered as an alternative site of aqueous drainage for its potential in providing a pathway through the uveoscleral outflow. In addition, if compared with the subconjunctival space, the suprachoroidal site is reported to show a more limited mytogenic activity for mesenchymal cells[41] and thus potentially decreased fibrosis.

The SOLX gold shunt (SOLX, Inc, Waltham, MA, USA) is derived from the human field, and is a nonvalved flat-plate implant made of 24-karat gold, concealing several microchannels.[41] The device is placed on top of the suprachoroidal space, under a scleral flap, and the flared distal ends are inserted in the anterior chamber.

In the study reported by Sapienza and colleagues,[42] six of nine treated eyes showed poor control of IOP, with vision loss in four of nine eyes 4 months postoperatively. Retinal detachment, hyphema, and vision loss were the most common complications.

INTRASCLERAL SHUNTS

A novel device has been recently introduced for treatment of human glaucoma. The Ex-Press glaucoma shunt (Optonol Ltd, Neve-Ilan, Israel) consists of a small, stainless steel, nonvalved implant, ranging from 2.64 to 2.96 mm in length and 50 to 400 μm in diameter (**Fig. 9**). The implant is inserted in the anterior chamber under a scleral flap, which is then secured with nylon sutures.

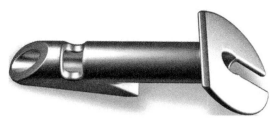

Fig. 9. Ex-Press glaucoma shunt (P model). (*From* McGrath LA, Lee GA, Goldberg I. Glaucoma surgery with the Ex-press glaucoma shunt. In: Samples JR, Ahmed IIK, editors. Surgical innovations in glaucoma. New York: Springer Science + Business Media; 2014. p. 199, with permission.)

The Ex-Press shunt gonioimplantation has been investigated in four cases of canine glaucoma, in combination with ECP.[43] At 1-year follow-up, two of four eyes were normotensive. The number of reported cases is still too limited to allow definitive conclusions.

COMPLICATIONS

Early and late complications are described following placement of GDDs in dogs. Hypotony, anterior uveitis, and occlusion of the tubular portion of the implant can occur within a few hours postoperatively. Hypotony is usually more commonly reported with nonvalved devices,[9] but poor flow control caused by excessive peritubular filtration at the anterior chamber site can also occur in valved devices.[44,45] Hypotensive retinopathy with multifocal retinal folds has been described in dogs and people undergoing glaucoma filtering surgery,[14,46] and shallow anterior chamber (15%, 17% of the cases), choroidal effusion (13%, 14%), and corneal decompensation (7%, 14%) have also been reported in a large study on human patients implanted with Ahmed and Baerveldt devices, respectively.[20] Inadequate placement of the tube may result in corneal endothelial damage and edema caused by its excessive length, its obstruction by the base of the iris when trimmed too short, or its displacement secondary to failure of the securing sutures.[18,19,47] Transient anterior uveitis is expected after implantation of the silicon tube in the anterior chamber, and it can lead to tube occlusion by intracameral fibrin.[7,9,12] Intracameral injections of TPA (25–37.5 μg) are usually effective in dissolving the fibrin within or surrounding the gonioimplant tube.[12,48] Hyphema and vitreous in the anterior chamber may also contribute to the plugging of the intracameral tube.

Late complications following GDD implantation in dogs include implant or tube erosion through the conjunctiva, tube migration, late-onset corneal decompensation, and filtration failure caused by fibrosis at the plate site or again at the intraocular tube. To provide protection against conjunctival erosion over the limbal portion of the tube, temporalis muscle fascia, partial-thickness scleral flaps, donor scleral, dura, fascia lata, porcine intestinal submucosa, and pericardium grafts have been reported in human and veterinary literature.[14,49,50] In the human literature, tube exposure is associated with increased risk of endophthalmitis[51]; however, the incidence of endophthalmitis in dogs with GDDs is low.[17,40]

Subconjunctival scarring and wound retraction with bleb fibrosis is the most common long-term complication in GDD procedures in dogs.[7,9,10] Bleb failure may occur within a few weeks to few months after surgery and is more common in animals than in humans (**Fig. 10**). In comparison with human and nonhuman primates, domestic animals show a far more labile blood ocular barrier, and a much more severe inflammatory reaction to ocular insults or procedures is expected.[52]

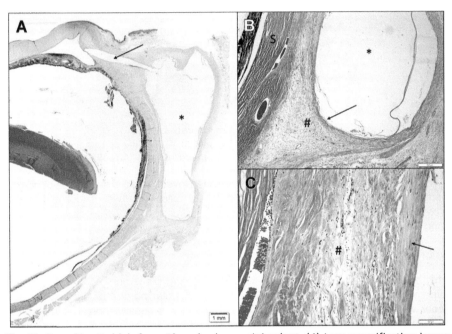

Fig. 10. Dog, fibrotic bleb from Ahmed valve gonioimplant. (*A*) Low magnification image showing the bleb that develops around the device (*) and the scleral track from the tube (*arrow*), extending into the anterior chamber. (*B, C*) The device (now removed) is surrounded by a layer of dense fibrous connective tissue (*arrow*) that becomes more loose and vascularized at the periphery (#). Note the relationship between bleb (*), surrounding fibrous connective tissue, and sclera (s). (*Courtesy of* Dr Leandro Teixeira, COPLOW, Madison, WI.)

Several different factors influence the creation of the bleb around the end plate, from proper surgical technique and wound healing processes, to timing and amount of AH outflow, material of the GDD, presence of pre-existent inflammation, upregulation of cytokines, and growth factors within the aqueous and chronic topical glaucoma treatment. The goal of a functional bleb is to allow the diverted AH to flow through the capsule via a process of passive diffusion and to be absorbed by conjunctival capillaries, thus lowering the IOP.[53] Recent studies on Molteno implants in people have described a functional bleb composed of an outer fibrovascular layer and an inner avascular layer of hypocellular moderately degenerative collagen.[54] Although the process is still not completely understood, it has been suggested that successful AH drainage depends on a dynamic balance between the healing inflammatory response in the outer layer and an apoptotic anti-inflammatory fibrodegenerative response to aqueous inflow in the inner layer of the bleb.[55] These studies have suggested that two-stage procedures, with early implant of the device and delayed drainage of AH in a preformed capsule at a later time, develop thinner functional capsules with less marked fibrovascular response.[54] A large study comparing the use of valved versus nonvalved implants in people with refractory glaucoma found similar failure rates at the 5-year follow-up in both groups.[56] However, as suggested in the study, the use of a valved device may be particularly advantageous in patients with markedly elevated IOP preoperatively, as it is usually the case in canine patients.

Proper surgical technique with gentle tissue manipulation and accurate hemostasis is warranted to minimize the inflammatory reaction in GDDs implantation. Wound healing following surgical procedures comprises a series of sequential events that are eventually responsible for fibroblast proliferation and migration. An immediate inflammatory response is started in the early postsurgical stage, when tissue damage and hemorrhages of the affected tissues cause release of cytokines and growth factors. Proliferation and tissue reparation represent the second phase, with migration of inflammatory cells and fibroblasts (attracted by growth factors from wound edges, subconjunctival, and episcleral tissues), and proliferation of new capillaries at the surgical site. This phase, leading to the formation of granulation tissue, begins in the few days postprocedure and lasts up to the second or third month. Finally, as a result of remodeling and final healing, collagen I is replaced by collagen III, with reabsorption of blood vessels and fibroblasts, and subsequent formation of a dense collagenous subconjunctival scar.[57] The process lasts several months, and the production of a functional filtering bleb depends on the ability to modulate its final outcome.

Several factors have been implicated in the pathogenesis of bleb failure, including transforming growth factor-β,[58] connective tissue growth factor,[59] vascular endothelium growth factor,[60] tumor necrosis factor-α, interleukin-6,[61] and matrix metalloproteinases and their tissue inhibitors.[62] These inflammatory mediators and cytokines are upregulated not only at the surgical site, but within the glaucomatous aqueous: increased levels of transforming growth factor-β_2 have been described in people[63] and dogs.[64] Glaucoma and vascular endothelium growth factor was upregulated in the AH of canine[65] and human glaucomatous patients and in the rabbit model of filtration surgery.[60] Rapid inflow of growth-factor-laden AH through the filtering device may enhance the recruitment and proliferation of episcleral fibroblasts and precipitate bleb fibrosis.[63] Because of this inflammatory priming at the surgical subconjunctival site, the placement of a second implant in the same area in case of bleb failure is not recommended.[63,66]

A whole body of literature has reported the occurrence of significant ocular surface changes associated with chronic use of topical antiglaucoma medications. Both active compounds (preserved latanoprost) and the preservative benzalkonium chloride are responsible for overexpression of proinflammatory mediators and cytokines in the conjunctival and ocular surface epithelia.[67,68] Conjunctival changes increase with the chronicity of medical therapy, and can reflect negatively on the outcome of filtering procedures. In veterinary ophthalmology, chronic topical medications for treatment and prophylactic use are a common feature in the management of glaucoma, and they may further contribute to bleb failure. Proper timing of surgical procedures with early intervention is currently advocated for human and canine glaucomatous patients, and could be shown to be beneficial in this regard.[27]

MMC and 5-FU are the most commonly used antimetabolites to inhibit bleb fibrosis in the human and veterinary fields of glaucoma surgery. MMC is an antibiotic, antimitotic molecule that inhibits DNA synthesis and causes fibroblast apoptosis. It is 100-fold more potent than 5-FU, and it is used intraoperatively as previously described. 5-FU is a pyrimidine analogue, with similar properties to MMC; however, it seems to be more selective in its toxicity toward fibroblasts, whereas MMC also affects the vascular endothelium, with formation of thin-walled avascular blebs.[69] Both agents are toxic to the corneal and conjunctival epithelium, and infections, bleb leaks, and endophthalmitis are reported complications in human literature. 5-FU may be used intraoperatively and in multiple subconjunctival injection at the implant site (0.1 mL, 50 mg/mL solution, 30G needle), typically at 1 week, 1 month, 3 months, and every 6 months post-GGD implantation. Protection of the corneal epithelium by lubricating ointment is warranted and sedation is usually required in canine patients.

The use of antimetabolites is controversial. Despite reports of their efficacy in successfully controlling bleb scarring,[70,71] the American Academy of Ophthalmology[33] and randomized clinical trials[72,73] have concluded that the use of antifibrotic agents presents no additional benefits in glaucoma filtering procedures. Few new potential antimetabolites, such as ilomastat, bevacizumab, and rapamycin, are currently investigated.[74–76] Recently, the addition of dried human amniotic membrane on top of Ahmed valves in rabbits has gained thinner and looser blebs.[77]

Contrasting reports on the efficacy of antimetabolites are also present in veterinary literature. Tinsley and colleagues[10,78] have reported in vitro (MMC and 5-FU) and in vivo (MMC) inhibition of fibroblast proliferation, with thinner capsules and IOP control in the short term. MMC treatment was also reported to contribute to the successful long-term outcome of Ahmed valve implantation in a case series of nine glaucomatous eyes.[14] Other studies have showed disappointing results, with consistent failure of effective fibrosis inhibition.[12,13,79] Described complications include conjunctival dehiscence and necrosis.[14] At this time, prudent use of antimetabolites should rely on the personal surgeon's choice, but more effective medications are strongly needed to better address bleb fibrosis.

END-STAGE GLAUCOMA PROCEDURES

Unfortunately, medical and surgical failure in canine glaucoma still represents a common frustrating reality. Once vision is lost, and uncontrolled elevated IOP is the source of ocular pain, buphthalmos, and corneal complications, end-stage procedures are recommended (see **Fig. 2**).

Enucleation is commonly performed in chronic glaucoma cases and the description of the technique can be found elsewhere.[80] Recently, several techniques to address intraoperative and postoperative pain have been described, including bupivacaine/lidocaine retrobulbar injection or intraorbital anesthetic-infused gelatin hemostatic sponges.[81,82] To improve cosmetic results, intraorbital polymethylmethacrylate or silicone prosthetics may be inserted in the orbit after globe removal. A new technique using polymethylmethacrylate implants with drilled interconnecting channels has proved cosmetically valuable and effective in allowing ingrowth of fibrovascular tissue, thus decreasing the risks of implant extrusion.[83]

Evisceration with intrascleral prosthesis provides a cosmetic solution in cases of primary and secondary nonneoplastic glaucoma (**Fig. 11**), provided that the ocular surface is healthy and intact. In this procedure a dorsal scleral incision is performed at

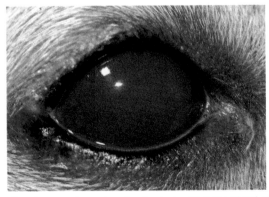

Fig. 11. Right eye of a glaucomatous dog, implanted with intrascleral silicone prosthesis.

approximately 4 to 5 mm from and parallel to the limbus; the choroidal and uveal tissues are dissected using a cyclodialysis spatula. The intraocular structures are removed, and a silicone prosthesis is inserted into the scleral shell via a Carter sphere introducer. Scleral and conjunctival incisions are then routinely closed with absorbable sutures. Prior ocular ultrasound is recommended, especially in case of cloudiness of the ocular media, to identify potential intraocular tumors. In a recent study, 8.21% of evisceration samples and 38.75% of scleral shells from previously eviscerated canine globes showed evidence of intraocular tumors.[84] The same study also highlighted a high percentage of severe corneal disease (46%) among the canine scleral shells, confirming corneal ulceration and perforation among the most common complications of this procedure.

Chemical Ablation of the Ciliary Body

Intravitreal injections of gentamicin and cidofovir are known to cause irreversible damage to the ciliary body with decrease or suppression of AH production. Chemical ablation is recommended when the patient poses potential anesthetic risks or when there are financial constraints. Cooperative patients may not require sedation, with analgesia provided by topical proparacaine solution and subconjunctival injection of 0.2 to 0.4 mL of 2% lidocaine in the dorsolateral quadrant.

The dose of intravitreal gentamicin varies according to the surgeon's preference (25–40 mg), but it is recommended that the total daily dose for the specific patient (6–8 mg/kg) not be exceeded.[85,86] Dexamethasone sodium phosphate (1 mg) may be added to control intraocular inflammation.[27] A 20- to 22-gauge needle is inserted 8 mm posterior to the dorsolateral limbus, directed toward the central vitreous space (**Fig. 12**). If possible, 0.5 to 0.6 mL of vitreous is aspirated. When the vitreous is too dense and cannot be aspirated, an aqueocentesis is performed. The selected dose of gentamicin is then injected in the vitreal cavity.

Recent reports show an improved success rate with this procedure, ranging from 86.4% to 100%,[85,87] mostly caused by increased doses of injected gentamicin. A negative correlation between success and patient weight is suggestive of a

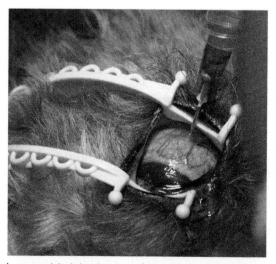

Fig. 12. Intravitreal gentamicin injection in a dog with chronic glaucoma.

dose-dependent effect of gentamicin, with doses less than 20 to 25 mg associated with failure to adequately control IOP postprocedure.[85,88,89]

The most common complications of chemical ablation include intraocular inflammation/hemorrhage, corneal opacity, cataracts, phthisis bulbi, and inadequate control of IOP.[27,88,89] Although the measurable levels of gentamicin present in the blood of treated animals are unlikely to be nephrotoxic or ototoxic in healthy dogs, caution has been recommended when administering intravitreal gentamicin in small patients.[85] Recently, a study has identified the presence of intraocular tumors in 40% of enucleated eyes that had been previously treated with intravitreal gentamicin injection (IGI)[90]; although the study could not prove a causal correlation between the injection of gentamicin and the development of tumors, it is concerning that a large portion of those tumors exhibited unusual malignant behavior. Thorough ocular examination, including ocular ultrasonography, should always be performed before proceeding for IGI in dogs.

Low and colleagues[91] have recently reported the results of intravitreal cidofovir injection for the treatment of chronic canine glaucoma. Cidofovir (562.5 µg, 0.15 mL) is injected 5 mm posterior to the limbus with a 30-gauge needle, in a similar fashion as IGI. Triamcinolone (1 mg) is then injected subconjunctivally. Because of the minimal volume of injected agent, delivered through a small-gauge needle, this procedure does not require sedation or anesthesia. Intravitreal cidofovir is recommended in high-risk anesthesia patients and patients suffering from renal disease where gentamicin may be contraindicated.

Despite the high success rate of 85% at 2 weeks postprocedure, the incidence of phthisis bulbi is quite elevated (70% at 6 months). Reported complications are similar to the complications secondary to IGI.

SUMMARY

Glaucoma represents a common cause of blindness in dogs, with often unavoidable failure of medical control. Surgical treatment is often necessary to provide IOP control, by increasing AH outflow and/or decreasing its production. As here reported, filtering procedures with gonioimplantation deviate the AH to a subconjunctival bleb, and from there the AH is absorbed into the local vessels. Recent improvements in techniques, materials, postoperative management, and patient selection have resulted in better long-term outcome of Ahmed gonioimplantation in canine primary glaucoma. Currently, the combination of cyclodestructive and filtering techniques offers attractive advantages, namely the additional control of potential IOP spikes postcyclophotoablation, while allowing more extensive cyclodestruction and long-term sight preservation. The consistent refinement of surgical options and a successful modulation of inflammation are the keys to effective GDD procedures in dogs.

However, inconsistencies in surgical results, caused by the frustrating wound healing response and eventual bleb fibrosis, are still a hard reality in canine filtering procedures. Surgical failure with relapsing glaucoma or irreversible ocular damage is still a common occurrence; end-stage procedures, such as enucleation, evisceration with intrascleral prosthesis, and pharmacologic ablation of the ciliary bodies, are then available to provide relief to blind and painful globes.

ACKNOWLEDGMENTS

The authors gratefully acknowledge the assistance of Dr Terah Webb and Jennifer Nadeau in editing the article.

REFERENCES

1. Plummer CE, Regnier A, Gelatt KN. The canine glaucomas. In: Gelatt KN, Gilger BC, Kern TJ, editors. Veterinary ophthalmology, vol. 2, 5th edition. Ames (IA): Wiley & Sons; 2013. p. 1050–145.
2. Gelatt KN. Canine glaucoma. In: Gelatt KN, editor. Veterinary ophthalmology. 2nd edition. Malvern (PA): Lea & Febiger; 1991. p. 396–428.
3. Lim KS, Allan BD, Lloyd AW, et al. Glaucoma drainage devices; past, present, and future. Br J Ophthalmol 1998;82(9):1083–9.
4. Wilson MR, Mendis U, Paliwal A, et al. Long-term follow-up of primary glaucoma surgery with Ahmed glaucoma valve implant versus trabeculectomy. Am J Ophthalmol 2003;136(3):464–70.
5. Wilson MR, Mendis U, Smith SD, et al. Ahmed glaucoma valve implant vs trabeculectomy in the surgical treatment of glaucoma: a randomized clinical trial. Am J Ophthalmol 2000;130(3):267–73.
6. Desai MA, Gedde SJ, Feuer WJ, et al. Practice preferences for glaucoma surgery: a survey of the American Glaucoma Society in 2008. Ophthalmic Surg Lasers Imaging 2008;42(3):202–8.
7. Gelatt KN, Gum GG, Samuelson DA, et al. Evaluation of the Krupin-Denver valve implant in normotensive and glaucomatous beagles. J Am Vet Med Assoc 1987; 191(11):1404–9.
8. Bedford PGC. A clinical evaluation of a one-piece drainage system in the treatment of canine glaucoma. J Small Anim Pract 1989;30(2):68–75.
9. Bentley E, Nasisse MP, Glover T, et al. Implantation of filtering devices in dogs with glaucoma: preliminary results in 13 eyes. Vet Comp Ophthalmol 1996;6(4): 243–6.
10. Tinsley DM, Betts DM. Clinical experience with a glaucoma drainage device in dogs. Vet Comp Ophthalmol 1994;4(2):77–84.
11. Garcia-Sanchez GA, Brooks DE, Gelatt KN, et al. Evaluation of valved and non-valved gonioimplants in 83 eyes of 65 dogs with glaucoma. Anim Eye Res 1998; 17:9–16.
12. Sapienza JS, van der Woerdt A. Combined transscleral diode laser cyclophotocoagulation and Ahmed gonioimplantation in dogs with primary glaucoma: 51 cases (1996-2004). Vet Ophthalmol 2005;8(2):121–7.
13. Bentley E, Miller PE, Murphy CJ, et al. Combined cycloablation and gonioimplantation for treatment of glaucoma in dogs: 18 cases (1992-1998). J Am Vet Med Assoc 1999;215(10):1469–72.
14. Westermeyer HD, Hendrix DV, Ward DA. Long-term evaluation of the use of Ahmed gonioimplants in dogs with primary glaucoma: nine cases (2000-2008). J Am Vet Med Assoc 2011;238(5):610–7.
15. Garcia-Sanchez GA, Whitley RD, Brooks DE, et al. Ahmed valve implantation to control intractable glaucoma after phacoemulsification and intraocular lens implantation in a dog. Vet Ophthalmol 2005;8(2):139–44.
16. Hakanson NW. Extraorbital diversion of aqueous humour in the treatment of glaucoma in the dog: a pilot study including two recipient sites. Vet Comp Ophthalmol 1996;6(2):82–8.
17. Gelatt KN, MacKay EO. Modified Ahmed anterior shunt to the parotid duct in the glaucomatous Beagle. Paper presented at: Proceedings of the American College of Veterinary Ophthalmologists. Montreal, October 11–15, 2000.
18. Cullen CL. Cullen frontal sinus valved glaucoma shunt: preliminary findings in dogs with primary glaucoma. Vet Ophthalmol 2004;7(5):311–8.

19. Cullen CL, Allen AL, Grahn BH. Anterior chamber to frontal sinus shunt for the diversion of aqueous humor: a pilot study in four normal dogs. Vet Ophthalmol 1998;1(1):31–9.

20. Christakis PG, Tsai JC, Kalenak JW, et al. The Ahmed versus Baerveldt study: three-year treatment outcomes. Ophthalmology 2013;120(11):2232–40.

21. Schwartz KS, Lee RK, Gedde SJ. Glaucoma drainage implants: a critical comparison of types. Curr Opin Ophthalmol 2006;17(2):181–9.

22. Britt MT, LaBree LD, Lloyd MA, et al. Randomized clinical trial of the 350-mm2 versus the 500-mm2 Baerveldt implant: longer term results: is bigger better? Ophthalmology 1999;106(12):2312–8.

23. Lloyd MA, Baerveldt G, Fellenbaum PS, et al. Intermediate-term results of a randomized clinical trial of the 350- versus the 500-mm2 Baerveldt implant. Ophthalmology 1994;101(8):1456–63 [discussion: 1463–4].

24. Kadri OA, Wilcox MJ. Surface tension controls capsule thickness and collagen orientation in glaucoma shunt devices. Biomed Sci Instrum 2001;37:257–62.

25. Ishida K, Netland PA, Costa VP, et al. Comparison of polypropylene and silicone Ahmed glaucoma valves. Ophthalmology 2006;113(8):1320–6.

26. Strubbe DT, Gelatt KN, MacKay EO. In vitro flow characteristics of the Ahmed and self-constructed anterior chamber shunts. Am J Vet Res 1997;58(11):1332–7.

27. Gelatt KN, Esson DW, Plummer CE. Surgical procedures for the glaucomas. In: Gelatt KNGP, editor. Veterinary ophthalmic surgery. Edinburgh (United Kingdom): W.B. Saunders; 2011. p. 263–303. Chapter 10.

28. Palmberg P. The failing filtering bleb. Ophthalmol Clin North Am 2000;13(3): 517–29.

29. Chang L, Crowston JG, Cordeiro MF, et al. The role of the immune system in conjunctival wound healing after glaucoma surgery. Surv Ophthalmol 2000; 45(1):49–68.

30. Fuller JR, Bevin TH, Molteno ACB, et al. Anti-inflammatory fibrosis suppression in threatened trabeculectomy bleb failure produces good long term control of intraocular pressure without risk of sight threatening complications. Br J Ophthalmol 2002;86(12):1352–4.

31. Molteno AC, Van Biljon G, Ancker E. Two-stage insertion of glaucoma drainage implants. Trans Ophthalmol Soc N Z 1979;31:17–26.

32. Starita RJ, Fellman RL, Spaeth GL, et al. Short- and long-term effects of postoperative corticosteroids on trabeculectomy. Ophthalmology 1985;92(7):938–46.

33. Minckler DS, Francis BA, Hodapp EA, et al. Aqueous shunts in glaucoma: a report by the American Academy of Ophthalmology. Ophthalmology 2008; 115(6):1089–98.

34. Cairo M, Sapienza JS. Outcome of a bleb diversion device in five dogs (five eyes) with uncontrolled primary glaucoma after prior Ahmed gonioimplantation. Paper presented at: European College of Veterinary Ophthalmologists. London (UK), May 15–18, 2014.

35. Esson DW, Gum GG, Brinkis J, et al. Evaluation of the effect of laser cyclophotocoagulation on the success of glaucoma drainage implant surgery in a rabbit model. Paper presented at: American College of Veterinary Ophthalmologists. Nashville, TN, 2005.

36. Warren JR, Munger RJ, Ring RD. Staged Ahmed valve and diode laser cyclophotocoagulation for the treatment of primary glaucoma in the dog. Paper presented at: American College of Veterinary Ophthalmologists. Kona (HI), October 22–27, 2007.

37. Busayawatanasood R, Sapienza JS. Evaluation for control of intraocular pressure in dogs with the use of a two-staged Ahmed valved gonioimplants followed by

endoscopic laser cyclophotocoagulation with or without phacoemulsification lens extraction. Paper presented at: American College of Veterinary Ophthalmologists. Hilton Head (SC), October 26–29, 2011.

38. Uram M. Endoscopic cyclophotocoagulation in glaucoma management. Curr Opin Ophthalmol 1995;11:19–29.

39. Czepiel TM, Labelle AL, Hamor RE. Clinical experience with a valved frontal sinus shunt for the treatment of canine glaucoma. Paper presented at: American College of Veterinary Ophthalmologists. Fort Worth (TX), October 8–11, 2014.

40. Cullen CL, Corcoran K, Bartoe JT, et al. Preliminary findings from the multicenter clinical study group evaluating the Cullen canine frontal sinus valved glaucoma shunt. Paper presented at: Proceedings of the American College of Veterinary Ophthalmologists. Coeur D'Alene, October 22–25, 2003.

41. Ichhpujani P, Moster MR. SolX suprachoroidal shunt. In: Samples JR, Ahmed I, editors. Surgical innovations in glaucoma. New York: Springer Science; 2014. p. 253–6.

42. Sapienza JS, Wolfer J, Lutz EA, et al. SOLX gold shunt gonioimplantation in dogs with primary glaucoma. Paper presented at: American College of Veterinary Ophthalmologists. Chicago (IL), November 4–7, 2009.

43. Lutz EA, Sapienza JS. Combined diode endoscopic cyclophotocoagulation and Ex-Press shunt gonioimplantation in four cases canine glaucoma. Paper presented at: American College of Veterinary Ophthalmologists. Chicago (IL), November 4–7, 2009.

44. Stein JD, McCoy AN, Asrani S, et al. Surgical management of hypotony owing to overfiltration in eyes receiving glaucoma drainage devices. J Glaucoma 2009; 18(8):638–41.

45. García-Feijoó J, Cuiña-Sardiña R, Méndez-Fernández C, et al. Peritubular filtration as cause of severe hypotony after Ahmed valve implantation for glaucoma. Am J Ophthalmol 2001;132(4):571–2.

46. Costa VP, Arcieri ES. Hypotony maculopathy. Acta Ophthalmol Scand 2007;85(6): 586–97.

47. Gelatt KN, Brooks DE, Miller TR, et al. Issues in ophthalmic therapy: the development of anterior chamber shunts for the clinical management of the canine glaucomas. Prog Vet Comp Ophthalmol 1992;2(2):59–64.

48. Martin C, Kaswan R, Gratzek A, et al. Ocular use of tissue plasminogen activator in companion animals. Prog Vet Comp Ophthalmol 1993;3(1):29–36.

49. Smith MF, Doyle JW, Ticrney JW Jr. A comparison of glaucoma drainage implant tube coverage. J Glaucoma 2002;11(2):143–7.

50. Tanji TM, Lundy DC, Minckler DS, et al. Fascia lata patch graft in glaucoma tube surgery. Ophthalmology 1996;103(8):1309–12.

51. Chen TC, Bhatia LS, Walton DS. Ahmed valve surgery for refractory pediatric glaucoma: a report of 52 eyes. J Pediatr Ophthalmol Strabismus 2005;42(5): 274–83 [quiz: 304–5].

52. Bito LZ. Species differences in the responses of the eye to irritation and trauma: a hypothesis of divergence in ocular defense mechanisms, and the choice of experimental animals for eye research. Exp Eye Res 1984;39(6):807–29.

53. Addicks EM, Quigley HA, Green W, et al. Histologic characteristics of filtering blebs in glaucomatous eyes. Arch Ophthalmol 1983;101(5):795–8.

54. Molteno ACB, Fucik M, Dempster AG, et al. Otago Glaucoma Surgery Outcome Study: factors controlling capsule fibrosis around Molteno implants with histopathological correlation. Ophthalmology 2003;110(11):2198–206.

55. Molteno ACB, Thompson AM, Bevin TH, et al. Otago Glaucoma Surgery Outcome Study: tissue matrix breakdown by apoptotic cells in capsules surrounding Molteno implants. Invest Ophthalmol Vis Sci 2009;50(3):1187–97.

56. Budenz DL, Barton K, Gedde SJ, et al. Five-year treatment outcomes in the Ahmed Baerveldt comparison study. Ophthalmology 2015;122(2):308–16.

57. Skuta GL, Parrish RK II. Wound healing in glaucoma filtering surgery. Surv Ophthalmol 1987;32(3):149–70.

58. Kay EP, Lee HK, Park KS, et al. Indirect mitogenic effect of transforming growth factor-beta on cell proliferation of subconjunctival fibroblasts. Invest Ophthalmol Vis Sci 1998;39(3):481–6.

59. Esson DW, Neelakantan A, Iyer SA, et al. Expression of connective tissue growth factor after glaucoma filtration surgery in a rabbit model. Invest Ophthalmol Vis Sci 2004;45(2):485–91.

60. Li Z, Van Bergen T, Van de Veire S, et al. Inhibition of vascular endothelial growth factor reduces scar formation after glaucoma filtration surgery. Invest Ophthalmol Vis Sci 2009;50(11):5217–25.

61. Cvenkel B, Kopitar AN, Ihan A. Inflammatory molecules in aqueous humour and on ocular surface and glaucoma surgery outcome. Mediators Inflamm 2010; 2010:939602.

62. McCluskey P, Molteno A, Wakefield D, et al. Otago Glaucoma Surgery Outcome Study: the pattern of expression of MMPs and TIMPs in bleb capsules surrounding Molteno implants. Invest Ophthalmol Vis Sci 2009;50(5): 2161–4.

63. Freedman J, Iserovich P. Pro-inflammatory cytokines in glaucomatous aqueous and encysted Molteno implant blebs and their relationship to pressure. Invest Ophthalmol Vis Sci 2013;54(7):4851–5.

64. Miller TR, Salmon JH, English RV, et al. Transforming growth factor β2 in the aqueous humor of normal dogs and dogs with glaucoma. Paper presented at: American College of Veterinary Ophthalmologists. Kona (HI), October 22–27, 2007.

65. Sandberg CA, Herring IP, Huckle WR, et al. Aqueous humor vascular endothelial growth factor in dogs with intraocular disease. Paper presented at: American College of Veterinary Ophthalmologists. Chicago (IL), November 4–7, 2009.

66. Sherwood MB, Esson DW, Sampson EM, et al. Glaucoma drainage implant surgery has a higher survival rate as a primary procedure in a rabbit model. Invest Ophthalmol Vis Sci 2005;46(5):66.

67. Mastropasqua L, Agnifili L, Mastropasqua R, et al. Conjunctival modifications induced by medical and surgical therapies in patients with glaucoma. Curr Opin Pharmacol 2013;13(1):56–64.

68. Liesegang TJ. Conjunctival changes associated with glaucoma therapy: implications for the external disease consultant and the treatment of glaucoma. Cornea 1998;17(6):574–83.

69. Smith S, D'Amore PA, Dreyer EB. Comparative toxicity of mitomycin C and 5-fluorouracil in vitro. Am J Ophthalmol 1994;118(3):332–7.

70. Perkins TW, Gangnon R, Ladd W, et al. Molteno implant with mitomycin C: intermediate-term results. J Glaucoma 1998;7(2):86–92.

71. Duan X, Jiang Y, Qing G. Long-term follow-up study on Hunan aqueous drainage implantation combined with mitomycin C for refractory glaucoma. Yan Ke Xue Bao 2003;19(2):81–5 [in Chinese].

72. Cantor L, Burgoyne J, Sanders S, et al. The effect of mitomycin C on Molteno implant surgery: a 1-year randomized, masked, prospective study. J Glaucoma 1998;7(4):240–6.

73. Costa VP, Azuara-Blanco A, Netland PA, et al. Efficacy and safety of adjunctive mitomycin C during Ahmed glaucoma valve implantation: a prospective randomized clinical trial. Ophthalmology 2004;111(6):1071–6.
74. Wong TT, Mead AL, Khaw PT. Prolonged antiscarring effects of ilomastat and MMC after experimental glaucoma filtration surgery. Invest Ophthalmol Vis Sci 2005;46(6):2018–22.
75. How A, Chua JL, Charlton A, et al. Combined treatment with bevacizumab and 5-fluorouracil attenuates the postoperative scarring response after experimental glaucoma filtration surgery. Invest Ophthalmol Vis Sci 2010;51(2):928–32.
76. Yan ZC, Bai YJ, Tian Z, et al. Anti-proliferation effects of Sirolimus sustained delivery film in rabbit glaucoma filtration surgery. Mol Vis 2011;17:2495–506.
77. Lee JW, Park WY, Kim EA, et al. Tissue response to implanted Ahmed glaucoma valve with adjunctive amniotic membrane in rabbit eyes. Ophthalmic Res 2014; 51(3):129–39.
78. Tinsley DM, Tinsley LM, Betts DM. In vivo clinical trial of perioperative mitomycin-C in combination with a drainage device implantation in normal canine globes. Vet Comp Ophthalmol 1995;5(4):231–41.
79. Glover TL, Nasisse MP, Davidson MG. Effects of topically applied mitomycin-C on intraocular pressure, facility of outflow, and fibrosis after glaucoma filtration surgery in clinically normal dogs. Am J Vet Res 1995;56(7):936–40.
80. Gelatt KN, Whitley RD. Surgery of the orbit. In: Gelatt KNGP, editor. Veterinary ophthalmic surgery. Edinburgh (United Kingdom): W.B. Saunders; 2011. p. 51–88.
81. Myrna KE, Bentley E, Smith LJ. Effectiveness of injection of local anesthetic into the retrobulbar space for postoperative analgesia following eye enucleation in dogs. J Am Vet Med Assoc 2010;237(2):174–7.
82. Ploog CL, Swinger RL, Spade J, et al. Use of lidocaine-bupivacaine-infused absorbable gelatin hemostatic sponges versus lidocaine-bupivacaine retrobulbar injections for postoperative analgesia following eye enucleation in dogs. J Am Vet Med Assoc 2014;244(1):57–62.
83. Oriá AP, de Souza MR, Dórea Neto FA, et al. Polymethylmethacrylate orbital implants with interconnecting channels. A retrospective study following enucleation in dogs and cats. Vet Ophthalmol 2015. [Epub ahead of print].
84. Naranjo C, Dubielzig RR. Histopathological study of the causes for failure of intrascleral prostheses in dogs and cats. Vet Ophthalmol 2014;17(5):343–50.
85. Rankin AJ, Lanuza R, KuKanich B, et al. Measurement of plasma gentamicin concentrations postchemical ciliary body ablation in dogs with chronic glaucoma. Vet Ophthalmol 2015. [Epub ahead of print].
86. Plumb DC. Plumb's veterinary drug handbook. 6th edition. Ames (IA): Blackwell Publishing Professional; 2008.
87. Goldenberg R, Evans PM, da Silva Curiel JMA, et al. Retrospective evaluation of success rate of pharmacological ciliary body ablation with gentamicin for the treatment of uncontrolled glaucoma in dogs. Paper presented at: American College of Veterinary Ophthalmologists. Fort Worth (TX), October 8–11, 2014.
88. Marchione B, da Silva Curiel JMA, Zhou Y, et al. Effectiveness of gentamicin for pharmacological ablation to treat end stage glaucoma in dogs. Paper presented at: American College of Veterinary Ophthalmologists. Hilton Head (SC), October 26–29, 2011.
89. Bingaman DP, Lindley DM, Glickman NW, et al. Intraocular gentamicin and glaucoma: a retrospective study of 60 dog and cat eyes (1985-1993). Vet Comp Ophthalmol 1994;4(3):113–9.

90. Duke FD, Strong TD, Bentley E, et al. Canine ocular tumors following ciliary body ablation with intravitreal gentamicin. Vet Ophthalmol 2013;16(2): 159–62.
91. Low MC, Landis ML, Peiffer RL. Intravitreal cidofovir injection for the management of chronic glaucoma in dogs. Vet Ophthalmol 2014;17(3):201–6.

Surgical Treatment of Canine Glaucoma

Cyclodestructive Techniques

Dineli Bras, DVM, MS[a],*, Federica Maggio, DVM[b]

KEYWORDS

- Canine • Glaucoma • Laser • Cyclophotocoagulation • Transscleral • Endoscopic

KEY POINTS

- Surgical treatment of glaucoma is directed toward altering aqueous humor production, drainage, or a combination of both.
- The most common surgical treatment performed to decrease aqueous humor production in primary or secondary glaucoma is diode cyclophotocoagulation.
- Diode laser energy can be applied via a transscleral approach (transscleral cyclophotocoagulation), or an endoscopic approach (endoscopic cyclophotocoagulation).
- Endoscopic cyclophotocoagulation provides direct visualization of the targeted ciliary body. The ability to observe tissue effect and titrate the energy, sparing adjacent tissues, results in fewer potential postoperative complications.
- Endoscopic cyclophotocoagulation combined with phacoemulsification and intraocular lens implantation can be performed in primary or secondary glaucoma cases.

 Videos on endoscopic cyclophotocoagulation for the surgical treatment of canine glaucoma accompany this article at http://www.vetsmall.theclinics.com/

INTRODUCTION

Glaucoma is a common cause of vision loss in cats and dogs. Increased intraocular pressure (IOP) is a significant risk factor in the pathogenesis of the disease in humans and a constant factor in canine glaucoma. Addressing increased IOP represents the only treatable and measurable component in terms of successful glaucoma treatment. IOP represents the balance between aqueous humor production and outflow. There are many pathophysiologic mechanisms that can threaten this balance, leading to

Disclosure: The authors have nothing to disclose.
[a] Ophthalmology Department, Centro de Especialistas Veterinarios de Puerto Rico (CEVET), Km 0.1 Carr. 873, Guaynabo, PR 00969, USA; [b] Ophthalmology Department, Tufts Veterinary Emergency Treatment and Specialties (Tufts VETS), 525 South Street, Walpole, MA 02081, USA
* Corresponding author.
E-mail address: dbras@cevet.net

Vet Clin Small Anim 45 (2015) 1283–1305
http://dx.doi.org/10.1016/j.cvsm.2015.06.007
0195-5616/15/$ – see front matter © 2015 Elsevier Inc. All rights reserved.

glaucoma. Initially, most dogs affected with glaucoma are managed medically. Long-term IOP control is often a challenge, requiring surgical intervention to maintain vision. Surgical treatment of glaucoma is directed toward altering aqueous humor production, drainage, or a combination of both. Damage to the secretory epithelium of the ciliary body leads to a decrease in aqueous humor production, whereas filtration surgery provides an alternate path for aqueous outflow.

Previously available surgical techniques for glaucoma carried a high long-term rate of failure, thus a conservative approach with long-term medical treatment has been recommended, followed by surgery in cases of refractory uncontrolled IOP. Surgical procedures in glaucomatous dogs are now more commonly recommended because of an increased knowledge of glaucoma pathogenesis and improvement of surgical techniques. There is preliminary information that early intervention on minimally affected eyes could provide a more successful outcome.[1] However, randomized, prospective, controlled studies with strict inclusion criteria comparing different treatment modalities are lacking. The decision to pursue surgical treatment of glaucoma depends on several factors including cause (primary vs secondary glaucoma), clinical stage (acute vs chronic), and the presence or potential for vision (**Fig. 1**). Most of the surgical procedures for visual patients involve the use of sophisticated techniques, with variable but usually significant financial impact for the owners. Demanding postsurgical topical therapy, close follow-up initially, and owner's expectations are also considered. Factors that influence the surgical treatment success include the surgeon's experience and skills as well as available instrumentation.

This article describes cyclophotocoagulation (CPC) methods to manipulate the aqueous production in primary and secondary glaucoma cases that are sighted or have potential to have vision restored postoperatively.

CYCLOPHOTOCOAGULATION

Destruction of the ciliary body (CB) has been used to treat glaucoma since the 1930s.[2] Multiple cyclodestructive modalities have been used, such as diathermy,[2] cryotherapy,[3–7] ultrasonography,[8] and photoablation.[9–11] CPC can be performed using different laser wavelengths and is the most commonly used cyclodestructive procedure.

CPC causes partial destruction of the CB through coagulation necrosis of the pigmented ciliary epithelium with subsequent thermal damage to the nonpigmented epithelium. Thermal damage is also responsible for vascular occlusion or nonperfusion of the ciliary processes (CPs).[12] The applied laser energy is well absorbed by uveal melanin, resulting in blanching, shrinking, and thereby damage to the secretory ciliary epithelium of the CP that produces aqueous humor.

The goal of CPC is to cause partial destruction of the CB through selective destruction of the ciliary epithelium. Possible undesired consequences such as marked disruption of the ciliary epithelium with severe architectural damage to the ciliary muscle, stroma, and adjacent sclera, and acute occlusive vasculopathy (in some cases permanent nonperfusion), have been reported.[12–15] There is agreement that the amount of energy delivered is correlated with tissue destruction and inflammation, and with postoperative complications. Balance between desired tissue destruction for adequate IOP control and overtreatment is the ideal surgical goal, although sometimes difficult to attain. Tailoring energy delivery and the subsequent amount of tissue destruction depends on tissue characteristics that may vary in each individual patient.

Lasers used for CPC are within the near-infrared electromagnetic spectrum and include neodymium-doped yttrium aluminum garnet (Nd:YAG; 1064-nm wavelength) and diode (810-nm wavelength). The transscleral use of an Nd:YAG laser either with noncontact or contact methods to achieve cyclodestruction has been described.[10,11,16] One study

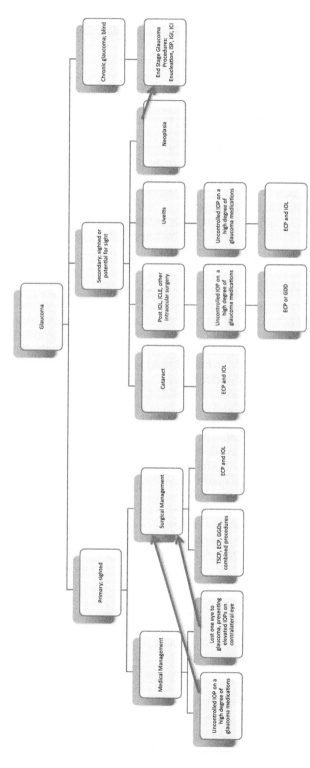

Fig. 1. Surgical treatment rationale for canine glaucoma. ECP, endoscopic cyclophotocoagulation; GDD, glaucoma drainage device; ICI, intravitreal cidofovir injection; ICLE, intracapsular lens extraction; IGI, intravitreal Gentocin injection; IOL, intraocular lens implant; ISP, intrascleral prosthesis; TSCP, transscleral cyclophotocoagulation.

showed promising results with an 83% efficacy in IOP control 12 to 24 weeks postoperatively in 37 dogs (56 eyes), but information about visual function was not reported.[16] Multiple complications were reported, including a 37%[16] to 75%[11] incidence of cataract formation, hemorrhage, phthisis bulbi, and uncontrolled IOP.[10,11,16] A histologic comparison of Nd:YAG laser and diode laser has shown similar cyclodestructive properties.[15]

Diode lasers have become the leading modality for CPC because of a more affordable cost, a better portability, and better absorption of their wavelength by melanin in the ciliary epithelium with less associated inflammation.[17–22]

Endoscopic CPC (ECP) studies in veterinary ophthalmology are lacking, but studies comparing transscleral CPC (TSCP) and ECP in pediatric glaucoma did not show a significant difference in surgical outcome, both offering a moderate long-term IOP control (66.7% and 62% success respectively).[23] At present, diode laser glaucoma therapy, TSCP, and ECP are used for the treatment of primary and secondary glaucoma in canine, feline, and equine patients.

A variety of treatment options are presently available, and it is necessary to analyze which procedure is optimal for each individual patient.

DIODE TRANSSCLERAL CYCLOPHOTOCOAGULATION

TSCP can be applied in noncontact or contact mode. Using noncontact mode, the distance to the target tissue influences the effects of the laser energy on the CB.[24] The amount of laser energy transmitted through the sclera varies between 35% and 70%, and the remainder is reflected or absorbed.[21] A contact mode application using scleral indentation enhances laser delivery and absorption by the pigmented epithelium, resulting in less total energy delivered to achieve the desired effect, and less collateral damage.[22]

Contact diode TSCP can be performed with minimal instrumentation; the diode laser console and the delivery device or glaucoma probe.

The diode laser console (DioVet 810-nm laser system, Iridex, Mountain View, CA) uses an aiming laser beam of 630 to 670 nm, (0–1 mW), and its treatment laser power ranges between 50 and 2000 mW. It has the capability to be used in a continuous or pulse mode with exposure durations between 10 and 9000 milliseconds and repeated intervals of 50 to 1000 milliseconds. The energy is delivered via a handpiece (G-probe, Iridex, Mountain View, CA) with a quartz glass fiber with a diameter of 600 μm. The fiber has a protruding, polished, hemispheric tip, and the probe has a conforming scleral footplate of 3 mm and a 4-mm extension on each end to allow precise, consistent probe placement in relation to the limbus. The hemispheric tip extends 0.55 mm beyond the footplate for scleral indentation to allow better laser penetration and to focus the laser energy on the target tissue, the CPs (**Fig. 2**).

SURGICAL PROCEDURE

Steps to perform TSCP

- Premedication with topical and systemic anti-inflammatories
- General anesthesia
- Select energy parameters (**Table 1**)
- Place G-probe 3 mm posterior to the limbus
- Treat superior and inferior quadrants avoiding 3 and 9 o'clock
- Aqueocentesis following procedure if IOP is >30 mm Hg

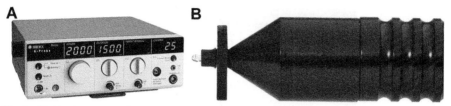

Fig. 2. DioVet laser console; a semiconductor 810-nm laser device with up to 2000 mW power (*A*). The G-probe laser delivery device has a footplate that ensures positioning of the probe 3 to 4 mm behind the limbus (*B*). (*Courtesy of* Iridex, Mountain View, CA.)

TSCP is a noninvasive laser technique in which the laser energy is transmitted to the CPs through the conjunctiva and sclera. Patients are premedicated with topical and systemic steroids, or other antiinflammatory medications of the surgeon's choosing. The procedure is performed under general anesthesia, and the animal is placed in lateral recumbency. An eyelid speculum is used for better perilimbal exposure, and stay sutures may be used for manipulation of the globe. The G-probe is positioned 3 mm posterior to the limbus (**Fig. 3**), and, while indenting the sclera, laser is applied to approximately 35 spots divided in the superior and inferior quadrant, avoiding the 3 and 9 o'clock positions. The nasal quadrants are to be avoided because the retina extends further forward nasally and risk of retinal detachment is increased.[25–27] Different diode TSCP surgical parameters in canine patients have been described (see **Table 1**).[24,28–30] Total energy delivered to the eye ranging from 50 to 300 J has been shown to cause coagulation necrosis of the CB and IOP reduction, but higher energy is associated with greater complications.[1,15,24,28–30] One study that evaluated 144 canine patients (176 eyes) reported a 53% efficacy in IOP control at 1 year when using the high-power/short-duration parameter (1200–2000 mW/1500 ms/30–40 spots) for a mean energy of 85 J per eye.[28] In a smaller study (18 dogs, 24 eyes), using the low-power/long-duration parameter (1000 mW/5000 ms/24 spots) with an average energy of 125 J per eye, a 92% success rate in IOP control was reported 1 year postoperatively.[29]

Another important aspect of TSCP is titrating the energy and the number of treatments to the eye. Because TSCP is applied without direct visualization of the CPs, effective laser treatment is identified by an audible pop that occurs when the threshold from coagulation to tissue vaporization is exceeded. The current treatment most commonly performed by veterinary ophthalmologists is to adjust energy levels to produce a pop in approximately 20% to 75% of the treatment sites.[24,28]

This concept needs further evaluation, because it is now known that the energy delivered to the eye should be minimized to reduce potential postoperative complications, and the success of IOP control is not influenced by pops during surgical treatment.[31] It should be recognized that a pop is an explosion of the CB tissue as a result of photodisruption and indicates overtreatment. This effect is associated with a greater quantity of tissue necrosis and a more intense inflammatory response.[12,37]

Table 1
Commonly used TSCP surgical parameters in dogs

	Power (mW)	Duration (ms)	Sites (n)
High power/short duration	1500	1500	35–50
Low power/long duration	1000	4000	35–50
Prophylactic therapy	Same as above	Same as above	15–25

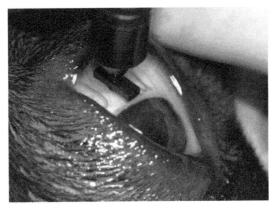

Fig. 3. G-probe positioned 3 mm posterior to the limbus so that the beam is directed through the sclera over the CB.

Avoiding pops should be considered and the energy should be titrated to maximize effect. Energy can be increased until a pop is heard, then decreased by 250 mW to avoid pops for the remainder of the treatment.

Energy levels may also have to be adjusted when treating blue-eyed dogs, in which higher energy levels may be required because there is less uveal pigment.[24] Although a significant difference in the amount and distribution of pigment in the CPs of blue-eyed and brown-eyed dogs has not been found,[33] the amount of pigment in the CB changes with different intensities of iris color, and increases with age in all breeds.[34]

At the conclusion of the procedure, an immediate increase in IOP is frequently seen. If IOP is greater than 30 mm Hg, passive aqueocentesis is performed using a 30-gauge needle. The target IOP after aqueocentesis is an IOP less than 20 mm Hg. IOP is monitored aggressively for the next 24 hours, with recommended follow-ups at 1 week, 2 weeks, 4 to 6 weeks, and every 3 months thereafter. Topical and systemic glaucoma and antiinflammatory therapy is maintained as indicated and according to the surgeon's preference.

POSTOPERATIVE MANAGEMENT

Medical management should be designed to control postoperative inflammation and IOP. Topical prednisolone acetate 1% is administered every 6 hours for the first 7 days, then tapered as needed to control inflammation. Systemic antiinflammatory therapy is administered for 2 weeks postoperatively.

Topical and systemic glaucoma medications are administered according to IOP measurements and tapered as IOP stabilizes postoperatively. Artificial tears are also recommended every 6 hours for the first 7 days, then as deemed necessary (**Table 2**).

Medications are modified according to clinical findings at complete ophthalmic evaluations scheduled at 1 week, 2 weeks, 4 to 6 weeks, and 2 to 3 months postoperatively, then every 3 months thereafter.

SUCCESS RATE

Evaluation of the effects of diode laser TSCP in the normal canine eye showed a decrease in IOP, and depigmented, atrophied CPs were evident at 28 days posttreatment.[14,24] Diode TSCP has been evaluated in glaucomatous canine eyes with an average of 50% efficacy of IOP control up to 1-year follow-up, but resulted in a poor

Table 2
Suggested TSCP postoperative management

| | Antiinflammatory Medications | | Glaucoma Medications | | Artificial Tears |
	Topical	Systemic	Topical	Systemic	Topical
—	Prednisolone Acetate 1%	Prednisone (0.5 mg/kg)/or Carprofen (2.2 mg/kg)	Dorzolamide or Dorzolamide/ Timolol	Methazolamide (2 mg/kg)	—
Immediate	Q6 h	Q12 h/Q12 h	Q8 h	Q8–12 h	Q6 h
1 wk	Q6 h	Q12–24 h/Q12 h	Q8 h	Q8–12 h	Q8 h
2 wk	Q8 h	Q48 h	Q8 h	Q12–24 h	Q12 h
4 wk	Q12 h	—	Q8 h	According to IOP	Q12 h
2–3 mo	Q24 h	—	Q8 h	According to IOP	Q12 h

Abbreviation: Q, every.

visual outcome and a high incidence of significant complications.[14,28] Some clinicians have found that a slower coagulation technique and lower power for a longer duration deliver a significant amount of energy while reducing the postoperative inflammatory response.[35] Hardman and Stanley[29] used this protocol for the treatment of primary glaucoma with 92% success in IOP control and fewer postoperative complications, but only 50% were sighted 1 year postoperatively. The same slow coagulation protocol was used for the treatment of aphakic glaucoma in dogs resulting in poor long-term IOP control.[30] Combined procedures using TSCP and a filtration device or trabeculectomy have also been described in canine patients with variable results.[32,36,37]

Newer TSCP surgical protocols in humans, micropulse TSCP, have provided a more consistent and predictable effect in reducing IOP with minimal ocular complications.[38] Micropulse technology uses a short wave of energy followed by a long pause of energy to reduce thermal buildup and deliver significantly less energy to the eye. Recent studies using TSCP micropulse in human patients showed an average of 70% success rate in IOP control, less postoperative inflammation, and fewer complications,[38,39] but there are no reports of this surgical technique in veterinary medicine.

COMPLICATIONS

Potential postoperative complications

- Immediate spike in IOP
- Conjunctival hyperemia
- Corneal ulceration
- Intraocular inflammation, with or without fibrin
- Intraocular hemorrhage
- Cataract
- Failure to control IOP
- Retinal detachment
- Phthisis bulbi

Conjunctival hyperemia, scleral thinning in the areas of the laser treatment, intraocular inflammation, corneal ulceration, fibrin, hemorrhage, cataract, retinal detachment, phthisis bulbi, and/or uncontrolled IOP are potential postoperative complications.[24,28–30] Severe complications are usually associated with higher energy levels delivered to the eye, whereas lesser complications and better prognosis for vision are associated with less energy.

ENDOSCOPIC CYCLOPHOTOCOAGULATION

Direct visualization CPC through an endoscopic approach (ECP), eliminates some of the concerns of TSCP. The energy can be titrated until the desired tissue shrinking and blanching is observed during ciliary epithelium destruction.

Two basic components are required for ECP: the endoscopy console and the endoscopic probe. The endoscopy console contains the video, illumination, and the laser source. The most common fiber-delivered laser source used in veterinary ophthalmology is the 810-nm diode laser.

There are integrated ophthalmic endoscopy systems that provide image and illumination (E4 console, Endo Optiks Little Silver, NJ) that can be combined with an existing external diode laser, or a console that provides image, illumination, and 810-nm diode laser source all together (E2 console, Endo Optiks, Little Silver, NJ) (**Fig. 4**).

The laser endoscope has 3 fiber groupings: the image guide, the light guide, and the semiconductor 810-nm diode laser guide (**Fig. 5**). These three exist as an endoprobe of 18, 19, 20, or 23 gauge, straight or curved, with a 110° to 140° field of view and depth of focus from 1 to 30 mm (**Figs. 6 and 7**). The light guide uses a 175-W xenon light source.

The laser endoscope is connected to the console that contains all of the instrumentation used for endoscopy, including the video camera, light source, video monitor, and video recorder. The surgeon controls the progress of surgery by viewing the video monitor rather than viewing through the operating microscope (**Fig. 8**, Video 1).

SURGICAL PROCEDURE

Steps to perform ECP

- Premedication with topical and systemic antiinflammatories and antibiotics.
- General anesthesia plus paralysis with a nondepolarizing neuromuscular blocking agent.
- Select surgical approach.
- Inflate the ciliary sulcus with viscoelastic.
- Select treatment extent and degrees of CPs to be treated (**Table 3**).
- Insert microendoscope through the incision.
- Start treatment at 0.25 W. Titrate energy to tissue effect; whitening and shrinking of the CP, avoiding pops.

ECP is an invasive cyclodestructive procedure in which laser energy is transmitted via direct endoscopic visualization of the CB. Patients are premedicated with topical prednisolone acetate 1%, diclofenac 0.1%, and a topical antibiotic (neomycin-polymyxin-gramicidin, tobramycin, or ofloxacin) every 6 hours starting the day before surgery. If part of the patient's ongoing medical therapy, prostaglandin analogues are

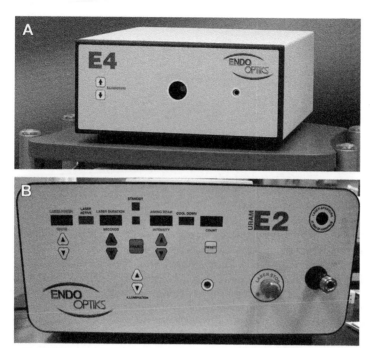

Fig. 4. Integrated ophthalmic endoscopy systems. (*A*) E4 image and light system. (*B*) E2 image, light, and 810-nm laser system. (*Courtesy of* Endo Optiks/Beaver Visitec Int, Waltham, MA.)

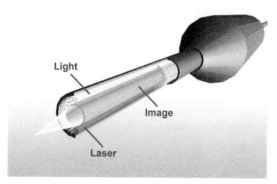

Fig. 5. Microendoscope containing light, laser, and camera. Multiple fibers create a wide cone of light matching the 110° to 140° field of view. (*Courtesy of* Martin Uram, MD, MPH, Retina Consultants, Little Silver, NJ.)

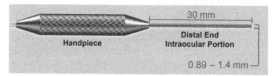

Fig. 6. Ophthalmic straight endoscope design. The distal portion of the probe is 30 mm in length, 0.8 to 1.4 mm outer diameter. (*Courtesy of* Martin Uram, MD, MPH, Retina Consultants, Little Silver, NJ.)

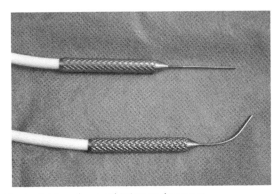

Fig. 7. Autoclavable straight and curved microendoscopes.

discontinued the night before surgery to improve pharmacologic mydriasis. Prednisolone acetate 1% and diclofenac 0.1% are administered every 15 minutes, beginning 2 hours before surgery. Atropine 1% is administered once for dilation. Systemic anti-inflammatory medication of the surgeon's choosing and intravenous cefazolin (20 mg/kg) are administered at induction. The procedure is performed under general anesthesia, and a nondepolarizing neuromuscular blocking agent is used to ensure adequate globe position and stability. The animal is positioned under an operating microscope for intraocular surgery.

CPs may be accessed from either a limbal or a pars plana approach (**Figs. 9** and **10**). The limbal approach is the most commonly used, and ECP in combination with phacoemulsification and intraocular lens (IOL) implantation is the recommended surgical protocol in canine and feline glaucoma. The amount of laser energy applied and the degrees of CB ablation are calibrated to fit each patient's needs (see **Table 3**).

SURGICAL APPROACH TO THE CILIARY PROCESSES
Limbal Approach

A limbal approach is feasible for all patients, whether they are phakic, pseudophakic, or aphakic (see **Fig. 9**). Placement of the incisions is the surgeon's preference. The

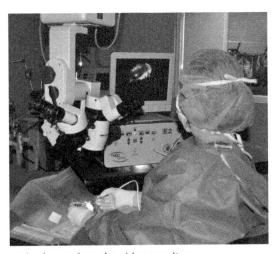

Fig. 8. ECP treatment is observed on the video monitor.

Table 3
Commonly used ECP surgical parameters in dogs and cats

	Power	Duration (ms)	Sites
E2 console	0.25 W	Continuous mode	270°–320°
E4 console	250 mW	9000	270°–320°
Prophylactic therapy	Same as above	Same as above	180°
Relaser	Same as above	Same as above	360°

incision should be at least 2 to 3 mm in length, and multiple incisions may be planned if treating greater than 180° of the ciliary ring. Even though the endoprobe is only 1 mm in diameter, a larger incision allows lateral movement of the probe and access to a larger area of the ciliary ring. Epinephrine (1:10,000) is administered intracamerally for pupil dilation and vasoconstriction. Intracameral 0.3 mL of lidocaine hydrochloride 2% can also offer mydriasis and intraocular analgesia.[40,41]

When combining ECP with phacoemulsification and IOL implantation, or intracapsular lens extraction (ICLE), the lens surgery is performed first, followed by sulcus inflation and ECP treatment (described later). Once the desired treatment area is completed, the IOL is placed in the capsule, and the incisions are closed, leaving 1 incision untied until irrigation aspiration of the viscoelastic in the anterior chamber is completed.

Pars Plana Approach (Pseudophakic, Aphakic)

A pars plana approach is only feasible in pseudophakic and aphakic patients because of the size of the lens and the high risk for lens trauma with this technique (see **Fig. 10**). Two to 3 sclerotomies are required for this procedure. Smith and colleagues[25] identified scleral penetration sites for the 4 quadrants of the canine eye. If working superiorly, a 5 to 6 mm (5 mm dorsonasal; 6 mm dorsotemporal) works well for most breeds.

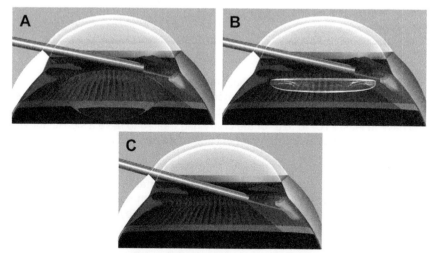

Fig. 9. Limbal approach in phakic (*A*), pseudophakic (*B*), and aphakic (*C*) patients. The laser endoscope is inserted through the limbal incision and through the pupillary space to access the CPs.

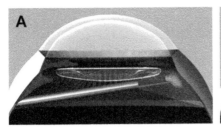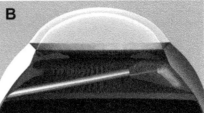

Fig. 10. Pars plana approach in pseudophakic (*A*) and aphakic (*B*) patients. The endoprobe is inserted from a sclerotomy site to access the CPs.

The nasal quadrant should be avoided in the Siberian husky because of a narrow pars plana nasally in this breed.[27]

For the 2-port procedure, 1 sclerotomy is used for vitrectomy, and the other for the endoprobe using an infusion sleeve around one of these instruments. A 3-port procedure uses a third sclerotomy for an infusion line. It is important to prevent hypotony during pars plana ECP in order to limit the risks for retinal detachment and spontaneous choroidal hemorrhage.

Vitrectomy, as described by Vainisi, and colleagues,[27] is performed before endoprobe insertion. Vitrectomy is only performed around the treatment site, around the CPs and instrument entry site before ECP treatment.

ENDOSCOPIC CYCLOPHOTOCOAGULATION TREATMENT AND TECHNIQUES

Treatment goals
• Treat entire CP: heads and tails
• Tissue shrinking and blanching
• Avoid tissue pop
• Greater than or equal to 270° for glaucoma treatment
• One-hundred and eighty degrees for prophylactic therapy

Species, breed, presumed cause of glaucoma, reliance on numerous glaucoma medications, lens status, and degree of IOP increase before surgery all influence the surgical protocol developed for each patient. In general, most cases with glaucoma should have at least 270° to 320° of the ciliary ring treated to have a significant effect in reducing the IOP. The extent of treatment should be planned according to each patient's criteria.

After the intraocular approach, the ciliary sulcus is inflated using a sodium hyaluronate viscoelastic. Sulcus inflation is the most important aspect of the surgical technique in order to have good access to the CPs. Sodium hyaluronate viscoelastics are the only appropriate viscoelastics for ECP,[42] and methylcellulose viscoelastics should be avoided because the laser energy is diverted. Injecting viscoelastic between the iris and lens, displacing the iris anteriorly and the lens posteriorly, allows good visualization of the CPs. Sulcus inflation with viscoelastic has to be repeated multiple times during surgery in order to avoid contact with the lens and posterior surface of the iris, especially in phakic patients (Video 2). In pseudophakic patients, sulcus inflation is easier, because the lens capsule or IOL implant can easily be displaced posteriorly. In aphakic patients, the goal is to displace the iris anteriorly to avoid touching the posterior surface of the iris with the endoprobe.

The laser endoscope is inserted through the incision to access the CPs. For most surgeons, a straight probe is easier to use and manipulate inside the eye than a curved probe. However, the straight probe can only treat 180° of the ciliary ring through 1 incision; therefore, at least 2 incisions should be performed to treat greater than 180°. Using a curved probe, up to 300° of the ciliary ring can be treated through 1 incision. Maintaining an image orientation corresponding with the anatomy is recommended. Keeping the posterior surface of the iris above and the CPs below on the image of the video monitor can be helpful. The probe is placed at a distance that allows visualization of at least 6 CPs (**Fig. 11**), but this may vary according to treatment technique and tissue effect response (**Box 1**).

The treatment goal is to treat the entire CP, but this may not be possible; therefore, the treatment zone is planned before surgery but determined during surgery. In an attempt to treat the entire CP, the anterior (heads) and posterior (tails) portions of the CP should be ablated. The valleys between each CP are also treated (**Fig. 12**). One-third of the posterior portion of the CP (near the pars plana) should be spared to prevent postoperative retinal edema. In phakic patients, the tails are not accessible without extensive lens damage, and only the heads can be treated; therefore, treating 320° to 360° of the ciliary ring should be considered. Treatment of the CP tails can be performed through a limbal approach in combination with phacoemulsification or ICLE, pseudophakic or aphakic patients, or via pars plana approach. The degrees of the treatment zone are then determined by the amount of CP ablation accomplished; the fewer the tails that can be treated, the higher the degrees of ciliary ring that should be targeted, and vice versa.

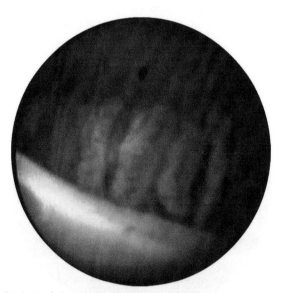

Fig. 11. Endoscopic view of the CPs displayed on the monitor. From top to bottom of the image: posterior surface of the iris, 6 CPs, and lens. The red aiming beam can be seen on the CP.

Box 1
ECP treatment technique

Microendoscope

- Curved probe (can treat up to 300° through 1 incision)
- Straight probe (can treat 180° through 1 incision)

Laser power density

- A function of laser power setting, duration of exposure, and distance
- Laser intensity varies with the distance of the endoprobe to the target
  - Small treatment area; close to CP, low power, short duration
  - Large treatment area; distant to CP, high power, long duration
  - Less intensity; distant to CP, low power, short duration
  - More intensity; closer to CP, high power, long duration

Methods

- Single CP treatment
- Painting or sweeping across the ciliary ring

Technique

- Limbal approach; combined ECP and IOL, pseudophakic
  - Over the capsule
  - Through the capsule

The desired tissue effect is CP shrinking and blanching (**Fig. 13**, Video 3). Laser power levels range between 100 mW and 1000 mW with continuous wave duration if using the E2 console, or at 9000 milliseconds if using the E4 console (see **Table 3**). Starting at 0.25 W of laser power, the laser energy is then adjusted until the desired

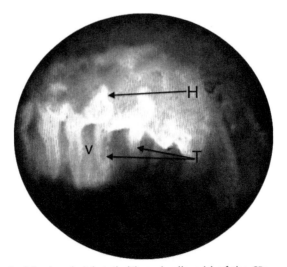

Fig. 12. Treatment of the heads (H), tails (T), and valleys (v) of the CPs.

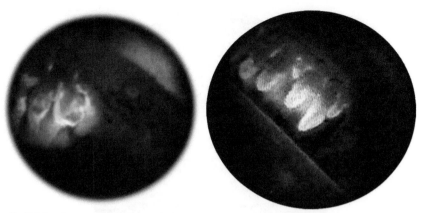

Fig. 13. Whitening and shrinking of the CP is observed with laser treatment.

tissue effect is reached. The amount of laser energy applied and the degrees of CB ablation are calibrated to fit each patient's needs, as previously described (see **Table 3**). The advantage of using a continuous mode of laser delivery is that the surgeon controls the amount of laser delivered with a footswitch pedal. A long, low-intensity application substantially controls what happens at the tissue level, minimizing the risk of overtreatment and undertreatment. The distance between the endoprobe and the CP also directly influences the degree of tissue effect (see **Box 1**), and overtreatment characterized by photodisruption (pop) must be avoided (Video 4). Laser energy setting and transmission are better preserved when the distance of the probe is 2 mm from the targeted tissue; this distance correlates with a field of view corresponding with 6 CPs.[43] If the probe is closer to the tissue, the energy delivered is higher than the assigned energy setting, whereas decreased energy transmission occurs at a distance greater than 2 mm from the tissue. These tissue variations can be visually assessed and corrected using ECP, whereas TSCP may result in overtreatment or undertreatment.

Color dilute dogs, carrying the recessive melanophilin gene (blue, recessive red, or Isabella color dogs), may require higher energies, because visible tissue effect is often difficult. Despite a pigmented appearance of the CB, an incomplete response to tissue blanching and shrinking occurs, and most surgeons increase the laser power to 1.0 W to obtain the desired tissue effect (**Fig. 14**, Video 5). In the author's experience, ECP in color dilute dogs is effective despite inconsistent real-time CP tissue blanching and shrinking. This clinical experience is supported by a report that showed histologic evaluation of cyclophotocoagulated lightly pigmented CPs, in which cyclodestructive properties were evident in all cases.[44] Because cyclodestruction occurs in lightly pigmented CPs despite the lack of real-time visible tissue response, overtreatment could be a common potential complication. Although there is no difference in pigment amount in the pigmented ciliary epithelium in dogs with blue or brown irises, the amount of pigment at the base of the CPs may differ.[29]

Different surgical techniques used to treat the CPs include a single-process technique versus a technique of sweeping or painting across the ciliary ring. As the CP heads shrink, the ciliary tails become visible and can then easily be treated (Video 6). In phakic patients with glaucoma, combining ECP and phacoemulsification offers the advantage of treating the CPs over the capsule (over-the-bag technique), and/or through the capsule (through-the-bag technique) before IOL implantation (**Fig. 15**).

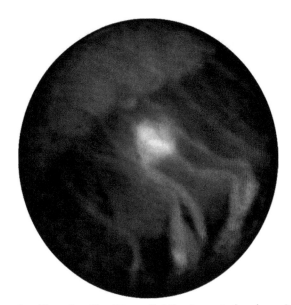

Fig. 14. CPs of a color dilute dog. The CPs are lightly pigmented and require high energy to obtain shrinking and blanching to obtain shrinking and blanching.

At the conclusion of phacoemulsification, the sulcus is inflated and treatment of the ciliary heads is performed. If further treatment to the tails is desired, the lens capsule is inflated with viscoelastic, and access and treatment to the entire CPs can easily be performed through the bag, but the laser energy needs to be increased for better tissue response.

Once the treatment is completed from a limbal approach, viscoelastic is removed from the anterior segment using irrigation/aspiration, leaving viscoelastic around the sulcus. Leaving viscoelastic material around the treatment area seems to help decrease inflammation postoperatively. When a pars plana approach is used, the viscoelastic material does not need to be removed. Incisions are closed routinely and 0.15 mL of dexamethasone sodium phosphate 4 mg/mL (individual vial dosing) is administered intracamerally. Real quantification of the total energy used during treatment is not possible because it is influenced not just by power and duration but also by other nonrecordable variables, like the distance of the laser source from the target and the angular direction of the beam.

Pearls for ECP

- Low-intensity, slow coagulation, thorough CP treatment (heads and tails)
- Treat greater than or equal to 270°
- Leave viscoelastic in the sulcus
- Intracameral 2% lidocaine to decrease postoperative discomfort
- Intracameral dexamethasone sodium phosphate at the conclusion of the procedure helps decrease postoperative inflammation
- Intense postoperative antiinflammatory treatment plays a significant role in surgical outcome
- Maintain IOP control during the first week postoperatively

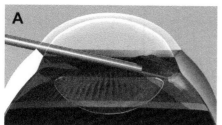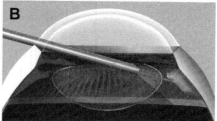

Fig. 15. Combined ECP and IOL implantation using the over-the-bag technique (*A*) and the through-the-bag (*B*) technique.

POSTOPERATIVE MANAGEMENT

Controlling postoperative inflammation is crucial. A high-frequency medical regimen is deemed necessary to improve postoperative outcome (**Table 4**). IOP control can be challenging in the first week after surgery. Even if IOP is less than 25 mm Hg, a topical carbonic anhydrase inhibitor (CAI) is recommended. Approximately 30% of patients undergoing ECP have increased IOPs (>25 mm Hg) postoperatively, some requiring aqueocentesis to decrease IOP.[45,46]

If IOP increases occur in the first week after surgery, topical and systemic CAI, a topical β-blocker, and a prostaglandin analogue are added to the medical regimen. These medications can then be tapered according to IOP levels at reevaluations. IOP is monitored aggressively for the next 24 hours, with recommended follow-ups at 1 week, 2 weeks, 4 to 6 weeks, and every 3 months thereafter.

Uncontrolled IOP during the first week after surgery should not be considered a postoperative failure because IOP usually stabilizes by the second week of surgery. Long term, a lower number of glaucoma medications are needed in most patients after ECP compared with the number of medications used before surgery.[45,46] Adjusting the medical regimen during the first week is of great significance for surgical outcome. Owners' compliance is also a critical factor that contributes to the success rate of the surgical procedure.

SUCCESS RATE

Because of direct visualization, there is less potential for overtreatment, and adjacent tissues are spared, leading to less postoperative inflammation and fewer complications.[47,48] Studies that describe histopathologic changes of the CB after treatment with ECP in other mammal species consistently report ciliary epithelium damage, sparing damage to the ciliary stroma, ciliary muscle, and adjacent tissue, unlike what has been shown with TSCP.[12,49,50] However, histologic studies of the chronic changes in the CB in dogs after ECP treatment are still lacking.

Numerous studies have reported ECP to be a successful surgical treatment of refractory glaucoma,[47,48,51–54] and when used in combination with cataract surgery.[55,56] Evaluation of ECP in the bovine and equine eye revealed adequate energy delivery and desired tissue effect.[57,58] ECP in feline and canine glaucoma has been performed since 2004, and reports describe promising results for the treatment of primary and secondary glaucoma.[45,46,59,60] ECP in feline glaucoma showed more than 90% success in long-term IOP control and sight preservation, with a decrease in glaucoma medications in 67% of the patients.[59] ECP for the treatment of canine primary and secondary glaucoma in 292 eyes revealed long-term IOP control and a decrease in

Table 4
Suggested ECP postoperative management

	Antiinflammatory Medications			Glaucoma Medications			Artificial Tears
	Topical		Systemic	Topical		Systemic	Topical
	Prednisolone Acetate 1%	Diclofenac[a] or Nepafenac	Prednisone (0.5 mg/kg)or Carprofen (2.2 mg/kg)	Dorzolamide or Dorzolamide/Timolol	Prostaglandin Analogue[a]	Methazolamide[a] (2 mg/kg)	
Immediate	Q2 h	Q2 h	Q12 h/Q12 h	Q8 h	—	± Q8–12 h	—
1 wk	Q4 h	Q4 h	Q12–24 h/Q12 h	Q8 h	± Q12 h	± Q8–12 h	Q6 h
2 wk	Q6 h	Q6 h	Q48 h/Q12 h	Q8 h	± Q12 h	± Q12–24 h	Q8 h
4 wk	Q8 h	Q8 h	—	Q8 h	—	According to IOP	Q12 h
2–3 mo	Q12 h	Q12 h	—	Q8 h	—	According to IOP	Q12 h

[a] If IOP is >30 mm Hg, diclofenac frequency is decreased and oral carbonic anhydrase inhibitor and prostaglandin analogues are added to the medical regimen.

glaucoma medications.[45] The efficacy in IOP control, sight preservation, and decrease in glaucoma medications after ECP was similar in cases with primary and secondary glaucoma. IOP was controlled in 80% of the patients 1 year postoperatively, and 70% were sighted. The success of IOP control in cases with primary glaucoma decreased to 50% 3 years postoperatively, with all maintaining vision. Although retrospective clinical results are promising, prospective, randomized controlled studies of the advantages of ECP compared with other procedures are still lacking.

COMPLICATIONS

Potential postoperative complications
• Intraocular inflammation, with or without fibrin
• Ectropion uvea
• Corneal edema
• Corneal ulceration
• Cataract
• Uncontrolled IOP
• Phthisis bulbi

The most common postoperative finding is intraocular inflammation. Minimal inflammation is seen in the first 2 days postoperatively. Inflammation worsens by the third day following surgery, so maintaining a high-frequency antiinflammatory protocol is important. Moderate inflammation occurs during the 3 to 5 days postoperatively, and slowly resolves over the subsequent 2 weeks. Severe inflammation and fibrin formation is usually a result of overtreatment.

There is a low incidence of corneal edema, corneal ulceration, and phthisis bulbi. Ectropion uvea occurs in all patients. A 30% incidence of cataract formation after ECP has been reported, hence the most commonly performed and recommended surgical protocol is to combine ECP with phacoemulsification and IOL implantation.[42,45,46]

If uncontrolled IOP is observed by the second week postoperatively, ECP can be repeated, and 360° of CPs should be treated.

SUMMARY

Advancements in the technology and surgical techniques of laser application seem promising in the treatment of glaucoma in veterinary medicine. CPC techniques in canine glaucoma can be modified according to each patient's need.

There are advantages and disadvantages for each CPC procedure (**Table 5**). Although TSCP is a noninvasive procedure that is easy to perform, ECP is invasive, requires expensive instrumentation, and poses a steeper learning curve than TSCP.

At present, recommended protocols for TSCP potentially cause overtreatment and damage to the adjacent tissues, resulting in a higher degree of complications. Reevaluation of this technique without audible pops should be considered, and may offer a better long-term outcome. Direct visualization of the targeted CB allows safer and more tailored treatment compared with TSCP techniques, offering a better prognosis for long-term vision and IOP control (see **Table 5**).

Table 5
Comparison of TSCP and ECP

	TSCP	ECP
Advantages	Noninvasive procedure Minimal learning curve	Direct visualization of target tissue Less energy required for treatment Treatment outcome can be controlled Can be performed in combination with cataract surgery or lens removal
Disadvantages	Blind laser delivery Overtreatment or undertreatment risk Damage to adjacent tissue Higher rate of serious complications	Invasive procedure Equipment expense Intense postoperative treatment More advanced/higher learning curve
Laser energy (W)	1–1.5	0.25
IOP control up to 1 y (%)	50–92[28–30]	81–84[45]
Vision up to 1 y (%)	50–53[28,29]	72–74[45]

CPC should be promptly recommended when progressive signs of glaucoma are seen and/or medical treatment fails to control IOP. As surgical experience improves, CPC techniques may be recommended earlier and could offer a better long-term prognosis for vision preservation.

SUPPLEMENTARY DATA

Supplementary data related to this article can be found online at http://dx.doi.org/10.1016/j.cvsm.2015.06.007.

REFERENCES

1. Plummer CE, Regnier A, Gelatt KN. The canine glaucomas. In: Gelatt KN, Gilger BC, Kern TJ, editors. Veterinary ophthalmology, vol. 2, 5th edition. Ames (IA): Wiley & Sons; 2013. p. 1050–145.
2. Vogt A. Versuche zur intraokularen druckherabsetzung mittelst diathermieschädigung des corpus ciliare Zyklodiathermiestichelung. Klin Monatsbl Augenheilkd 1936;97:672–3.
3. Brightman A, Vestre W, Helper L, et al. Cryosurgery for the treatment of canine glaucoma. J Am Anim Hosp Assoc 1982;18:319–22.
4. Meredith R, Gelatt KN. Cryotherapy in veterinary ophthalmology. Vet Clin North Am 1980;10:837–46.
5. Robert S, Severin G, Lavach J. Evaluation of a liquid nitrogen system. J Am Anim Hosp Assoc 1984;20:823–33.
6. Vestre W, Brightman A. Ciliary body temperatures during cyclocryotherapy in the clinically normal dog. Am J Vet Res 1983;44:187–94.
7. Vestre W, Brightman A. Effects of cyclocryosurgery on the clinically normal canine eye. Am J Vet Res 1983;44:187–94.
8. Coleman D, Lizz FL, Driller J, et al. Therapeutic ultrasound in the treatment of glaucoma. II. Clinical applications. Ophthalmology 1985;92:347–53.

9. Beckman H, Sugar H. Neodymium laser cyclophotocoagulation. Arch Ophthalmol 1973;90:27–8.
10. Nassise M, Davidson M, McLachian N, et al. Neodymium:yttrium, aluminum, and garnet laser energy delivered transsclerally to the ciliary body of dogs. Am J Vet Res 1988;49:1972–8.
11. Sapienza J, Miller T, Gum G, et al. Contact transscleral cyclophotocoagulation using a neodymium:yttrium aluminum garnet laser in normal dogs. Prog Vet Comp Ophthalmol 1992;2:147–53.
12. Lin S, Chen M, Lin M, et al. Vascular effects on ciliary tissue from endoscopic versus trans-scleral cyclophotocoagulation. Br J Ophthalmol 2005;90:496–500.
13. Cavens VJK, Gemensky-Metzler A, Wilkie DA, et al. The long-term effects of semiconductor diode laser transscleral cyclophotocoagulation on the normal equine eye and intraocular pressure. Vet Ophthalmol 2012;15(6):369–75.
14. Nadelstein B, Wilcock B, Cook C, et al. Clinical and histopathologic effects of diode laser transscleral cyclophotocoagulation in the normal canine eye. Vet Comp Ophthalmol 1997;7:155–62.
15. Quinn R, Tingey D, Parkinson K, et al. Histopathologic and thermographic comparisons of ND: YAG and diode laser contact transscleral cyclophotocoagulation in enucleated canine eyes. Vet Ophthalmol 1994;24:72.
16. Nassise M, Davidson M, English R, et al. Treatment of glaucoma by use of transscleral neodymium:yttrium aluminum garnet laser cyclocoagulation in dogs. J Am Vet Med Assoc 1990;197:350–3.
17. Frankhauser F, Frankhauser-Kwasniewska S, England C, et al. Laser cyclophotocoagulation in glaucoma therapy. Ophthalmol Clin North Am 1993;6:449–71.
18. Gilmour MA. Lasers in ophthalmology. Vet Clin Small Anim 2001;32:649–72.
19. Pastor S, Singh K, Lee D, et al. Cyclophotocoagulation: a report by the American Academy of Ophthalmology. Ophthalmology 2001;108:2130–8.
20. Smith R, Stein M. Ocular hazards of transscleral laser radiation. Am J Ophthalmol 1968;66(1):21–32.
21. Vogel A, Dlugos C, Nuffer R, et al. Optical properties of human sclera, and their consequences for transscleral laser applications. Lasers Surg Med 1991;11:331–40.
22. Whingham H, Brooks D, Andrew S, et al. Treatment of equine glaucoma by transscleral neodymium:yttrium aluminum garnet laser cyclophotocoagulation: a retrospective study of 23 eyes of 16 horses. Vet Ophthalmol 1999;2:243–50.
23. Kraus CL, Tychsen L, Leder GT, et al. Comparison of the effectiveness and safety of transscleral cyclophotocoagulation and endoscopic cyclophotocoagulation in pediatric glaucoma. J Pediatr Ophthalmol Strabismus 2014;51(2):120–7.
24. Cook C. Surgery for glaucoma. Vet Clin North Am Small Anim Pract 1997;27(5):1109–29.
25. Smith P, Penner L, MacKay E, et al. Identification of sclerotomy sites for posterior segment surgery in the dog. Vet Comp Ophthalmol 1997;7:180–91.
26. Sullivan T, Davidson M, Nassise M, et al. Canine retinopexy-a determination of surgical landmarks and comparison of cryoapplication, and diode laser methods. Prog Vet Comp Ophthalmol 1997;7:89–95.
27. Vainisi SJ, Wolfer JC, Hoffman AR. Surgery of the canine posterior segment. In: Gelatt KN, Gilger B, Kern T, editors. Veterinary ophthalmology, vol. 2, 5th edition. Ames (IA): Wiley-Blackwell; 2013. p. 1393–431.
28. Cook C, Davidson M, Brinkmann M, et al. Diode laser transscleral cyclophotocoagulation for the treatment of glaucoma in dogs: results of six and twelve months follow-up. Vet Comp Ophthalmol 1997;7:148–54.

29. Hardman C, Stanley R. Diode laser transscleral cyclophotocoagulation for the treatment of primary glaucoma in 18 dogs: a retrospective study. Vet Ophthalmol 2001;4(3):209–15.

30. O'Reilly A, Hardman C, Stanley R. The use of transscleral cyclophotocoagulation with a diode laser for the treatment of glaucoma occurring post intracapsular extraction of displaced lenses: a retrospective study of 15 dogs (1995-2000). Vet Ophthalmol 2003;6(2):113–9.

31. Rebolleda G, Munoz F, Murube J. Audible pops during cyclodiode procedures. J Glaucoma 1999;8:177–83.

32. Pizzirani S, Desai S, Pirie C, et al. Age related changes in the anterior segment of the eye in normal dogs. Vet Ophthalmol 2010;13(6):421.

33. Newkirk KM, Haines D, Calvarese S, et al. Distribution and amount of pigment within the ciliary body and iris of dogs with blue and brown irides. Vet Ophthalmol 2010;13(2):76–80.

34. Gaasterland D. Diode laser cyclophotocoagulation. Technique and results. Glaucoma Today 2009;7(2):35–8.

35. Amagai Y, Kaoru K, Matsuda H, et al. Diode laser transscleral cyclophotocoagulation in combination with trabeculectomy for surgical therapy of canine refractory glaucoma. J Vet Med Res 2014;1(2):1010.

36. Bentley E, Miller P, Murphy C, et al. Combined cycloablation and gonioimplantation for treatment of glaucoma in dogs: 18 cases (1992-1998). J Am Vet Med Assoc 1999;215(10):1469–72.

37. Sapienza J, van der Woerdt A. Combined transscleral cyclophotocoagulation and Ahmed gonioimplantation in dogs with primary glaucoma: 51 cases (1996-2004). Vet Ophthalmol 2005;8(2):121–7.

38. Aquino M, Barton K, Tan A, et al. Micropulse versus continuous wave transscleral diode cyclophotocoagulation in refractory glaucoma: a randomized exploratory study. Clin Experiment Ophthalmol 2015;43(1):40–6.

39. Tan A, Chockalingam M, Aquino M, et al. Micropulse transscleral diode laser cyclophotocoagulation in the treatment of refractory glaucoma. Clin Experiment Ophthalmol 2010;38(3):266–72.

40. Park SA, Park YW, Son WG, et al. Evaluation of the analgesic effect of intracameral lidocaine hydrochloride injection on intraoperative and postoperative pain in healthy dogs undergoing phacoemulsification. Am J Vet Res 2010;71(2):216–22.

41. Park SA, Kim N, Park YW, et al. Evaluation of mydriatic effect of intracameral lidocaine hydrochloride injection in eyes of clinically normal dogs. Am J Vet Res 2009;70(12):1521–5.

42. Uram M. Endoscopy surgery in ophthalmology. Philadelphia: Lippincott Williams and Wilkins; 2003.

43. Yu JY, Kahook M, Lathrop K, et al. The effect of probe placement and type of viscoelastic material on endoscopic cyclophotocoagulation laser energy transmission. Ophthalmic Surg Lasers Imaging 2006;39(2):133–6.

44. Fritz K, Ko P, Newkirk K, et al. The use of intravenous indocyanine green (ICG) dye as an adjunctive photodynamic agent when performing canine endoscopic cyclophotocoagulation (ECP). Vet Ophthalmol 2012;16(1):E7.

45. Lutz EA, Webb TE, Bras ID, et al. Diode endoscopic cyclophotocoagulation in dogs with primary and secondary glaucoma: 292 cases (2004-2013). Vet Ophthalmol 2013;16(6):40.

46. Bras ID, Robbin TE, Wyman M, et al. Diode endoscopic cyclophotocoagulation in canine and feline glaucoma. Vet Ophthalmol 2005;8(6):449.

47. Uram M. Endoscopic cyclophotocoagulation in glaucoma management. Curr Opin Ophthalmol 1995;11:19–29.
48. Uram M. Endoscopic cyclophotocoagulation in glaucoma management: indications, results, and complications. Ophthalmic Practice 1995;13:173–85.
49. Pancheva MB, Kahook M, Schuman J, et al. Comparison of acute structural and histopathological changes of the porcine ciliary processes after endoscopic cyclophotocoagulation and transscleral cyclophotocoagulation. Clin Experiment Ophthalmol 2007;35:270–4.
50. Pantcheva MB, Kahook MY, Schuman J, et al. Comparison of acute structural and histopathological changes in human autopsy eyes after endoscopic cyclophotocoagulation and trans-scleral cyclophotocoagulation. Br J Ophthalmol 2007; 91(2):248–52.
51. Berke S. Endolaser cyclophotocoagulation in glaucoma management. Tech Ophthalmol 2006;4:74–81.
52. Francis B, Kawji A, Dustin L, et al. Endoscopic cyclophotocoagulation (ECP) in the management of uncontrolled glaucoma with prior aqueous tube shunt. J Glaucoma 2011;20(8):523–7.
53. Uram M. Ophthalmic laser microendoscopy ciliary process ablation in the management of neovascular glaucoma. Ophthalmology 1992;99:1823–8.
54. Uram M. Diode laser endocyclodestruction. Ophthalmic Surg 1994;25:268–9.
55. Francis B, Berke S, Dustin L, et al. Endoscopic cyclophotocoagulation combined with phacoemulsification versus phacoemulsification alone in medically controlled glaucoma. J Cataract Refract Surg 2014;40:1313–21.
56. Uram M. Combined phacoemulsification, endoscopic cyclophotocoagulation, and intraocular lens insertion in glaucoma management. Ophthalmic Surg 1995;26:346–52.
57. Harrington J, McMullen R Jr, Cullen J, et al. Diode laser endoscopic cyclophotocoagulation in the normal equine eye. Vet Ophthalmol 2013;16(2):97–110.
58. Harrington J, McMullen R Jr, Cullen J, et al. Evaluation of diode endoscopic cyclophotocoagulation in bovine cadaver eyes. Am J Vet Res 2012;73(9):1445–52.
59. Bras ID, Webb TE. Diode endoscopic cyclophotocoagulation in feline glaucoma. Vet Ophthalmol 2009;12(6):407.
60. Lutz EA, Sapienza J. Diode endoscopic cyclophotocoagulation in pseudophakic and aphakic dogs with secondary glaucoma. Vet Ophthalmol 2008;11(6):423.

Feline Glaucoma

Gillian J. McLellan, BVMS, PhD, MRCVS[a,b,c,]*,
Leandro B.C. Teixeira, DVM, MS[c,d]

KEYWORDS

- Cat • Feline • Uveitis • Neoplasia • Primary glaucoma • Congenital glaucoma
- Secondary glaucoma • Treatment

KEY POINTS

- Feline glaucoma is most commonly secondary to other ocular or systemic disease.
- Clinical signs of glaucoma are more insidious in onset and subtle in cats than in dogs.
- The clinical management of feline glaucoma is complicated by unwelcome side effects and by poor compliance with frequent, long-term application of topical medications.

AQUEOUS HUMOR DYNAMICS IN CATS

As in dogs and most other vertebrate species, maintenance of normal intraocular pressure (IOP) in cats relies on a delicate balance between aqueous humor outflow and production. In cats, more than 97% of aqueous humor produced at the level of the nonpigmented epithelium of the ciliary processes exit the eye by the conventional route: through the pupil from the posterior to anterior chamber, then via the trabecular meshwork, located within a long and relatively wide ciliary cleft, and collector channels of the angular aqueous plexus into the intrascleral venous plexus (**Fig. 1**), and ultimately, the general circulation.[1] Only a very small proportion (<3%) of aqueous humor outflow occurs by the uveoscleral route in cats: through the iris and ciliary body stroma to the suprachoroidal circulation and vortex veins, and through the sclera to the episcleral tissues.[2]

EPIDEMIOLOGY AND CAUSES OF GLAUCOMA IN CATS

Compared with the situation in dogs, glaucoma is a relatively uncommon clinical diagnosis in the cat, accounting for less than 0.3% feline diagnoses in the Veterinary

The authors have nothing to disclose.
[a] Department of Ophthalmology and Visual Sciences, University of Wisconsin-Madison, 1300 University Avenue, Madison, WI 53706, USA; [b] Department of Surgical Sciences, University of Wisconsin-Madison, 2015 Linden Drive, Madison, WI 53706, USA; [c] McPherson Eye Research Institute, University of Wisconsin-Madison, Madison, WI 53706, USA; [d] Department of Pathobiological Sciences, University of Wisconsin-Madison, 2015 Linden Drive, Madison, WI 53706, USA
* Corresponding author. Department of Surgical Sciences, School of Veterinary Medicine, 2015 Linden Drive, Madison, WI 53706.
E-mail address: mclellan@vetmed.wisc.edu

Vet Clin Small Anim 45 (2015) 1307–1333
http://dx.doi.org/10.1016/j.cvsm.2015.06.010
0195-5616/15/$ – see front matter © 2015 Elsevier Inc. All rights reserved.

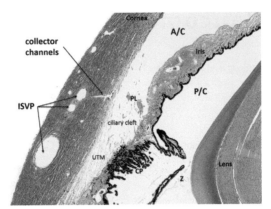

Fig. 1. Structures relevant to aqueous humor outflow in the anterior segment of a normal cat. A/C, anterior chamber; CP, ciliary processes; ISVP, intrascleral venous plexus; P/C, posterior chamber; PL, pectinate ligament; UTM, uveal trabecular meshwork; Z, lens zonule. Hematoxylin and Eosin.

Medical Database.[3] However, this figure may underestimate the actual prevalence of glaucoma, and it is likely that many feline cases go unrecognized. In a prospective study that screened ostensibly normal cats 7 years of age and older, 0.9% had abnormally high IOP.[4] Glaucoma also appears to be a rather common indication for enucleation in cats, representing 29% of feline globe submissions to the Comparative Ocular Pathology Laboratory of Wisconsin (COPLOW).[5]

> Primary glaucoma is rare in cats. Most cases of feline glaucoma are secondary to other underlying ocular or systemic disease.

In a recent, unpublished review of more than 3200 feline submissions to COPLOW that had a histologic diagnosis of glaucoma, more than half had evidence of ocular neoplasia, and less than one-fourth had histologic findings consistent with underlying lymphoplasmacytic uveitis (**Fig. 2**). Specific causes of glaucoma in cats are summarized in **Table 1** and discussed in detail in later sections.

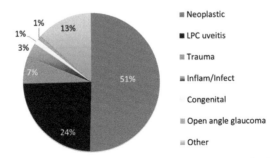

Fig. 2. Relative distribution of the causes of feline glaucoma identified in 3212 glaucomatous eyes submitted to the COPLOW over an approximately 30-year period from 1983 to 2015. Chronic lymphoplasmacytic (LPC) uveitis and neoplasia are leading causes of glaucoma, together accounting for 75% of feline glaucoma diagnoses. Inflamm/Infect, glaucoma secondary to intraocular inflammation, with or without confirmed infection.

Table 1
Causes of glaucoma in cats, with possible locations of aqueous humor outflow obstruction

Primary Glaucoma	
Open angle glaucoma	Uncommon, older cats of any breed may be bilateral, or unilateral/asymmetric in presentation
	Location of outflow obstruction: vascular channels associated with aqueous outflow
Congenital glaucoma	Sporadic in any breed; recessively inherited in Siamese
	May be associated with other congenital ocular abnormalities
Angle closure glaucoma	Very rare, presumed congenital
	Reported in association with gonioscopic abnormalities (pectinate ligament dysplasia)
Secondary Glaucoma	
Neoplasia	Most common cause of glaucoma in cats
	Outflow blocked by obliteration of outflow pathways by infiltrates of neoplastic cells (eg, feline diffuse anterior uveal melanoma and lymphoma)
Uveitis	Commonly seen with chronic lymphoplasmacytic uveitis
	Outflow may be blocked by cellular infiltrates in outflow pathways, extensive peripheral anterior synechiae, or posterior synechiae with iris bombé
Trauma	May be known or suspected history of blunt or penetrating trauma
	Outflow obstructed by inflammatory infiltrates, hemorrhage, or anatomic disruption of outflow pathways
Intraocular hemorrhage	Hyphema
	Erythrocytes or associated inflammation may obstruct aqueous outflow (eg, due to trauma, severe uveitis, or arterial hypertension)
Lens-associated glaucoma	Rare in cats
	Intumescent cataract rarely accompanies diabetes in cats and lens luxation seldom results in glaucoma
FAHMS	Occasionally seen in older cats
	Condensation of anterior vitreous diverts and traps aqueous humor in vitreous
	Diffusely shallow anterior chamber (vitreous, block)
Orbital space-occupying lesions	Uncommon cause of glaucoma, increase in IOP is usually modest
	Decreased aqueous humor outflow may result from increase in episcleral venous pressure
Steroid-induced ocular hypertension/glaucoma	Some cats susceptible to substantial increases in IOP following corticosteroid treatment. Reversible with prompt withdrawal of therapy

Note: Within individual patients, aqueous humor outflow may be obstructed at multiple sites.

Glaucoma in cats is invariably due to impaired aqueous humor outflow. Often outflow is impaired at multiple locations within the eye by pathologic processes that contribute to obstruction of aqueous humor flow through the pupil; closure of the iridocorneal angle; infiltration, collapse, or compression of the ciliary cleft and trabecular meshwork; or congenital or acquired abnormalities affecting the aqueous collector channels and scleral venous plexus. The complex nature of the underlying pathologic abnormality in many feline glaucoma patients contributes to the difficulty in treating glaucoma in this species. In order to create a rational treatment plan, tailored to the individual cat, the clinician must first identify the predominant mechanisms of outflow obstruction and any underlying disease in each case.

The importance of pursuing an etiologic diagnosis cannot be overstated, because this information is critical in determining which treatments are indicated (or contraindicated), the likely response of the patient to treatment, and the prognosis for retaining vision or even for survival of the animal.

PRIMARY GLAUCOMA IN CATS

By definition, the primary glaucomas have no other identifiable antecedent ocular disease. Primary glaucoma with goniodysgenesis appears to be quite rare in cats compared with dogs[6] and has only been reported sporadically. Although domestic shorthair and longhair cats are most frequently affected, the veterinary literature does suggest that certain cat breeds are predisposed to primary glaucoma, including the Siamese, Burmese, and Persian.[7–9] Open-angle glaucoma, and, less often, glaucoma associated with narrow to closed angles, and with pectinate ligament dysplasia, have been reported in middle-aged and older adult cats.[8–12]

Feline Open Angle Glaucoma

Although not commonly seen in practice, a form of open angle, open cleft glaucoma has been identified in feline eyes submitted for histologic evaluation.[13,14] The disease is characterized by an insidious, gradually progressive globe enlargement in middle-aged and older adult cats, with a mean age of around 10 years.[14] The disease may be unilateral or bilateral, but is frequently asymmetric in presentation, and several months or even years may elapse between diagnosis of glaucoma in the first affected eye and subsequent diagnosis in the contralateral eye. IOPs may be only moderately elevated, or may fluctuate widely, limiting the value of tonometry in diagnosis or monitoring of disease progression or response to therapy. Optic nerve damage and loss of retinal ganglion cells from the inner retina result in diminished pupillary light reflexes and pupil dilation. Optic disc cupping, although a consistent histopathologic feature, can be difficult to fully appreciate on ophthalmoscopy, particularly if the disease is bilateral in presentation. Histopathology of enucleated globes has identified characteristic myxomatous change within the vascular channels associated with aqueous outflow, including the scleral venous plexus and the vortex veins (**Fig. 3**).[13,14] No other lesions are recognizable within the iridocorneal angle or trabecular meshwork; thus, it is proposed that resistance to aqueous outflow may be posttrabecular at the level of the scleral venous plexus and vortex veins. However, the precise nature and significance of the myxomatous changes surrounding these vessels remain unclear, and no specific treatment has been established. Response to conventional medical therapies, such as topical carbonic anhydrase inhibitors (CAIs), seems to be highly variable between individuals, and loss of vision with subsequent enucleation is a common outcome in affected cats.

Feline Congenital Glaucoma

Congenital and early-onset glaucomas are seen sporadically in cats with various ocular malformations, which may include lens abnormalities (such as microphakia, macrophakia, ectopia lentis) or anterior uveal abnormalities (such as iridoschisis, pectinate ligament dysplasia, multiple iridociliary cysts, and persistent pupillary membranes).[8,15]

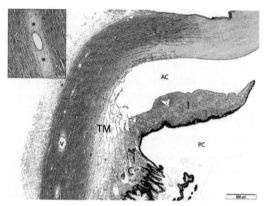

Fig. 3. Feline open angle glaucoma. Open ciliary cleft and normal trabecular meshwork. Inset shows high magnification of scleral vessels (v). Note the deposition of a myxomatous matrix (*asterisk*) surrounding the scleral vessels. AC, anterior chamber; C, ciliary body; I, iris; PC, posterior chamber; TM, trabecular meshwork. Hematoxylin and Eosin. Bar marker = 500 microns.

A research colony has been established from a pedigree of Siamese cats with a rare form of congenital glaucoma that shows simple autosomal-recessive inheritance.[16] These cats have bilaterally symmetric, slowly progressive glaucoma that can be recognized early in life by elongated ciliary processes, globe enlargement, and spherophakia (**Fig. 4**).[17] In kittens with this form of congenital glaucoma, there is an arrest in early postnatal development of the aqueous outflow pathways, resulting in IOP that is significantly higher than normal cats by 8 weeks of age[18,19] and gradually increases throughout the first 6 months of life in glaucomatous kittens. The underlying genetic mutation has now been identified (manuscript in process), but its prevalence within the breed has not yet been determined. Review of isolated case reports in the veterinary literature suggests that this form of glaucoma may have been present in the Siamese cat breed in the United States and Europe for many years.[20–22]

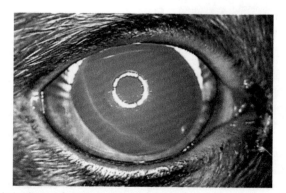

Fig. 4. Characteristic clinical features of recessively inherited congenital glaucoma in a Siamese cat. In this subject, in addition to globe enlargement, there are iris hypoplasia, prominent, elongated ciliary processes, and spherophakia. Haab striae, which represent tears in Descemet membrane, due to globe stretching are visible. Note the very limited degree of corneal edema in this subject. (*From* McLellan GJ and Miller PE. Feline glaucoma - a comprehensive review. Vet Ophthalmol 2011;14(Suppl 1):18; with permission.)

SECONDARY GLAUCOMA IN CATS

The secondary glaucomas constitute most cases of feline glaucoma and are most often diagnosed in adult cats. Secondary glaucoma results from antecedent ocular or systemic disease processes, most commonly neoplasia and uveitis (see **Fig. 2**, **Table 1**).[3,7,8,23,24] Secondary glaucoma is more often unilateral in presentation but, particularly when associated with systemic disease processes, can affect both eyes.

Glaucoma Secondary to Neoplasia

Intraocular neoplasia is a leading cause of glaucoma in cats and accounted for more than half of the feline glaucoma cases in the authors' recent review of the COPLOW archive.[3,8,10,23] In terms of incidence, anterior uveal melanoma (**Fig. 5**) and lymphoma (**Fig. 6**) predominate, although other tumor types, including post-traumatic ocular sarcoma[25,26] and iridociliary epithelial tumors,[27] may also be associated with secondary glaucoma in cats. Diffuse anterior uveal melanoma in particular seems to be a common cause of feline glaucoma and more than 10% of all feline submissions were diagnosed with glaucoma secondary to melanoma.[5]

Neoplasia may contribute to the development of glaucoma by several mechanisms, including diffuse infiltration and obliteration of the outflow pathways in the trabecular meshwork and ciliary cleft, or neovascular glaucoma associated with preiridal fibrovascular membranes and subsequent angle closure.[28]

Glaucoma Secondary to Uveitis

Intraocular inflammation, in particular lympho-plasmacytic uveitis, is a major cause of glaucoma in cats.[29] Chronic lymphoplasmacytic uveitis was identified as the cause of glaucoma in around one-fourth of cats in the authors' previously unreported large series of cases (see **Fig. 1**), and lymphoplasmacytic uveitis with glaucoma accounted for 10% of all feline submissions to the same diagnostic ocular pathology laboratory.[5]

Many different pathogenic mechanisms can contribute to the development of glaucoma in cats with intraocular inflammation.[5,7,8,10,23,30] Inflammatory infiltrates can obliterate the aqueous outflow pathways (**Fig. 7**), but the extent of these infiltrates

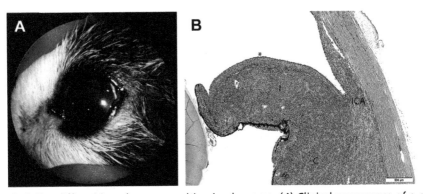

Fig. 5. Feline diffuse iris melanoma resulting in glaucoma. (*A*) Clinical appearance of a cat with secondary glaucoma secondary to diffuse infiltration of the anterior uveal tract with darkly pigmented melanocytes, resulting in pupil distortion. (*B*) Photomicrograph from another cat with a less pigmented neoplasm illustrates that the iris surface (*asterisk*), iris stroma (I), ciliary body (C), and iridocorneal angle (ICA) are infiltrated by a population of poorly pigmented neoplastic melanocytes that are obliterating the aqueous outflow pathways. Hematoxylin and Eosin. Bar marker = 500 microns.

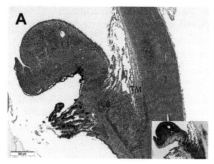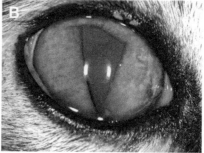

Fig. 6. Ocular lymphoma resulting in secondary glaucoma. (*A*) Neoplastic lymphocytes are diffusely infiltrating the iris stroma (I), ciliary body (*B*), and trabecular meshwork (TM). Note that the ciliary cleft is still open but the trabecular meshwork and the scleral veins (sv) are obliterated by the neoplastic cells. Hematoxylin and Eosin. Bar marker = 500 microns. (*Inset*) Uveal lymphoma in cats is often of B-lymphocyte origin shown by the positive immunohistochemical labeling for CD20. (*B*) Glaucoma secondary to uveal lymphoma. Neoplastic infiltrates often result in thickening and congestion of the iris and distortion of the pupil that may mimic uveitis. (*Courtesy of* John S. Sapienza, DVM, DACVO, Long Island Veterinary Specialists, Plainview, NY.)

can be highly variable, and chronic lymphoplasmacytic uveitis frequently leads to formation of preiridal fibrovascular membranes and extensive peripheral anterior synechiae that effectively close the opening to the ciliary cleft obstructing aqueous outflow. Chronic inflammation can also contribute to condensation, degeneration, and prolapse of vitreous as well as lens luxation (see later discussion).

Trauma

Both penetrating trauma (with subsequent inflammation, infection, or intraocular fibrosis) and blunt force trauma (that can cause intraocular hemorrhage or distortion of anterior segment anatomy, eg, angle recession) can result in secondary glaucoma.

In cats with penetrating ocular trauma (most often a cat claw injury), intractable uveitis and glaucoma may occur secondary to a phacoclastic uveitis or septic

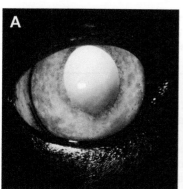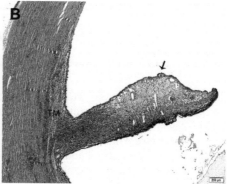

Fig. 7. (*A*) Features of chronic lymphoplasmacytic uveitis, including rubeosis iridis and keratic precipates, in a cat with secondary glaucoma. (*B*) Large numbers of lymphocytes and plasma cells infiltrating the iris stroma (I) and trabecular meshwork (TM) blocking aqueous outflow. Also note a preiridal fibrovascular membrane (*arrow*) on the anterior iris surface that contributes to peripheral anterior synechiae and angle closure. Hematoxylin and Eosin. Bar marker = 200 microns.

implantation syndrome resulting from lens trauma and intralenticular abscessation,[10,28,30,31] and in the longer-term, lens trauma may be associated with the development of post-traumatic ocular sarcoma that can, in turn, present as glaucoma.[32]

Angle recession may contribute to aqueous outflow obstruction and has been identified histologically in glaucomatous feline eyes,[10,28,33] but its role in the pathogenesis of glaucoma in cats has not yet been definitively established. In human patients with angle recession, it has been postulated that blunt force trauma deforms the globe, with a rebound effect on the lens that exerts traction on the ciliary body. In cats, however, a history of trauma is generally lacking, and concurrent lymphoplasmacytic uveitis is often seen in those eyes in which angle recession is identified.[5]

Intraocular Hemorrhage

Intraocular hemorrhage, in particular related to systemic hypertension in older cats, but also due to trauma, systemic bleeding disorders, intraocular neoplasia, and paraneoplastic disease, can lead to secondary glaucoma. Cats with single episodes of hemorrhage resulting in only a partial hyphema are unlikely to develop glaucoma, and blood cells are generally cleared from the anterior chamber over a matter of days. Development of acute, painful glaucoma secondary to intraocular hemorrhage is of particular concern in animals with "8-ball hyphema" caused by episodes of rebleeding that completely fill the anterior chamber with blood.

Management of glaucoma secondary to hyphema is especially challenging in cats with potentially life-threatening comorbidities. Therapy is generally limited to topical corticosteroids and CAIs, with attention to systemically administered analgesia as necessary. Although some advocate the judicious use of short-acting topical mydriatics to help limit the formation of synechiae in patients with hyphema, unless extensive posterior synechiae are identified, use of mydriatics is generally contraindicated in patients once glaucoma has become established secondary to hyphema.

Lens-Associated Secondary Glaucoma in Cats

Lens luxation in cats is only rarely considered primary and seldom plays a direct role in the pathogenesis of glaucoma in this species.[34]

> Unlike the situation in dogs with primary anterior lens luxation, acute glaucoma is seldom recognized, and anteriorly luxated lenses in cats are unlikely to be considered a surgical emergency.

Feline lens luxation is more often recognized secondary to chronic uveitis (**Fig. 8**) and glaucoma, resorbing cataract, or occasionally, as a result of senile degeneration of lens zonules in aged cats.[34]

Intumescent cataract and phacomorphic glaucoma resulting from this lens swelling is also rare in cats, perhaps related to the elliptical or slit-shape of the feline pupil that renders it resistant to conventional mechanisms of lens-associated pupil block.

Feline Aqueous Humor Misdirection Syndrome

In this unusual form of insidious glaucoma in older cats, a uniformly shallow anterior chamber leads to a very characteristic, striking clinical appearance (**Fig. 9**).[23,35,36] In addition to a shallow anterior chamber, affected eyes with Feline Aqueous Humor Misdirection Syndrome (FAHMS) often exhibit mydriasis.[3] As this form of glaucoma

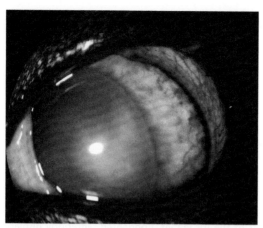

Fig. 8. Anterior lens luxation in a cat with chronic lymphoplasmacytic uveitis. As in many cats with lens luxation, this cat showed no signs of secondary glaucoma.

is frequently asymmetric, or unilateral at the time of initial presentation, anisocoria is often a feature of the disease. This feline condition bears some clinical resemblance to vitreous block glaucoma in people, but the degree of IOP elevation in affected cats is typically only modest, although occasionally, pronounced IOP elevation can be documented.[36]

Ocular ultrasonography and histopathology in affected cats reveal condensation and thickening of the anterior vitreous face, anterior displacement of the iris and lens by an expanded vitreous, and clear spaces in the vitreous cavity (**Fig. 10**). In FAHMS, it has been postulated that aqueous humor is misdirected posteriorly, rather than anteriorly through the pupil, and becomes trapped in the vitreous cavity leading to vitreous block glaucoma as anteriorly displaced vitreous becomes further compressed and tightly apposed against the lens and ciliary processes. This vitreous block glaucoma causes a cilio-vitreal-lenticular block that prevents flow of aqueous humor from the ciliary processes into the posterior chamber, further diverting aqueous humor into the vitreous cavity in a vicious cycle. Anterior displacement of the lens zonules and

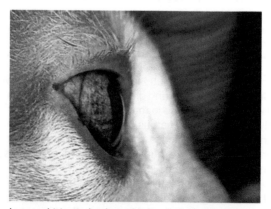

Fig. 9. FAHMS. The lens and iris are both pushed anteriorly, leading to a uniformly shallow anterior chamber, which is a striking feature of this syndrome.

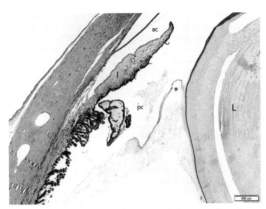

Fig. 10. FAHMS. Condensation and forward bowing of the anterior vitreous face (*asterisk*) and anterior displacement of the iris leaflet. Condensed, anteriorly displaced vitreous presents an Alcian blue-positive (proteoglycans) and a PAS-positive component. AC, anterior chamber; I, iris; L, lens; PC, posterior chamber. Alcian blue/PAS stain. Bar marker = 500 microns.

ciliary processes intensifies pupil block. With progressive increase in IOP and forward displacement of the iris-lens diaphragm, collapse of the ciliary cleft, compression of the trabecular meshwork, and narrowing of the iridocorneal angle ensues.[3,36]

Despite a strong rationale for surgical intervention in FAHMS, including phacoemulsification and anterior vitrectomy to relieve underlying mechanisms of pupil and vitreous block, postoperative outcomes are often disappointing. The slowly progressive nature of disease, and its tendency to affect mainly elderly animals that may have other serious systemic disease, favor conservative management. Topical CAIs, when tolerated, may be associated with preservation of limited vision in at least one eye for periods of up to several years.[36] In some affected cats, spontaneous restoration of anterior chamber depth, with normalization of IOP, has been observed.[3]

CLINICAL SIGNS AND DIAGNOSIS OF FELINE GLAUCOMA

> Diagnosis of glaucoma in cats should be based on observation of clinical signs that are often very subtle. Marked IOP fluctuation in affected animals means that the diagnosis or exclusion of glaucoma should not rely solely on IOP values.

In cats with glaucoma, moderate elevations in IOP are associated with few overt clinical signs. As the disease is insidious and gradually progressive, cats are often not presented for clinical evaluation until late in the disease process.[7,8,23,24] In one published retrospective study, 73% of glaucomatous cats were blind at the time of initial presentation.[23] Observant owners may notice relatively subtle anisocoria, with more pronounced anisocoria, due to relative pupil dilation in the affected eye constituting a common presenting complaint in cats with glaucoma (**Fig. 11**).

Acutely painful, fulminant, congestive glaucoma is rarely recognized in cats. The presence of overt clinical signs of discomfort is variable but affected cats seldom show obvious signs of severe ocular pain, even in the face of very high IOP, and glaucomatous cats generally maintain a normal appetite and relatively normal

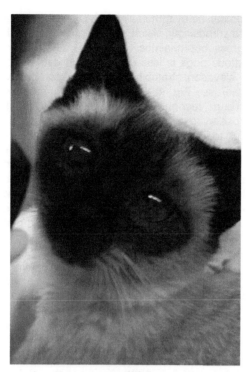

Fig. 11. Primary glaucoma in a Siamese cat. Subtle anisocoria may be the only sign of feline glaucoma that is noted by observant cat owners.

activity level. In some animals, underlying ocular disease such as uveitis can contribute to ocular discomfort. Globe enlargement can be dramatic, especially in young animals, and may lead to exposure keratopathy and painful corneal ulceration (**Fig. 12**).

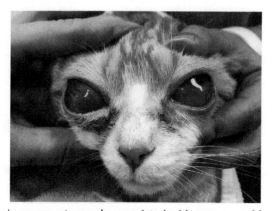

Fig. 12. Glaucoma in young cats may be associated with pronounced buphthalmos, dense edema, and corneal ulceration due to exposure, as seen in both eyes of this 7-month-old domestic shorthair cat with congenital glaucoma related to anterior segment dysgenesis. Remarkably, the left eye in this patient retained light perception. (*Courtesy of* Jacqueline W. Pearce, DVM, MS, DACVO, University of Missouri, Columbia, MO.)

In comparison to the canine eye, the feline eye is relatively resistant to glaucomatous damage. Perhaps surprisingly, vision may be preserved in chronically glaucomatous cats despite gross buphthalmos.[9,17] Dense, diffuse corneal edema that is common in glaucomatous dogs is less often seen in cats at comparable levels of IOP. With chronic IOP elevation, stretching of the globe can lead to tears in Descemet membrane (Haab striae) (see **Fig. 4**). Panretinal degeneration, which is a common feature of glaucoma in dogs, recognized as sectoral retinal thinning and altered tapetal reflectivity, is seldom observed in cats, even those with advanced disease. Optic disc cupping can be difficult to identify by ophthalmoscopy in cats, especially those with bilateral disease, because the feline optic nerve head (ONH) lacks myelin and appears depressed relative to the plane of the surrounding retina, even in normal animals. Subtle changes in the ophthalmoscopic appearance of the ONH of cats with glaucoma include a dark or pale gray appearance; a peripapillary pigmented or hyperreflective halo; and altered course of retinal vasculature so that blood vessels are no longer observed crossing the neuroretinal rim of the ONH for a short distance, or increased prominence of the pores in the lamina cribrosa through which optic nerve axons exit the eye (the so-called laminar dot sign) (**Fig. 13**). Optical coherence tomography (OCT) provides confirmation of ONH changes and thinning of the retinal nerve fiber layer in cats with glaucoma (see **Fig. 13C, D**), but availability of this advanced imaging technology is limited to a few research institutions.

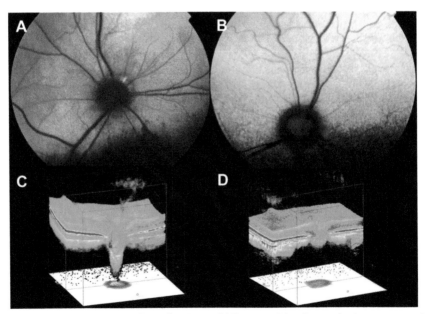

Fig. 13. Fundus photographs show the ONH of (*A*) a cat with advanced primary congenital glaucoma and (*B*) a normal cat. (*C*) optic nerve cube scan obtained by spectral Domain OCT (Cirrus; Carl Zeiss Meditec Inc, Dublin, CA, USA), acquired in a cat with glaucoma that demonstrates dramatic posterior displacement of the lamina cribrosa, compared to (*D*) OCT scan acquired in a normal cat. (*From* McLellan GJ, Rasmussen CA. Optical coherence tomography for the evaluation of retinal and optic nerve morphology in animal subjects: practical considerations. Vet Ophthalmol 2012;15(Suppl 2):17; with permission.)

Measuring Intraocular Pressure in Cats

As IOP is the main target for therapy in cats with glaucoma, a reliable and accurate method for estimating IOP is essential when diagnosing this disease and assessing treatment efficacy. However, documentation of high IOP alone is neither necessary nor sufficient to diagnose glaucoma, and other clinical features of glaucoma are expected.

In normal cats, IOP can be influenced by handling and restraint, time of day, age, and reproductive status.[4,37,38] The inherent limitations of tonometry, and degree of IOP variability, must be clearly understood; the following sections detail important considerations when interpreting tonometry readings.

Fluctuations in Intraocular Pressure Should Be Expected, Even in Normal Cats

In normal cats, there is a pronounced circadian fluctuation (about 4–5 mm Hg) in IOP, which is generally highest at night and tends to be 1 to 1.5 mm Hg lower in the mid to late afternoon than in the morning.[37] Fluctuations in IOP within and between days are greatly accentuated, and are less consistent, in cats with glaucoma.[39] As with measurement of blood pressure, IOP can be affected by stress in cats. Tonometry should be performed early in the examination procedure if glaucoma is suspected. If high values are obtained, then tonometry should be repeated after allowing the patient to acclimate for a few minutes, to ensure that IOP is persistently elevated. Significantly higher IOP has been observed in estrus female cats than other groups,[38] but this may be of limited clinical significance in veterinary practice, as most adult feline patients will have been spayed or neutered.

The Age of the Patient Can Influence Intraocular Pressure

Age has a significant influence on IOP in normal cats, being considerably lower in geriatric animals than in young cats, higher in adolescent than in adult cats, and much lower in young kittens within the first few weeks of life than in adolescent and adult cats.[4,19] In young kittens, at the time of eyelid opening, neither aqueous humor production nor outflow have reached adult levels; IOP is very low, and the anterior chamber is shallow, with near apposition between the iris and cornea. Over the first 3 months of life in cats, the anatomy and physiology of the anterior segment and aqueous outflow pathways undergo a process of maturation, and IOP approaches adultlike values by 10 to 12 weeks of age.[19,40] Aged cats, with no other signs of ocular disease, also tend to have very low IOPs (often ≤7 mm Hg).[4] This study concluded that an IOP of 25 mm Hg or greater, measured with the Tono-Pen XL in older cats, or marked asymmetry in IOP (≥12 mm Hg difference between eyes), warrants a thorough examination for ocular disease, including glaucoma.[4]

Prior Drug Administration May Alter Intraocular Pressure

Prior application of mydriatic, including tropicamide, may lead to substantial increases in IOP in both normal and glaucomatous cats.[41–43] As discussed later, topical or systemic administration of corticosteroids may also increase IOP in cats.

Tonometers Provide Only an Estimate of Intraocular Pressure and Have Important Limitations

Aside from these physiologic and pharmacologic effects on IOP, there are significant limitations of some of the most commonly used tonometer designs in cats (**Table 2**). Pronounced differences in values obtained by different tonometers mean that a consistent tonometer type and model should be used for clinical monitoring of IOP in cats, and the model used should be clearly recorded. Veterinary

Table 2
Summary of published studies evaluating different tonometer types in cats

Tonometer Type	Tonometric Principle	IOP in mm Hg (Mean ± Standard Deviation) in Normal Cats	Limitations/Comments	Refs.
Schiøtz tonometer	Indentation	21.6 ± 5 (n = 37)	5.5 g weight; 1955 human conversion table	46
Pneumotonometer	Applanation	Not established	Underestimates IOP >20 mm Hg, overestimates IOP <15 mm Hg	47
Mackay-Marg	Applanation	19.7 ± 5.6 (n = 41)	Underestimates higher IOPs	48
Tono-Pen	Applanation	22.6 ± 4 (n = 37)	Underestimates higher IOPs	48
Tono-Pen XL/Vet	Applanation	18.4 ± 0.6 (SEM: n = 33)	Markedly underestimates higher IOPs	44,45,47,49
Perkins	Applanation	15.1 ± 1.7[a]	Not tested outside normal physiologic range; upper maximal scale measurement limits IOP readings to about 50 mm Hg	50
TonoVet	Rebound (induction–Impact)	20.74 ± 0.5 (n = 76)	Accurate in cats (but less precise at high IOP). Does not require topical anesthetic, well tolerated	44,45

Note: Mean IOP is presented ± standard deviation unless indicated otherwise.
Abbreviations: n, number of animals used to determine reference range where applicable; SEM, standard error of mean.
[a] Perkins tonometer values presented were calculated from calibration curve.
Adapted from McLellan GJ, Miller PE. Feline glaucoma–a comprehensive review. Vet Ophthalmol 2011;14(Suppl 1):28; with permission.

clinicians should also be aware of any limitations of the tonometer type used. Although most of the tonometer types commonly used in veterinary practice demonstrated acceptable accuracy within the normal physiologic range in cats, it is noteworthy that most applanation tonometers dramatically underestimate higher IOPs when compared with manometry. Despite their widespread application in clinical veterinary practice, the systematic underestimation of IOP in glaucomatous cats by most applanation tonometers may have contributed to an underestimation of the true prevalence of glaucoma in the feline population. The TonoVet rebound tonometer is more accurate than the Tono-Pen, particularly at IOPs greater than 30 mm Hg (**Fig. 14**). The TonoVet does not require application of topical anesthetic, is well-tolerated by cats, and may be considered most suitable among current, commercially available tonometers, for diagnosis and monitoring of glaucoma in cats.[44,45]

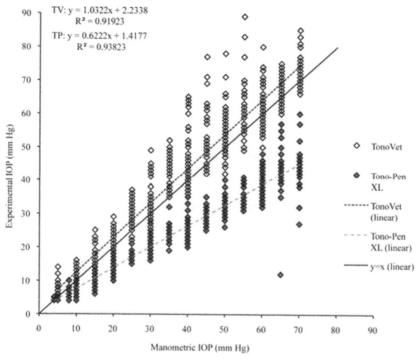

Fig. 14. The TonoVet tonometer (TV) is more accurate than the Tono-Pen XL (equivalent to the Tono-Pen Vet) tonometer (TP) at high IOPs in the feline eye. (*From* McLellan GJ, Kemmerling JP, Kiland JA. Validation of the TonoVet rebound tonometer in normal and glaucomatous cats. Vet Ophthalmol 2013;16(2):113; with permission.)

Gonioscopy

The anterior chamber is deeper and the opening of the iridocorneal angle in cats is considerably wider than in humans and dogs. The individual fibers of the pectinate ligament, that span the anterior opening of the ciliary cleft, are very fine and relatively sparse in normal cats (**Fig. 15**), in comparison to the typical appearance of the canine drainage angle. The iridocorneal angle and opening of the ciliary cleft are best evaluated by gonioscopy, using a goniolens. However, it is possible to evaluate a significant portion of the feline drainage angle by direct observation using focal illumination and magnification, or even using an indirect ophthalmoscope and condensing lens held at an extreme angle to view the pectinate ligament and opening of the ciliary cleft. Although developmental abnormalities of the pectinate ligament are very uncommon in cats, gonioscopy may aid in the identification of closure of the iridocorneal angle (collapse of the opening of the ciliary cleft), neoplastic infiltrates, or neovascularization in cats with secondary glaucoma.

Ancillary Diagnostic Tests

In addition to thorough general physical examination, additional ancillary testing may be appropriate in individual cases. Serologic testing for infectious causes of uveitis may be considered appropriate in some cats with secondary glaucoma, but may fail to reveal an underlying cause in many patients with chronic lymphoplasmacytic uveitis. Ocular ultrasonography may be helpful in evaluating patients for the presence of

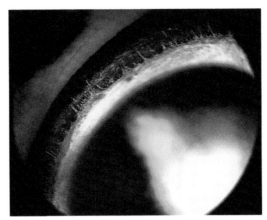

Fig. 15. Appearance of a normal cat iridocorneal angle on gonioscopy. Note that the opening to the normal feline ciliary cleft is wide and is spanned by delicate, widely spaced pectinate ligament fibers.

intraocular mass lesions. Cytologic evaluation of aqueous humor samples obtained by paracentesis may aid in a diagnosis of suspected uveal lymphoma. Thoracic radiography or abdominal ultrasonography may be indicated when ocular neoplasia with potential for systemic involvement or metastasis is suspected.

CLINICAL MANAGEMENT OF GLAUCOMA IN CATS

> Treatment should be directed at the underlying disease process leading to secondary glaucoma, whenever possible.
>
> Glaucoma therapy in cats must be tailored to the individual, and response to therapy must be closely monitored.

The following are important considerations when selecting an appropriate management strategy for feline glaucoma patients:

- *Establish the underlying cause whenever possible.* A diagnosis of primary glaucoma is uncommon and should be a diagnosis made by exclusion. Always consider, and offer, referral for specialist evaluation and further diagnostics, including imaging, particularly when the underlying cause of glaucoma is not immediately apparent.
- *Take steps to exclude intraocular neoplasia.* Enucleation or even exenteration will generally be appropriate if neoplasia is identified or strongly suspected. Ocular lymphoma may be diagnosed cytologically following aqueous humor paracentesis and may respond to chemotherapy in some cases. When enucleation is elected, enucleated globes should ALWAYS be submitted for histopathologic evaluation.
- *Determine the specific mechanisms for IOP elevation in each case.* By identifying the location of the block to aqueous outflow, therapy may be better targeted. Some drug classes may be contraindicated, such as those that induce miosis

(eg, prostaglandin analogues, timolol, or pilocarpine) and may intensify pupil block in patients with uveitis, FAHMS, or lens luxation.

- *Consider whether the pathogenic mechanisms are reversible or irreversible.* In acute uveitis, for example, alleviating miosis early in the disease process may limit the formation of extensive posterior synechiae, iris bombé, and subsequent collapse of the ciliary cleft, but with chronicity, this sequence of changes may become irreversible.
- *Identify and address any concurrent systemic health concerns.* Associated systemic disease or comorbidities may impact the prognosis, priority assigned to management of glaucoma, and the management plan ultimately selected by the owner.
- *Consider the potential for vision in the affected eye or eyes* and whether the contralateral eye is also at risk in patients presenting with unilateral glaucoma. In the management of irreversibly blind, glaucomatous eyes, with no menace response, dazzle, or direct pupillary light reflex, the cost-to-benefit analysis often favors enucleation, particularly if the eye is painful.
- *Establish the likelihood of owner and patient compliance.* Long-term topical treatment can present a considerable practical challenge in cats.
- *Discuss owner financial constraints* because these are an important consideration, particularly for surgical options, and may significantly limit the potential for referral and the range treatments that can be considered.

MEDICAL THERAPY FOR FELINE GLAUCOMA

Cat owners are more likely than the owners of dogs with glaucoma to encounter difficulties in the frequent application of topical medications to their pets' eyes, so ensuring compliance with prescribed treatment regimens may prove challenging.

Nasolacrimal drainage of topically applied medications often results in an aversive taste response in cats.

To minimize nasolacrimal drainage of medication to the pharynx, owners should be instructed to attempt manual occlusion of the lacrimal puncta, by gentle digital pressure through the eyelids at the medial canthus immediately following instillation of eye drops.

Unfortunately, there is lack of published, randomized, controlled, prospective clinical trials that examine the efficacy of antiglaucoma medications in cats in a clinical setting. When interpreting the findings of the few published studies that have been conducted in either normal cats or cats with primary, congenital glaucoma, the heterogeneity of response between and within species and even within individual patients (that may experience diurnal and nocturnal fluctuations in IOP), and between different forms of glaucoma, must be taken into account. In particular, the extrapolation of results of studies conducted in normal subjects may not be appropriate, given that the response to the same drug or procedure may be very different in individual glaucomatous cats that have varying pathologic conditions affecting their aqueous humor outflow pathways.

INTRAOCULAR PRESSURE–LOWERING DRUGS

A summary of glaucoma medications that have been studied in cats is provided in **Table 3**. It should be noted that not all medications may be commercially available.

Table 3
Intraocular pressure–lowering drugs that have been investigated in cats

Class	Examples	Route	Frequency	Mechanism	IOP-Lowering Effect	Adverse Effects	Contraindications
Carbonic anhydrase inhibitor	Dorzolamide 2% Brinzolamide 1%	Topical	Q8–12 h	↓ Production	Potent (dorzolamide > brinzolamide)	May be transient salivation; innappetance in some cats Topical irritation (brinzolamide < dorzolamide)	None
β-Blocker	Timolol 0.5% Betaxolol 0.5% (Betaxolol is more β2-selective)	Topical	Q12 h	↓ Production	Minimal to modest	Mild: bradycardia, miosis	Avoid in animals with feline asthma, cardiovascular disease, or pupil block glaucoma
Adrenergic agonist	Epinephrine 1%–2%; dipivefrin 0.1%	Topical	Q6–12 h	↑ Outflow ↓ Production	Modest, not studied in cats with glaucoma	Not reported but local irritation might be anticipated	Do not use dipivefrin with cholinesterase inhibitors
Cholinergic	Pilocarpine 2%	Topical	Q6–12 h	↑ Outflow	Minimal to modest	Miosis Systemic toxicity may be seen	Uveitis, FAHMS, pupil block, & lens-associated glaucoma
Prostaglandin analogue	Latanoprost 0.005%	Topical	Q12–24 h	Not determined	Efficacy varies between individuals; may increase or decrease IOP	Intense miosis	Uveitis, FAHMS, pupil block & lens-associated glaucoma

Note: Given the preponderance of secondary glaucoma in cats, it is important to determine and, where possible, directly address the underlying cause of glaucoma and to carefully evaluate individual response to therapy and treatment efficacy in each patient.

Carbonic Anhydrase Inhibitors

> Topical CAIs are generally considered the first-line treatment choice for cats with glaucoma, regardless of the underlying pathogenesis of glaucoma.

CAIs have no effect on pupil size, do not potentiate pupil block, or intensify any pre-existing uveitis. CAIs reduce active aqueous humor secretion by the ciliary epithelium. Topical dorzolamide 2% has been shown to significantly lower IOP in both normal and glaucomatous cats when given 2 to 3 times daily.[39,51] Brinzolamide 1% did not significantly lower IOP in normal cats when applied twice daily,[52] but did significantly lower IOP and blunt circadian fluctuation in IOP in glaucomatous cats when administered 3 times daily.[53] Topical CAIs are preferred over systemic CAIs because of their enhanced safety profile, but may be associated with hypersalivation and inappetance in some cats. Systemic CAIs, such as acetazolamide, methazolamide, and dichlorphenamide, are also very effective in reducing aqueous humor production in cats, but their application is severely limited by their systemic toxicity in this species.

DRUGS WITH VARIABLE RESPONSE
β-Blockers

Topical β-blockers have, at best, a modest IOP-lowering effect in cats.

Timolol may cause bradycardia and bronchoconstriction and is therefore contraindicated in cats with feline asthma or cardiac disease. Although clinically significant bradycardia is unlikely in otherwise healthy cats, heart rate should be monitored in cats undergoing topical therapy with Timolol.

β-Blockers should be used only with caution in cats with uveitis or pupil block glaucoma because they may cause miosis.

Timolol is a nonselective β-adrenergic blocker that reduces aqueous humor production.[54] Although one study in normal cats reported a reduction in IOP in the treated eye, about 6 hours after topical application of a single dose of timolol maleate 0.5%, reduction in IOP in the contralateral, untreated eye was also observed.[55] In a more recent study in glaucomatous and normal cats, that used a 0.5% gel-forming solution once daily, no consistent reduction in IOP was observed.[56] In both studies, miosis was observed in the timolol-treated eye.[55,56] In combination therapy, no significant additive IOP-lowering effect was observed in normal cats receiving timolol 0.5% together with dorzolamide 2%, relative to the effect of treatment with dorzolamide 2% alone.[51] β-1-Selective blockers in particular (such as betaxolol) may have lower efficacy in cats, because β-2 receptors predominate in the anterior segment tissues of this species.[57] β-Blockers may also be less effective during sleep, because of lower sympathetic tone. Because cats nap frequently, and their IOP tends to be highest during the night, this characteristic could impact IOP-lowering efficacy in felines.

Prostaglandin Analogues

Prostaglandin analogues should be used with extreme caution in animals with significant anterior uveitis; these drugs induce intense miosis in animals and therefore their use should be avoided in subjects at risk of pupil block or in which posterior synechiae are expected/partially present. Prostaglandin analogues that are currently available commercially, including latanoprost, travoprost, and bimatoprost, have no significant IOP-lowering effect in normal cats.[58–60] Species differences in prostanoid receptor distribution have been proposed as the reason these prostaglandin analogues are not effective in lowering IOP in normal cats, despite being highly effective in dogs and humans and widely used in the management of primary glaucoma these species. These prostaglandin analogues are all F Prostanoid (FP) receptor agonists, and their lack of efficacy in normal cats has been attributed to a relative lack of FP receptors in the feline ciliary body of cats, in which EP receptors are predominantly responsible for relaxation of ciliary muscle.[61,62] However, a recent study found that latanoprost 0.005% significantly and substantially lowered IOP in cats with inherited congenital glaucoma following a single topical application, but this effect was diminished following chronic twice-daily administration of the drug.[63] Cats, like dogs, exhibit intense miosis when treated with commercially available prostaglandin analogues,[58–60] because of the presence of FP receptors in their iris sphincter muscle.[64,65] Further unpublished studies indicate that latanoprost administration may alter the morphology of the anterior segment, lowering IOP as a result of an increase in width of the ciliary cleft in glaucomatous cats.[66] The reasons for the discrepancy in IOP reduction between normal and glaucomatous cats, mechanisms of action and for the apparent tachyphylaxis, with moderation of response over time, have not yet been definitively established. In some cats with glaucoma and in some normal cats,[63] latanoprost may actually lead to an increase in IOP.

> It is clear that responses to topical FP receptor agonist can vary between individuals. The use of latanoprost in the long-term management of feline glaucoma requires further study before it can be recommended as a first-line therapy in this species.

Cholinergics

Because of their limited effect on IOP and their miotic effect, cholinergic drugs are contraindicated in animals with a tendency to pupil block and should be used with caution in subjects with uveitis.

These miotic drugs reduce IOP by increasing conventional aqueous outflow. Topical administration of a single dose of the direct-acting cholinergic, pilocarpine at 2% concentration, reduced IOP by about 15% in the treated eye but caused miosis in both the treated and the untreated eye of normal cats.[67] This contralateral effect, observed following unilateral application, indicates that systemic, adverse cholinergic effects might be anticipated during long-term treatment. However, in a more recent study in normal and glaucomatous cats, only slight miosis was observed under dim light conditions (as might be experienced in the nocturnal phase, when IOP peaks in cats) in cats treated with 2% pilocarpine. Furthermore, the IOP-lowering effect of this drug was inconsistent and, at best, modest.[66] Demecarium bromide 0.125%, a cholinesterase inhibitor, is a more potent and longer-lasting miotic, but to the authors' knowledge, its effects have not been specifically evaluated in cats.

Adrenergic Agonists

> Because of their systemic adverse effects, including lowering of heart rate and vomiting, α2-adrenergic agonists are not recommended for the management of glaucoma in cats.

The nonspecific adrenergic agonist, epinephrine, reduced IOP in normal cats by about 27% when applied twice daily, by both reducing aqueous production and increasing outflow facility.[68] Ocular surface irritation might be expected, based on reported adverse effects in human patients, but was not evaluated in that feline study. Efficacy of dipivefrin, a prodrug of epinephrine, might be expected to be similar to epinephrine, but has not been specifically investigated in cats. These drugs cause mild pupil dilation and do not exacerbate uveitis.

In contrast, the α-2 agonist apraclonidine, although it also reduced IOP in normal cats by an average of 24% within 6 hours of treatment, resulted in miosis that persisted up to 24 hours. Evidence of systemic toxicity following topical application of 0.5% apraclonidine, consisting of a mean reduction in heart rate of about 12%, and propensity to cause vomiting (noted in 8/9 cats treated with the drug) precludes use of the commercially available formulation of aproclonidine in cats.[69]

Topical Corticosteroids in Feline Glaucoma

Topical corticosteroid therapy (usually with either 0.1% dexamethasone or 1% prednisolone) is a mainstay of therapy for chronic uveitis as well as nonherpetic ocular surface disease in cats. However, topical administration of corticosteroids can increase IOP by about 5 to 10 mm Hg in some normal cats.[70–72] Even more dramatic, steroid-induced increases in IOP, exceeding 50 mm Hg within a few weeks, have been documented in cats with pre-existing compromise in their aqueous humor outflow pathways.[72] Corticosteroid-induced IOP responses show considerable variability between individuals and can be difficult to predict. This phenomenon is unlikely to be a major concern in cats with normal aqueous humor outflow pathways, in which true steroid-induced ocular hypertension appears to be very rare, but the potential for steroid-induced increase in IOP should be an important clinical consideration when treating glaucoma associated with ocular inflammation in cats.

> IOP should be monitored closely in all cats that are being treated long term with topical corticosteroids.

If steroid-induced IOP elevation is promptly recognized, then a change in the route of administration or selection of a different topical or systemic anti-inflammatory drug may help mitigate this effect.

SURGICAL MANAGEMENT OF GLAUCOMA IN CATS
Cyclodestructive Procedures

> Laser cyclophotocoagulation and cyclocryotherapy incite significant inflammation and are contraindicated in cats with glaucoma secondary to uveitis or neoplasia.

Cyclophotocoagulation or cyclocryotherapy seems to be considerably less successful in regulating IOP in glaucomatous cats than in dogs, and often repeated treatments are required. In an experimental study, cyclophotocoagulation with neodymium-doped yttrium aluminum garnet laser led to a mean reduction in IOP of about 30% in normal cats.[73] Unpredictable and disappointing outcomes in feline clinical patients may reflect a relative lack of melanin pigment that absorbs commonly used diode laser wavelengths, within the ciliary body stroma of some cats. Accurate transscleral laser delivery may also be confounded by marked interindividual variation in the location of the ciliary processes relative to the limbus in glaucomatous compared with normal cats, due to disproportionate stretching of ocular tissues in glaucoma. Preoperative ultrasound biometry that can be used to identify the location of the ciliary body in individual glaucomatous cats could feasibly increase the success rate of surgical, cyclodestructive procedures. Although the alternate technique of endocyclophoto-coagulation, might better target laser damage to the ciliary epithelium, iatrogenic lens trauma should be a significant concern in this species with the potential for subsequent malignant transformation of lens epithelium.[32]

Anterior Chamber Shunt Procedures

Gonio-implantation surgery in glaucomatous cats can be very challenging, and treatment failure is common.

Because chronic uveitis is commonly associated with development of secondary glaucoma, pre-existing inflammation often contributes to shunt failure related to anterior tube occlusion. Buphthalmos is common in cats with glaucoma and, combined with the relatively confined orbit and tight eyelids in this species, substantially complicates the surgical placement of conventional drainage implants and limits formation of an adequate filtering bleb.

Pharmacologic Ablation of the Ciliary Body Epithelium

> Pharmacologic ablation of the ciliary body, by intravitreous injection of gentamicin or other cyclodestructive agents, cannot be recommended for the treatment of end-stage feline glaucoma.

The procedure carries a relatively low rate of success, of only about 66% in one limited study.[74] Malignant intraocular neoplasia is a common cause of secondary glaucoma in cats and may not be clinically suspected before pharmacologic ablation. Corneal opacification following pharmacologic ablation will also limit ongoing monitoring and may mask progression of disease. In a recent retrospective study, malignant intraocular neoplasms (3 sarcomas and 2 uveal melanomas) were identified in 5 of 8 feline eyes enucleated following intravitreal gentamicin injections.[75] In those cases, it was not possible to determine whether intravitreal gentamicin injections had actually been administered to cats with glaucoma secondary to an occult intraocular neoplasm, if neoplasia arose independently of the injection, or whether the injection incited neoplastic transformation.[32,75]

ENUCLEATION AND EVISCERATION FOR FELINE GLAUCOMA

For irreversibly blind eyes, or those in which there is a suspicion of intraocular neoplasia based on clinical findings, enucleation must be considered, and enucleated globes should always be submitted for histopathological diagnosis.[5] Enucleation is strongly preferred over evisceration with intrascleral prosthesis (ISP) placement in cats, because the success rate of ISP placement in this species is lower than in dogs.[76,77] In a published study, the most common reason for corneoscleral shell failure, following prior evisceration and ISP placement in cats, was recurrence of intraocular neoplasia, which was diagnosed in about two-thirds of specimens. These neoplasms were generally malignant and potentially life-threatening[78] (**Fig. 16**). The

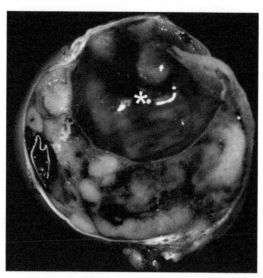

Fig. 16. Regrowth of uveal melanoma, surrounding site of an intrascleral prosthesis (*asterisk*), within the previously eviscerated corneoscleral shell of a cat eye. (*Courtesy of* Richard R. Dubielzig, DVM, DACVP, Comparative Ocular Pathology Laboratory of Wisconsin, Madison, WI.)

risk of late complications following placement of intraorbital prostheses at the time of enucleation may also be greater in cats than in dogs and may necessitate removal of the orbital prosthesis in some cats.[79,80]

Irreversibly blind glaucomatous cats, even those with bilateral disease, tolerate enucleation extremely well.

In summary, glaucoma in cats typically follows an insidious, gradually progressive clinical course and is most often secondary to other ocular or systemic disease. Treatment of glaucoma presents a clinical challenge in cats. Systemic and local side effects are common, and most cats are poorly tolerant of frequent application of topical medications. Poor patient and owner compliance with prescribed therapy is a common scenario. In some cats, adverse effects of medications used, and stress they experience as a result of frequent medication, may be more severe than minimal signs of ocular discomfort or illness observed before initiating therapy. The cost-to-benefit ratio should be given careful consideration for each individual patient and may favor a more conservative approach of monitoring or palliative therapy rather than aggressive vision-sparing medical or surgical therapy, especially in older cats. Enucleation is generally the most appropriate treatment for cats with irreversibly blind, painful eyes, particularly when intraocular neoplasia is suspected or cannot be excluded.

REFERENCES

1. Tripathi RC. Ultrastructure of the exit pathway of the aqueous in lower mammals (a preliminary report on the "angular aqueous plexus"). Exp Eye Res 1971;12: 311–4.
2. Bill A. Formation and drainage of aqueous humour in cats. Exp Eye Res 1966;5: 185–90.
3. McLellan GJ, Miller PE. Feline glaucoma–a comprehensive review. Vet Ophthalmol 2011;14(Suppl 1):15–29.

4. Kroll MM, Miller PE, Rodan I. Intraocular pressure measurements obtained as part of a comprehensive geriatric health examination from cats seven years of age or older. J Am Vet Med Assoc 2001;219(10):1406–10.

5. Dubielzig RR, Ketring KL, McLellan GJ, et al. The glaucomas. Veterinary ocular pathology. A comparative review. Oxford (United Kingdom): Saunders Elsevier; 2010. p. 419–48.

6. Gelatt KN, Brooks DE, Samuelson DA. Comparative glaucomatology. I: The spontaneous glaucomas. J Glaucoma 1998;7(3):187–201.

7. Ridgway MD, Brightman AH. Feline glaucoma: a retrospective study of 29 clinical cases. J Am Anim Hosp Assoc 1989;25:485–90.

8. Walde I, Rapp E. Feline glaucoma. Clinical and morphological aspects (a retrospective study of 38 cases). Eur J Compan Anim Pract 1993;4:87–105.

9. Hampson EC, Smith RI, Bernays ME. Primary glaucoma in Burmese cats. Aust Vet J 2002;80(11):672–80.

10. Wilcock BP, Peiffer RL Jr, Davidson MG. The causes of glaucoma in cats. Vet Pathol 1990;27(1):35–40.

11. Stadtbaumer K, Peiffer RL, Nell B. Goniodysgenesis associated with primary glaucoma in an adult European shorthair cat: clinical and histopathological findings. Paper presented at: Annual Meeting of the European College of Veterinary Ophthalmologists and the European Society of Veterinary Ophthalmology. Oporto, Portugal, June 15–19, 2005.

12. Trost K, Peiffer RL Jr, Nell B. Goniodysgenesis associated with primary glaucoma in an adult European short-haired cat. Vet Ophthalmol 2007;10(Suppl 1):3–7.

13. Jacobi S, Dubielzig RR. Feline primary open angle glaucoma. Vet Ophthalmol 2008;11(3):162–5.

14. Teixeira LB, Linder T, Dubielzig RR. Spontaneous post-trabecular open angle glaucoma in cats. Paper presented at: Assoc Res Vis Ophthalmol. Denver, CO, May 3–7, 2015.

15. Brown A, Munger R, Peiffer RL Jr. Congenital glaucoma and iridoschisis in a Siamese cat. Vet Comp Ophthalmol 1994;4(3):121–4.

16. Rutz-Mendicino MM, Snella EM, Jens JK, et al. Removal of potentially confounding phenotypes from a Siamese-derived feline glaucoma breeding colony. Comp Med 2011;61(3):251–7.

17. McLellan GJ, Betts D, Sigle K, et al. Congenital glaucoma in the Siamese cat—a new spontaneously occurring animal model for glaucoma research. Paper presented at: 35th Annual Meeting of the American College of Veterinary Ophthalmologists. Washington, DC, October 20–23, 2004.

18. McLellan GJ, Kuehn MH, Ellinwood NM, et al. A feline model of primary congenital glaucoma—histopathological and genetic characterization. Paper presented at: Assoc Res Vis Ophthalmol Annual Meeting. Fort Lauderdale, FL, April 30–May 4, 2006.

19. Adelman S, McLellan GJ, Ellinwood NM, et al. Early life intraocular pressures in normal cats and cats with primary congenital glaucoma. Paper presented at: American College of Veterinary Ophthalmologists. Puerto Rico, November 4–9, 2013.

20. Coop MC, Thomas JR. Bilateral glaucoma in the cat. J Am Vet Med Assoc 1958; 133:369–70.

21. Aguirre GD, Bistner SI. Microphakia with lenticular luxation and subluxation in cats. Vet Med Small Anim Clin 1973;68:498–500.

22. Molleda JM, Martin E, Ginel PJ, et al. Microphakia associated with lens luxation in the cat. J Am Anim Hosp Assoc 1995;31:209–12.

23. Blocker T, van der Woerdt A. The feline glaucomas: 82 cases (1995-1999). Vet Ophthalmol 2001;4(2):81–5.

24. Dietrich U. Feline glaucomas. Clin Tech Small Anim Pract 2005;20:108–16.

25. Dubielzig RR, Everitt J, Shadduck JA, et al. Clinical and morphologic features of post-traumatic ocular sarcomas in cats. Vet Pathol 1990;27(1):62–5.

26. Dubielzig RR, Hawkins KL, Toy KA, et al. Morphologic features of feline ocular sarcomas in 10 cats: light microscopy, ultrastructure, and immunohistochemistry. Vet Comp Ophthalmol 1994;4(1):7–12.

27. Dubielzig RR, Steinberg H, Garvin H, et al. Iridociliary epithelial tumors in 100 dogs and 17 cats: a morphological study. Vet Ophthalmol 1998;1:223–31.

28. Dubielzig RR, Ketring KL, McLellan GJ, et al. The uvea. Veterinary ocular pathology. A comparative review. Oxford (United Kingdom): Saunders Elsevier; 2010. p. 245–322.

29. Peiffer RL Jr, Wilcock BP. Histopathologic study of uveitis in cats: 139 cases (1978-1988). J Am Vet Med Assoc 1991;198(1):135–8.

30. McCalla TL, Moore CP, Collier LL. Phacoclastic uveitis with secondary glaucoma in a cat. Compan Anim Pract 1988;2(11):13–7.

31. Bell CM, Pot SA, Dubielzig RR. Septic implantation syndrome in dogs and cats: a distinct pattern of endophthalmitis with lenticular abscess. Vet Ophthalmol 2013; 16(3):180–5.

32. Zeiss CJ, Johnson EM, Dubielzig RR. Feline intraocular tumors may arise from transformation of lens epithelium. Vet Pathol 2003;40(4):355–62.

33. Peiffer RL Jr, Wilcock BP, Yin H. The pathogenesis and significance of pre-iridal fibrovascular membrane in domestic animals. Vet Pathol 1990;27(1):41–5.

34. Olivero DK, Riis RC, Dutton AG, et al. Feline lens displacement: a retrospective analysis of 345 cases. Prog Vet Comp Ophthalmol 1991;1(4):239–44.

35. La Croix N, van der Woerdt A, Silverman RH, et al. Feline malignant glaucoma/ aqueous misdirection: 16 cases. Paper presented at: 34th Ann Meeting Am Coll Vet Ophthalmol. Coeur d'Alene, Idaho, October 22–26, 2003.

36. Czederpiltz JM, La Croix NC, van der Woerdt A, et al. Putative aqueous humor misdirection syndrome as a cause of glaucoma in cats: 32 cases (1997-2003). J Am Vet Med Assoc 2005;227(9):1434–41.

37. Del Sole MJ, Sande PH, Bernades JM, et al. Circadian rhythm of intraocular pressure in cats. Vet Ophthalmol 2007;10(3):155–61.

38. Ofri R, Shub N, Galin Z, et al. Effect of reproductive status on intraocular pressure in cats. Am J Vet Res 2002;63(2):159–62.

39. Sigle KJ, Camano-Garcia G, Carriquiry AL, et al. The effect of dorzolamide 2% on circadian intraocular pressure in cats with primary congenital glaucoma. Vet Ophthalmol 2011;14(Suppl 1):48–53.

40. Richardson TM, Marks MS, Ausprunk DH, et al. A morphologic and morphometric analysis of the aqueous outflow system of the developing cat eye. Exp Eye Res 1985;41(1):31–51.

41. Stadtbaumer K, Kostlin RG, Zahn KJ. Effects of topical 0.5% tropicamide on intraocular pressure in normal cats. Vet Ophthalmol 2002;5(2):107–12.

42. Stadtbaumer K, Frommlet F, Nell B. Effects of mydriatics on intraocular pressure and pupil size in the normal feline eye. Vet Ophthalmol 2006;9(4):233–7.

43. Espinheira Gomes F, Bentley E, Lin T-L, et al. Effects of unilateral topical administration of 0.5% tropicamide on anterior segment morphology and intraocular pressure in normal cats and cats with primary congenital glaucoma. Vet Ophthalmol 2011;14(Suppl 1):75–83.

44. Rusanen E, Florin M, Hassig M, et al. Evaluation of a rebound tonometer (Tonovet) in clinically normal cat eyes. Vet Ophthalmol 2010;13(1):31–6.

45. McLellan GJ, Kemmerling JP, Kiland JA. Validation of the TonoVet((R)) rebound tonometer in normal and glaucomatous cats. Vet Ophthalmol 2013;16(2):111–8.
46. Miller PE, Pickett JP. Comparison of the human and canine Schiotz tonometry conversion tables in clinically normal cats. J Am Vet Med Assoc 1992;201(7): 1017–20.
47. Stoiber J, Fernandez V, Lamar PD, et al. Ex vivo evaluation of Tono-Pen and pneumotonometry in cat eyes. Ophthalmic Res 2006;38(1):13–8.
48. Miller PE, Pickett JP, Majors LJ, et al. Evaluation of two applanation tonometers in cats. Am J Vet Res 1991;52(11):1917–21.
49. Passaglia CL, Guo X, Chen J, et al. Tono-Pen XL calibration curves for cats, cows and sheep. Vet Ophthalmol 2004;7(4):261–4.
50. Andrade SF, Cremonezi T, Zachi CA, et al. Evaluation of the Perkins handheld applanation tonometer in the measurement of intraocular pressure in dogs and cats. Vet Ophthalmol 2009;12(5):277–84.
51. Dietrich UM, Chandler MJ, Cooper T, et al. Effects of topical 2% dorzolamide hydrochloride alone and in combination with 0.5% timolol maleate on intraocular pressure in normal feline eyes. Vet Ophthalmol 2007;10(Suppl 1):95–100.
52. Gray HE, Willis AM, Morgan RV. Effects of topical administration of 1% brinzolamide on normal cat eyes. Vet Ophthalmol 2003;6(4):285–90.
53. McLellan GJ, Lin T-L, Hildreth S, et al. Diurnal intraocular pressure and response to topically administered 1% brinzolamide in a spontaneous feline model of primary congenital glaucoma. Paper presented at: Annual Meeting of the Association for Research in Vision and Ophthalmology. Fort Lauderdale, FL, May 3–7, 2009.
54. Liu HK, Chiou GC, Garg LC. Ocular hypotensive effects of timolol in cat eyes. Arch Ophthalmol 1980;98(8):1467–9.
55. Wilkie DA, Latimer CA. Effects of topical administration of timolol maleate on intraocular pressure and pupil size in cats. Am J Vet Res 1991;52(3):436–40.
56. McLellan GJ, Voss AM, Bowie OR, et al. Effect of timolol maleate on intraocular pressure, pupil diameter, and heart rate in normal and glaucomatous cats. 44th Trans. Am. Coll. Vet Ophthalmol. Paper presented at: 44th Annual Meeting of the Am. Coll. Vet. Ophthalmol. Rio Grande, Puerto Rico, November 4–9, 2013.
57. Colasanti BK, Trotter RR. Effects of selective beta 1- and beta 2-adrenoreceptor agonists and antagonists on intraocular pressure in the cat. Invest Ophthalmol Vis Sci 1981;20(1):69–76.
58. Studer ME, Martin CL, Stiles J. Effects of 0.005% latanoprost solution on intraocular pressure in healthy dogs and cats. Am J Vet Res 2000;61(10):1220–4.
59. Bartoe JT, Davidson HJ, Horton MT, et al. The effects of bimatoprost and unoprostone isopropyl on the intraocular pressure in normal cats. Vet Ophthalmol 2005; 8(4):247–52.
60. Regnier A, Lemagne C, Ponchet A, et al. Ocular effects of topical 0.03% bimatoprost solution in normotensive feline eyes. Vet Ophthalmol 2006;9(1):39–43.
61. Chen J, Woodward DF. Prostanoid-induced relaxation of precontracted cat ciliary muscle is mediated by EP2 and DP receptors. Invest Ophthalmol Vis Sci 1992; 33(11):3195–201.
62. Bhattacherjee P, Williams BS, Paterson CA. Responses of intraocular pressure and the pupil of feline eyes to prostaglandin EP1 and FP receptor agonists. Invest Ophthalmol Vis Sci 1999;40(12):3047–53.
63. McDonald JE, Kiland JA, Kaufman PL, Bentley E, Ellinwood NM, Effect of topical latanoprost 0.005% on intraocular pressure, pupil diameter in normal and glaucomatous cats. Vet Ophthalmol 2015; Jul 16 [Epub ahead of print].

64. Bhattacherjee P, Paterson CA. Studies on prostanoid receptors in ocular tissues. J Ocul Pharmacol 1994;10(1):167–75.
65. Sharif NA, Kaddour-Djebbar I, Abdel-Latif AA. Cat iris sphincter smooth-muscle contraction: comparison of FP-class prostaglandin analog agonist activities. J Ocul Pharmacol Ther 2008;24(2):152–63.
66. Delgado C, Lovstad J, Kuehn CE, et al. Effect of topical pilocarpine and latanoprost on IOP and anterior segment morphology in normal and glaucomatous cats. Paper presented at: 43rd Ann. Meeting. Am. Coll. Vet Ophthalmol. Portland, OR, October 17–20, 2012.
67. Wilkie DA, Latimer CA. Effects of topical administration of 2.0% pilocarpine on intraocular pressure and pupil size in cats. Am J Vet Res 1991;52(3):441–4.
68. Wang YL, Toris CB, Zhan G, et al. Effects of topical epinephrine on aqueous humor dynamics in the cat. Exp Eye Res 1999;68(4):439–45.
69. Miller PE, Rhaesa SL. Effects of topical administration of 0.5% apraclonidine on intraocular pressure, pupil size, and heart rate in clinically normal cats. Am J Vet Res 1996;57(1):83–6.
70. Zhan GL, Miranda OC, Bito LZ. Steroid glaucoma: corticosteroid-induced ocular hypertension in cats. Exp Eye Res 1992;54(2):211–8.
71. Bhattacherjee P, Paterson CA, Spellman JM, et al. Pharmacological validation of a feline model of steroid-induced ocular hypertension. Arch Ophthalmol 1999; 117(3):361–4.
72. Gosling AA, Kiland JA, Rutkowski LE, et al. Effects of topical corticosteroid administration on intraocular pressure in normal and glaucomatous cats. Paper presented at: 45th Annual Meeting Am. Coll. Vet. Ophthalmol. Fort Worth, TX, October 8–11, 2014.
73. Rosenberg LF, Burchfield JC, Krupin T, et al. Cat model for intraocular pressure reduction after transscleral Nd:YAG cyclophotocoagulation. Curr Eye Res 1995; 14(4):255–61.
74. Bingaman DP, Lindley DM, Glickman NW, et al. Intraocular gentamicin and glaucoma: a retrospective study of 60 dog and cat eyes (1985-1993). Vet Comp Ophthalmol 1994;4(3):113–9.
75. Duke FD, Strong TD, Bentley E, et al. Feline ocular tumors following ciliary body ablation with intravitreal gentamicin. Vet Ophthalmol 2013;16:188–90.
76. Koch SA. Intraocular prosthesis in the dog and cat: the failures. J Am Vet Med Assoc 1981;179(9):883–5.
77. McLaughlin SA, Ramsey DT, Lindley DM, et al. Intraocular silicone prosthesis implantation in eyes of dogs and a cat with intraocular neoplasia: nine cases (1983-1994). J Am Vet Med Assoc 1995;207(11):1441–3.
78. Naranjo C, Dubielzig RR. Histopathological study of the causes for failure of intrascleral prostheses in dogs and cats. Vet Ophthalmol 2014;17(5):343–50.
79. Nasisse MP, van Ee RT, Munger RJ, et al. Use of methyl methacrylate orbital prostheses in dogs and cats: 78 cases (1980-1986). J Am Vet Med Assoc 1988; 192(4):539–42.
80. Hamor RE, Roberts SM, Severin GA. Use of orbital implants after enucleation in dogs, horses, and cats: 161 cases (1980-1990). J Am Vet Med Assoc 1993; 203(5):701–6.

Canine Secondary Glaucomas

Stephanie Pumphrey, DVM

KEYWORDS

- Glaucoma • Dog • Uveitis • Lens luxation • Cataract • Hyphema
- Retinal detachment

KEY POINTS

- Secondary glaucomas are diagnosed frequently in dogs. Common causes include uveitis, lens luxations, cataracts and cataract surgery, retinal detachments, and neoplasia.
- Secondary glaucoma may be suspected based on patient signalment, examination findings, bilateral involvement, or poor response to treatment of glaucoma.
- Treatment strategies differ from those used for primary glaucomas. Prompt referral and aggressive management are crucial for successful outcomes.
- Prognosis for vision is guarded but may be better than for primary glaucoma in cases in which an underlying cause can be identified and corrected.

As information accumulates regarding underlying pathologic changes in dogs and cats with so-called primary glaucoma, the categorization of glaucomas into primary and secondary types has become more problematic. It is now understood that congenital malformations like pectinate ligament dysplasia and goniodysgenesis may not be sufficient to produce glaucoma, and that inflammation, pigment dispersion, vascular changes, and other alterations within the eye may provide the trigger for development of overt disease even in cases of apparent primary glaucoma.[1–5] However, increases in intraocular pressure (IOP) in dogs and cats frequently occur as a direct consequence of other well-defined ocular diseases. This article provides an overview of these secondary glaucomas in dogs.

Secondary glaucomas are common in dogs and cats. Seven percent of canine patients examined by the ophthalmology service at one teaching hospital were diagnosed with secondary glaucoma.[6] Gelatt and MacKay[7] found a prevalence at least equal to that of primary glaucoma, whereas Strom and colleagues[8] documented 1.78 cases of secondary glaucoma for every 1 case of primary glaucoma treated at their institution. Average age at time of onset for dogs with secondary glaucoma in

Disclosure: The author has nothing to disclose.
VCA South Shore, 595 Columbian Street, South Weymouth, MA 02190, USA
E-mail address: stephanie.pumphrey@vca.com

Vet Clin Small Anim 45 (2015) 1335–1364
http://dx.doi.org/10.1016/j.cvsm.2015.06.009
0195-5616/15/$ – see front matter © 2015 Elsevier Inc. All rights reserved.

the second study population was 7.7 years, which is similar to the average age of onset for primary glaucoma in the same study.[8] Canine breeds overrepresented in the studies available to date include Cairn Terriers, Jack Russell or Parson Russell Terriers, Poodles, Cocker Spaniels, Rhodesian Ridgebacks, Australian Cattle Dogs, and Boston Terriers.[6,8] In cats, based on the retrospective studies available to date, secondary glaucoma seems to be markedly more common than primary glaucoma, with 95% to 98% of feline glaucomas categorized as secondary.[9,10] Secondary glaucoma in cats is discussed by McLellan and Teixeira.[11]

Secondary glaucomas occur due to obstruction of aqueous humor flow by 1 or more mechanisms. Both the pupil and the iridocorneal angle (ICA) may be directly occluded or may be subject to closure by compression caused by displacement of adjacent structures. Flow may be obstructed at the pupil due to blockade by the lens, vitreous, inflammatory material or other debris, or neoplasms; or due to development of synechiae. Similarly, flow may be obstructed at the ICA or trabecular meshwork due to the presence of inflammatory material, blood, debris from uveal cysts, neoplasms or other cellular proliferations, or iatrogenically introduced material such as viscoelastics; due to occlusion by preiridal fibrovascular membranes (PIFMs); or due to formation of peripheral anterior synechiae (PAS). Dogs with underlying goniodysgenesis may be more vulnerable to secondary angle occlusion than anatomically normal dogs.[6]

PIFMs in particular may be underappreciated contributors to the development of secondary glaucoma. More substantial PIFMs may be apparent clinically as rubeosis iridis (growth of new blood vessels on the surface of the iris), whereas delicate or thin PIFMs may only be detected on histopathologic evaluation of the eye (**Fig. 1**). They develop in response to hypoxic conditions or other proangiogenic stimuli and have been documented in a wide range of ocular diseases in dogs and humans, including uveitis, retinal detachment, ocular neoplasia, hyphema, cataract, and lens luxation.[12–16] Vascular endothelial growth factor (VEGF) is thought to be a major mediator of PIFM development. Increased levels of VEGF in aqueous humor and positive immunohistochemical staining for VEGF in histologic samples have been reported for dogs with uveitis, retinal detachment, lens luxation, intraocular neoplasia, hyphema, and various forms of secondary glaucoma.[12,13] Anti-VEGF therapies represent a promising treatment option for many secondary glaucomas, although their efficacy has not been shown definitively in humans and information is lacking on their use in veterinary patients.[17]

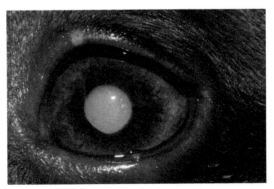

Fig. 1. A PIFM, represented clinically as rubeosis iridis, can be seen on the pupillary portion of the iris in this dog with a hypermature cataract, lens-induced uveitis, and an IOP of 28 mm Hg.

Secondary glaucoma may be suspected clinically based on ophthalmic examination findings such as flare, hyphema, iris changes, lens luxations, cataracts, or obvious intraocular masses. However, presence of increased IOP in a very young or very old animal, an animal with other signs of systemic illness, or a dog belonging to a breed not thought to be at risk of primary glaucoma should also increase suspicion of secondary glaucoma, as should documentation of concurrent bilateral increases in IOP. Bilateral involvement on initial presentation with primary glaucoma is rare, whereas 21% of dogs with secondary glaucoma had bilateral involvement in one study.[6]

Animals with secondary glaucoma may require more diagnostic testing than animals with primary glaucoma, and a thorough physical examination is crucial. High-resolution ocular ultrasonography (20 MHz) and ultrasonography biomicroscopy (35–50 MHz) are frequently helpful when evaluating a dog with suspected secondary glaucoma, particularly in cases in which dense corneal edema, hyphema, or other abnormalities preclude visualization of the interior of the eye. Other animals may benefit from additional imaging such as thoracic radiographs or abdominal ultrasonography; serology; cytology; or other laboratory testing.

Management of secondary glaucoma can be complicated. Treatment must be modified to account for the clinical features present in a given patient. Many of the medications used to treat primary glaucoma also have utility in the management of secondary glaucoma, although some commonly used topical medications, including prostaglandin analogues, β-blockers, demecarium bromide, and pilocarpine, are contraindicated in certain disease processes due to their ability to induce miosis, which can worsen pupillary block and further increase IOP. Conversely, mydriatics such as atropine or tropicamide, which tend to increase IOP and are typically detrimental in primary glaucoma, may be of use in specific patients with secondary glaucomas.

Selected surgical procedures and in-hospital therapies, such as removal of a luxated or cataractous lens or instillation of tissue plasminogen activator (tPA) into the anterior chamber, can also play important roles in treating secondary glaucoma. However, definitive information regarding outcomes for filtering or cycloablative surgeries in canine secondary glaucomas is limited.[18–24] Some of these procedures may be ineffective or even deleterious in the context of secondary glaucoma. For example, anterior chamber shunts may become occluded by fibrin, inflammatory cells, neoplastic cells, or other debris, and cycloablative procedures may worsen inflammation or trigger recurrent hyphema.

Prognosis for vision and/or globe retention in certain types of secondary glaucoma may be better than for primary glaucoma, particularly in cases in which an underlying cause can be found and addressed in a timely fashion (eg, treatment of uveitis or surgical removal of an anteriorly luxated lens). Prompt recognition of secondary glaucoma and rapid referral to a veterinary ophthalmologist will therefore increase the likelihood of a positive outcome.

In cases that result in a blind and painful eye, some of the definitive treatments used for primary glaucoma may not be appropriate for patients with secondary glaucomas. Cycloablative intravitreal injections of gentamicin or cidofovir may fail to achieve therapeutic goals in cases in which a tumor or other disorder is present, may worsen inflammation or lead to hemorrhage, and have been theorized to contribute to development of intraocular tumors.[25] Evisceration may also lead to poor outcomes (ie, need for eventual enucleation of the scleral shell and prosthesis), particularly in the context of neoplasia.[26] With rare exceptions, evisceration and intravitreal cycloablative injections should not be performed when secondary glaucoma is suspected, and enucleation with submission of the globe for histopathology should be the procedure of choice for blind and painful eyes.

UVEITIS

Glaucoma secondary to uveitis is common, accounting for up to 45% of secondary glaucomas in dogs.[6] Seventeen percent of dogs with uveitis in one study developed glaucoma within 5 years of diagnosis.[6] Potential underlying causes of uveitis are numerous and are not reviewed extensively here, but may include infectious, neoplastic or paraneoplastic, inflammatory, immune-mediated, vascular, iatrogenic, or idiopathic conditions. Reflex uveitis secondary to corneal disease may also lead to transient or permanent increases in IOP; anecdotally, brachycephalic breeds such as Shih Tzus and Boston Terriers seem to be most vulnerable to this occurrence (**Fig. 2**). Uveitides associated with lens trauma, cataracts, and cataract surgery are discussed separately later, as are selected immune-mediated and idiopathic uveitides.

Key Findings

Alterations to the clarity and composition of the aqueous humor are a hallmark of uveitis. Flare, hypopyon, hyphema, fibrin, or cellular infiltrates may all be noted. The iris may also change in shape, color, or texture. Possible iris changes include rubeosis iridis, inflammatory nodules, stromal hemorrhage, hyperpigmentation or depigmentation, iris bombe, and stromal edema (**Fig. 3**). Uveitis normally induces miosis, whereas increased IOP typically produces mydriasis caused by insults to the vascular and nerve supply to the iris. Patients presenting with glaucoma secondary to uveitis can therefore display a wide range of pupillary sizes, caused by the contradictory effects of inflammation and increased IOP on the iris. Presence of posterior synechiae and prior use of mydriatic drugs such as atropine or tropicamide may also affect pupillary size, and synechiae and iris infiltrates can lead to dyscoria (**Fig. 4**). Blepharospasm, photophobia, scleral injection or ciliary flush, corneal edema, keratic precipitates, corneal neovascularization, and vitreal infiltrates are also common signs of uveitis.

Pathogenesis

Uveitis has the potential to induce glaucoma via several mechanisms. Glaucoma may occur concurrently with uveitis, or may occur months to years after the uveitic episode secondary to damage from the initial inflammatory insult. In active uveitis, inflammatory debris such as white blood cells or fibrin can obstruct the pupil, ICA, or trabecular meshwork. PAS may form and block the ICA, whereas posterior synechiae can prevent egress of aqueous humor through the pupil, leading in some cases to iris bombe.

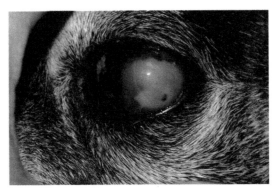

Fig. 2. Hypopyon, a corneal defect, and heavy corneal edema can be seen in this Boston Terrier with severe reflex uveitis. IOP was 69 mm Hg and the eye was nonvisual.

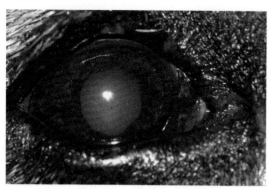

Fig. 3. Iris bombe and a fixed, miotic pupil have occurred secondary to posterior synechia formation in this uveitic dog with secondary glaucoma. Aqueous flare makes interior structures appear hazy.

Iris bombe can in turn alter aqueous humor flow in the anterior chamber, further worsening IOP. PIFMs are common and may occlude the pupil or ICA. Breakdown of lens zonules secondary to chronic or past inflammation can also cause lens instability or lens luxation.

Additional Diagnostics

Because the causes of uveitis are so diverse, a detailed discussion of diagnostics is beyond the scope of this article. Diagnostics are designed to eliminate potential underlying causes and should start with a thorough general physical examination. Serum chemistries, complete blood count, and urinalysis are warranted in most patients. Imaging, such as thoracic radiographs, abdominal ultrasound, and ocular ultrasonography, should be considered. Appropriate infectious disease testing will depend on patient signalment, ocular and physical examination findings, and geographic location, as well as the patient's recent travel history.

The role of aqueous humor cytology is controversial.[27] Aqueous humor cytology may be most useful when lymphoma is suspected.[28,29] Aqueous humor sampling for bacterial culture and sensitivity may also be rational if endophthalmitis is

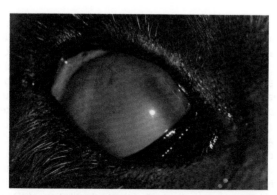

Fig. 4. Dyscoria, a swollen iris, aqueous flare, and heavy corneal edema with neovascularization are present in this German shepherd dog with uveitis and secondary glaucoma. Note the relative miosis caused by inflammation and formation of posterior synechiae.

suspected. Risk of iatrogenic trauma to the eye must be weighed against likely diagnostic utility when aqueocentesis is considered. Aspiration of material from the vitreous and/or subretinal space for cytology and culture likewise carries significant risk of complications, such as retinal detachment and hemorrhage, but may be indicated when posterior segment signs are present and life-threatening systemic conditions such as fungal disease or neoplasia are suspected.[30]

Treatment

Medical management of uveitic glaucoma can be difficult because many common therapeutic agents are associated with potential risks. For example, both steroids and nonsteroidal antiinflammatory drugs have the ability to increase IOP in susceptible dogs and may blunt the effectiveness of glaucoma medications, but their use is almost always necessary in uveitic glaucoma.[31–36]

Control of inflammation is critical and may require systemic as well as topical antiinflammatories. Attention to medication interactions and potential systemic side effects is important when using these medications. Options include topical and systemic corticosteroids and nonsteroidal antiinflammatory drugs (NSAIDs), and systemic immunomodulators such as tetracyclines, cyclosporine, azathioprine, or mycophenolate. Note that cyclosporine and tacrolimus do not reach therapeutic intraocular concentrations when applied topically and are therefore not suitable topical treatments for uveitis.[37,38] Depending on the underlying cause, chemotherapeutic agents, antibiotics, antifungals, or antiparasitics may also be required to achieve control of inflammation. If IOP fails to decrease in response to treatment in a patient with uveitic glaucoma, the possibility of corticosteroid-induced or NSAID-induced ocular hypertension should be considered.[39]

Mydriatic agents like atropine or tropicamide are also frequently used in managing uveitis, but they may increase IOP significantly in normal and glaucomatous animals.[40–43] However, mydriatics can also prevent formation of posterior synechiae, break down newly formed synechiae, release pupillary block, and promote restoration of the blood-aqueous barrier.[44] Judicious use of mydriatics may therefore help normalize IOP in selected patients with secondary glaucoma. However, because these drugs have the potential to cause significant harm in this context, they must be used with caution and patients must be monitored closely. Tropicamide is a weaker mydriatic and a poor cycloplegic but has a shorter duration of action than atropine, and therefore may be a safer, if potentially less effective, choice in dogs with uveitic glaucoma.

Conversely, use of miotics may also be undesirable in uveitic glaucoma. Latanoprost and related prostaglandin analogues are powerful antihypertensives in dogs but are also potent miotics in this species. Although these drugs can be helpful in reducing IOP, the potential detrimental effects of inducing miosis, including promotion of synechia formation and pupillary block, must also be considered. Use of prostaglandin analogues in uveitic glaucoma is additionally controversial due to their potential to worsen inflammation. However, this potential seems to be more of a theoretical than an actual concern, and in humans the available evidence is solidly in favor of using these drugs when necessary in patients with uveitic glaucoma.[45–47] Evidence is more limited in dogs but also supports their use.[48,49]

In humans, uveitic glaucoma often fails to respond to medical management alone, and the same may be true in veterinary patients.[50] Specific surgical interventions can be targeted toward findings in individual patients. Instillation of tPA into the anterior chamber can reduce IOP by inducing dissolution of fibrin and other proteinaceous debris or by breaking down synechiae.[51–53] Manual synechiolysis may be performed but carries the risk of intraocular hemorrhage, lens trauma, and cataract formation. Similarly, procedures such as iridotomies, designed to bypass pupillary block, are often limited in their effectiveness due to intraoperative complications (particularly hemorrhage) and failure of the iridotomy site to remain patent in the long term.[54]

Cyclodestructive and filtering procedures as described for primary glaucomas may fail to perform in cases of uveitic glaucoma. Attempting endocyclophotocoagulation (ECPC) or transscleral cyclophotocoagulation (TSCPC) in an actively inflamed eye may carry an increased risk of hyphema or retinal detachments, whereas anterior chamber shunts may occlude with inflammatory debris. These procedures may be more successful in quiet eyes in which past uveitic episodes have led to a delayed glaucoma due to fibrosis or the presence of synechia.

Prognosis

Prognosis for vision and for globe retention should be considered guarded in cases of uveitic glaucoma. Aggressive early intervention and identification and treatment of underlying causes may promote better outcomes.

CATARACTS AND CATARACT SURGERY

Glaucoma is a recognized early-term and late-term complication of phacoemulsification and other surgical procedures for cataract removal. However, glaucoma may also occur in dogs with cataracts that have not undergone surgery. Recent studies are not in agreement regarding frequency of this complication, with 5.1% to 16.8% of dogs developing glaucoma after cataract surgery and up to 20% of dogs with untreated cataracts developing glaucoma.[7,55–57] Underlying pathophysiology likely differs between surgical and nonsurgical patients. However, for both groups, regular monitoring, along with appropriate long-term use of antiinflammatories, may help to prevent glaucoma.

Key Findings

Patients may have a history of cataract surgery or a cataract may be present on examination. Synechiae or signs of uveitis, as described earlier, including miosis, flare, fibrin deposition, keratic precipitates, increased iris pigmentation, pigment deposition on the lens capsule, and rubeosis iridis, may be present. In diabetic dogs or patients with rapidly developing cataracts, anterior chamber depth may be decreased, and in patients with anterior capsule ruptures or larger equatorial lens capsule ruptures lens material may be present in the anterior chamber (smaller equatorial or posterior capsular ruptures may only become apparent on ultrasonographic examination of the anterior segment).

Pathogenesis

Uveitis accounts for many cases of glaucoma in pets with cataracts or with a history of cataract surgery, and pathogenesis in these cases is similar to that described earlier for other uveitic glaucomas. Lens-induced uveitis (LIU) is now thought to occur in all patients with significant cataracts, although etiology is not clear and may vary between patients (**Fig. 5**).[58–60] LIU may be particularly severe in diabetics, in certain breeds, in patients with cataracts that have developed rapidly, and in dogs with hypermature cataracts. These patients often present with prominent keratic precipitates and inflammatory cell clumps in the aqueous (**Fig. 6**).[58] Long-standing cataracts and LIU may also lead to breakdown of zonular fibers and subsequent lens instability.

Patients with rapidly developing cataracts, particularly diabetics, are at additional risk of glaucoma due to the potential for lens capsule rupture and/or pupillary block. Marked lens intumescence is present in these patients due to an osmotic gradient

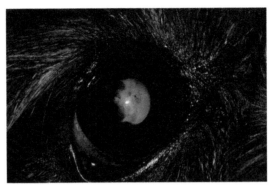

Fig. 5. A diabetic miniature schnauzer with chronic LIU and secondary glaucoma. The iris is heavily pigmented and posterior synechiae are present. The pupil is miotic due to synechiae.

drawing water into the lens, which promotes rupture or tearing of the lens capsule, most commonly equatorially (**Fig. 7**).[61,62] Labrador retrievers may be at increased risk.[61,62] Patients with lens capsule ruptures often present with severe uveitis, and 20% of eyes with capsular ruptures were glaucomatous on initial evaluation in one study.[61] Intumescent cataracts, by occupying more space within the globe than a normal lens, may also cause pupillary block and narrow the ICA (**Fig. 8**). This situation is sometimes termed phacomorphic glaucoma.

Glaucoma after cataract surgery must be differentiated from postoperative hypertension (POH). POH is a temporary and reversible increase in IOP occurring in the hours to days following cataract surgery. POH is extremely common, although its pathogenesis is not well understood.[63,64] Possible mechanisms include changes in ICA and ciliary cleft morphology and angle occlusion by inflammatory material or surgical viscoelastics.[63–65] The relationship between POH and glaucoma is not clear in most studies done to date, although Labrador retrievers with POH seem to be at increased risk of subsequent glaucoma.[66]

Postoperative glaucoma may occur secondary to pupillary obstruction by synechia formation, fibrin, vitreous, proliferating lens epithelial cells, or other material. This type of glaucoma has been suggested to occur most commonly in the immediate

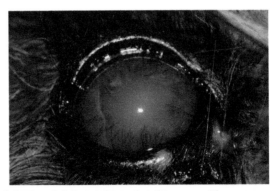

Fig. 6. Another diabetic miniature schnauzer, this one with severe granulomatous LIU, including keratic precipitates, dense corneal edema, heavy aqueous flare, and corneal neovascularization. This eye was enucleated due to vision loss and intractable glaucoma.

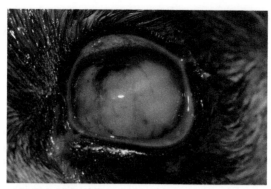

Fig. 7. A lens capsule rupture has occurred in this terrier mix with diabetes mellitus and rapidly developing cataracts. Flare and corneal edema partially obscure the view of interior structures, but hyphema and pigment dispersion can be seen, along with herniation of the lens nucleus into the anterior chamber on the right-hand side of the frame. The curved line to the right of center is the torn equatorial margin of the lens capsule.

postoperative period.[54] Postoperative pupillary occlusion may also lead to redirection of aqueous humor into the vitreous, producing a so-called malignant glaucoma. Infectious endophthalmitis is a rare near-term postoperative complication but can be serious and can lead to refractory glaucoma. Similarly, toxic anterior segment syndrome (TASS), a marked inflammatory response to endotoxin, preservatives, or other inflammatory mediators in the absence of documented infection, can produce a severe postoperative uveitis and secondary glaucoma.[67] TASS has been linked with contaminated irrigation fluids, viscoelastics, and intraocular lenses and with improperly cleaned and sterilized surgical instruments and equipment.[67]

In the longer term, however, angle occlusion may be responsible for the majority of postoperative glaucomas. Angle occlusion may occur due to PIFMs, PAS, pigment dispersion, complications associated with retinal detachments, or other postoperative changes.[54,68] Preexisting goniodysgenesis may be a risk factor for postoperative glaucoma, and pathogenesis may vary depending on breed.[68] Boston Terriers, Cocker Spaniels, Cocker-Poodle Crosses, Shih Tzus, Jack Russell Terriers, Bichon Frises, and Labrador Retrievers appear to have a greater chance of developing postoperative glaucoma than other breeds.[57,66,68] Other identified risk factors include increased patient age, hypermature cataracts, increased phacoemulsification time, failure to place

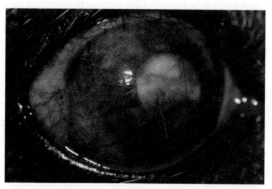

Fig. 8. Chronic phacomorphic glaucoma in a diabetic miniature dachshund. The intumescent lens has pushed the iris forward and the anterior chamber is almost nonexistent.

an intraocular lens, and intraoperative hemorrhage.[55–57,69] Dogs with overt preoperative LIU have not been proven to have a higher incidence of postoperative glaucoma than those without overt LIU, although LIU is considered to be a risk factor by most ophthalmologists.[57,69] Diabetes also does not seem to increase risk of preoperative or postoperative complications, aside from those associated with lens intumescence.[69]

Additional Diagnostics

All dogs with cataracts should be offered prompt referral to a veterinary ophthalmologist, particularly if signs of uveitis are present or if cataracts have developed rapidly. Patients with rapidly developing cataracts should be screened for diabetes mellitus and should be evaluated using high-resolution ultrasonography to document existing lens capsule ruptures. Preoperative gonioscopy may also provide some information regarding risk of postoperative glaucoma.[68]

Patients presenting with postoperative glaucoma must receive a careful ophthalmic examination, as treatment will depend on pathogenesis. If endophthalmitis is suspected, aqueous humor cytology and bacterial culture may be warranted.

Treatment

Patients with LIU, intumescent cataracts, or lens capsule ruptures benefit most from aggressive antiinflammatory therapy followed by phacoemulsification as soon as appropriate. Glaucoma may be managed with topical carbonic anhydrase inhibitors, and with intravenous mannitol as needed. Use of latanoprost and other miotics may worsen pupillary block, and the miosis produced by these medications is also incompatible with performing lens extraction surgery.

Patients with postoperative glaucoma should be treated according to pathogenesis. Topical carbonic anhydrase inhibitors, β-blockers, and intravenous mannitol are appropriate in many situations. As in other secondary glaucomas, miotics, such as latanoprost, must be used with care if pupillary block is a concern. Intracameral tPA injection or topical mydriatics may be helpful if fibrin is present or if synechia are of recent origin.[51–53] Explantation of intraocular lenses and irrigation of the anterior chamber with antibiotics may be appropriate if endophthalmitis or TASS are suspected or fibrin formation is extensive. Synechiolysis, iridotomy, or anterior vitrectomy procedures are a consideration in cases of pupillary block or malignant glaucoma, although they may provide only temporary relief.[54] Iridencleisis was reportedly successful in maintaining vision and IOP over a 6-month period in 1 dog with postoperative pupillary occlusion and iris bombe.[70] Glaucomas developing months to years after cataract surgery may behave more like the primary glaucomas, and may be amenable to many of the same medical and surgical treatments.[20–24,69] ECPC may prove an effective treatment for these patients.[22]

Prognosis

Prognosis for vision and for globe retention is guarded in these patients. From 62% to 75% of dogs with postoperative glaucoma reportedly lose vision.[55,69] Prognosis may be favorable for dogs with intumescent cataracts or lens capsule ruptures that receive timely medical and surgical management.[61]

LENS INSTABILITY AND LENS LUXATION

Lens instability may occur as a primary disease process or may arise secondary to other diseases. Specific canine breeds, including many of the terrier breeds,

Shar-Peis, Border Collies, and Chinese Crested Dogs, show a predisposition for zonular fiber breakdown in the absence of other ocular diseases. This type of lens instability occurs most frequently in young dogs and is typically bilateral, although often not simultaneous.[71] A mutation in the ADAMTS17 gene has been identified in many of the affected breeds and is thought to be causative.[72,73] Lens instability may also occur secondary to chronic uveitis, trauma, hypermature cataracts, or advanced age. In addition, lens luxations can be seen secondary to globe enlargement caused by primary glaucoma; this particular phenomenon will not be covered here.

Key Findings

Dogs with anterior lens luxations often present with markedly elevated IOP and dense corneal edema, which may complicate initial diagnosis. This is particularly true if an anterior luxation is present. Many of these patients are quite uncomfortable and may be difficult to examine. Signalment is key and suspicion should be high for any painful, red, or cloudy eye in a susceptible breed.

In patients with a clear cornea, the lens may often be visualized in the anterior chamber. Use of a slit beam may help highlight the altered lens-iris relationship. Focal corneal edema may be present where the luxated lens makes contact with the corneal endothelium (**Fig. 9**). Posterior luxations or subluxations may be more difficult to appreciate clinically, particularly for nonspecialists. In humans, angle closure caused by lens subluxation is often misdiagnosed as primary glaucoma.[74] Findings in cases of posterior luxation or subluxation may include changes or inconsistencies in the depth of the anterior chamber, iridodonesis or phacodonesis (fluttering or trembling of the iris or lens), vitreal strands in the pupil or anterior chamber, or presence of an aphakic crescent (**Fig. 10**). A posteriorly luxated lens may be visible in the dependent portion of the posterior segment, particularly if it is cataractous. A focal region of edema may be present in the ventral cornea in patients with a previously anteriorly luxated lens that has moved posteriorly.

Pathogenesis

In the case of an anterior luxation, the pupil is blocked by formed vitreous adherent to the posterior aspect of the lens or by the lens itself. This condition tends to lead to a rapid, marked increase in IOP. The pathogenesis of glaucoma in dogs with subluxations or posterior luxations is less clear. Chronic instability and iris microtrauma, leading to

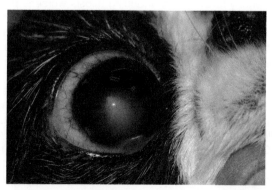

Fig. 9. This Japanese Chin has an anterior lens luxation and a region of focal corneal edema where the lens contacts the corneal endothelium. In this dog severe iris hypoplasia likely helped blunt IOP increase secondary to pupillary block.

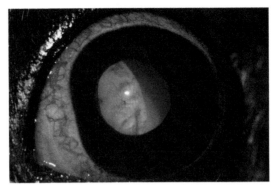

Fig. 10. An aphakic crescent is present in this Boston Terrier with glaucoma secondary to lens subluxation. A posterior luxation was present in the fellow, normotensive eye.

inflammation and subsequent PIFM formation, likely plays a role in the development of glaucoma in these patients.[75] Pupillary block or angle compression caused by an anteriorly displaced but not yet fully luxated lens, development of PAS, or occlusion of the pupil or ICA by strands of liquefied vitreous may also promote the onset of glaucoma in patients with subluxations or posterior luxations. In patients with lens instability secondary to uveitis or a hypermature cataract, the underlying disease state may contribute as much to the development of glaucoma as the lens instability itself.

Additional Diagnostics

Careful ocular examination is necessary to rule out underlying causes for lens instability, such as uveitis or preexisting glaucoma. In cases in which visualization of the lens is prevented by dense corneal edema, anterior segment ultrasonography may be required for diagnosis.

Treatment

Emergency treatment of glaucoma secondary to lens instability requires careful and considered use of topical medications. Any medication with the potential to induce miosis, including pilocarpine, timolol or other β-blockers, demecarium bromide, and latanoprost or other prostaglandin analogues, is absolutely contraindicated in the presence of an anteriorly luxated lens. Inducing miosis worsens pupillary block and traps the lens in the anterior chamber. Topical carbonic anhydrase inhibitors and intravenous mannitol are rational choices to try to reduce IOP. In selected cases of pupillary block, mydriatics may be warranted to try to release or break the block, but these drugs must be used with care and in a controlled clinical setting due to their ability to increase IOP.

Miotics may be used in dogs with subluxations and posterior luxations as long as excessive amounts of liquefied vitreous are not transiting the pupil. These medications may be helpful in preventing future anterior luxations in these patients. Latanoprost is an excellent first-line choice given its potent effects on IOP and the marked miosis it tends to induce. Owners must be counseled on the importance of rigid compliance with twice a day dosing, as rebound mydriasis, which may allow anterior lens movement, tends to occur when the drug is withdrawn. Other topical glaucoma treatments may be added as needed.

Definitive treatment of an anterior lens luxation requires removal or repositioning of the lens, and must be done on an emergent basis if the potential for vision exists.

Surgical removal is accomplished by means of an intracapsular lens extraction (ICLE) or by phacoemulsification followed by extraction of the lens capsule through a small incision. A sutured sulcus intraocular lens may or may not be placed.[76] Medical management with antihypertensives and antiinflammatories is continued. Recently it has been proposed that ECPC at the time of lens removal may lead to better outcomes than lens removal alone.[77]

Transcorneal repositioning or reduction is achieved via changes in head position and manipulation of the globe; once the lens is posterior to the iris, miotics are applied to maintain the lens in the posterior segment.[78] Although transcorneal repositioning sounds simple, its success depends on the underlying state of the vitreous and on an accurate analysis of the position of the pupillary margin with relation to the lens, which typically requires a slit lamp for evaluation. If miotics are applied prematurely or with the pupillary margin still posterior to the lens, or if significant liquefied vitreous still occupies the pupil, the procedure will fail and the glaucomatous crisis may be worsened. For this reason, transcorneal repositioning should be performed by a veterinary ophthalmologist. Furthermore, if repositioning fails, ICLE is necessary and also requires a veterinary ophthalmologist.[78]

In patients with subluxations or posterior luxations, long-term medical management with miotics, additional antihypertensives, and antiinflammatories may be possible.[75,79] Surgical removal of a subluxated or posteriorly luxated lens is a consideration but may cause more harm than good, particularly if surgical removal requires disruption of the vitreous. In visual eyes with subluxations or posterior luxations, cycloablative and filtering procedures such as ECPC or TSCPC or anterior chamber shunt placement may be considered, although shunts may become occluded with liquefied vitreous or with inflammatory material.[77] In one study, TSCPC was minimally effective in treating glaucoma that developed after ICLE in dogs.[19]

Prognosis

Prognosis has generally been considered guarded for dogs with anterior luxations. In the largest study to date, only 47% of dogs undergoing ICLE remained visual and normotensive at 1 year after surgery.[80] Dogs with preoperative glaucoma were significantly less likely to have favorable outcomes than dogs with normal IOP before surgery.[80] In contrast, 70% of dogs that underwent ICLE with placement of a sutured sulcus lens in another study were visual at time of last follow-up, with 20% developing glaucoma.[76] It should be noted that most dogs in the latter study did not have increased IOP at the time of surgery and were not considered to have undergone emergency surgery; the stated goal of this study was to assess dogs that were considered good candidates for surgery.[76] This study may provide a rationale for earlier surgical intervention in dogs with lens instability.

Dogs with posterior luxations and subluxations that were managed medically with demecarium bromide did not show any difference from dogs that received no treatment with respect to time of onset of glaucoma or vision loss. In this study, 58% of eyes were visual at 2 years from the time of diagnosis.[79] Success rates for transcorneal repositioning in dogs with anterior luxations were comparable with those for ICLE and medical management: 54.5% of dogs were visual at time of last follow-up and median time to vision loss was 12 months.[78]

NEOPLASIA

Intraocular neoplasia can be divided broadly into 2 types: primary and metastatic. Melanoma was the most common primary intraocular tumor associated with glaucoma in dogs in one study.[8] Metastatic lesions constitute about 4% of canine ocular neoplasias and involvement may be bilateral.[81] A recent review of canine ocular neoplasia provides an excellent overview of this broad subject.[82]

Key Findings

Intraocular neoplasia may present as an obvious mass in the iris or ciliary body, or as diffuse or sectorial iris color change (**Fig. 11**). Dyscoria or anisocoria may be present (**Fig. 12**). Alternatively, ocular tumors, particularly posterior segment neoplasms and metastases from distant sites, may first manifest as hyphema, uveitis, or glaucoma without other obvious signs (**Fig. 13**). Round cell neoplasias often mimic uveitis, with or without hypopyon, hyphema, or iris changes. Neoplasia should also be suspected in cases of unexplained hyphema or in patients that fail to respond to treatment for uveitis or glaucoma.[83]

Pathogenesis

Twenty-six percent of canine eyes with intraocular neoplasia submitted for histopathology have evidence of glaucoma.[81] Neoplasms may efface or occlude the ICA or pupil via a direct mass effect, or may displace the iris and produce PAS or ciliary cleft collapse. Metastatic neoplasias may carpet the uveal tract and angle with neoplastic cells.[81] Exfoliated neoplastic cells may migrate to the ICA or trabecular meshwork, preventing normal aqueous drainage. Inflammatory infiltrates, red blood cells, or PIFMs associated with tumors can also lead to angle blockage or synechia formation.

Additional Diagnostics

Preliminary diagnosis of intraocular neoplasms is often made based on observation alone. However, eyes with unexplained hyphema or uveitis in which intraocular structures cannot be clearly visualized should be evaluated using ocular ultrasonography. Additional imaging, including thoracic radiographs and abdominal ultrasonography, is also warranted. Cytology is seldom helpful except in cases of suspected round cell neoplasia.[27–29] Moreover, aqueocentesis or attempted aspiration of intraocular masses may lead to uveitis, hyphema, or further increases in IOP.

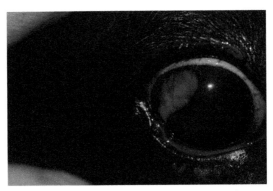

Fig. 11. A Labrador retriever with a large, minimally pigmented iris mass and secondary glaucoma. Histopathology was not performed, but clinically the mass was suspected to represent metastasis from a primary lung tumor.

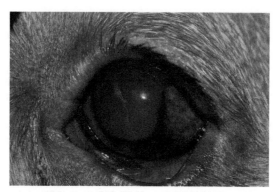

Fig. 12. Dyscoria, a mass effect in the lateral iris, and hyphema are manifestations of multi-centric lymphoma in this mixed-breed dog with secondary glaucoma.

Treatment

Although small anterior uveal neoplasms may be amenable to surgical resection or laser ablation, most neoplasms extensive enough to cause glaucoma are best treated with enucleation. The exception to this may be lymphoma and other round cell tumors, which can respond to chemotherapy.

Prognosis

Melanoma and ciliary body adenoma are the two most common primary intraocular tumors in dogs. Prognosis for the globe is poor in cases in which glaucoma has already occurred, but prognosis for life is favorable, because these tumors have low metastatic rates in dogs.[84,85] Prognosis for both the globe and for life is poor in cases of metastatic tumors, again with the possible exception of lymphoma and other round cell tumors, in which prognosis for life is guarded to poor but in which resolution of ocular signs may be seen with chemotherapy. Dogs with intraocular lymphoma, however, are highly likely to have concurrent central nervous system involvement.[27]

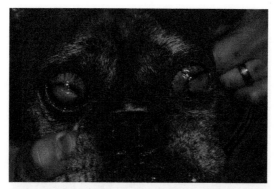

Fig. 13. Both eyes were severely buphthalmic in this boxer. Lymphadenopathy was also present and lymph node cytology was diagnostic for lymphoma. Intraocular structures could not be visualized, but high-resolution ocular ultrasonography (images not available) showed a marked thickening of the choroid, suspected to be tumor infiltrate.

HYPHEMA

Hyphema is a common clinical finding in dogs. Common causes for hyphema include uveitis, trauma, systemic hypertension, thrombocytopenia, coagulation disorders, vascular disease, neoplasia, retinal detachments, intraocular surgery, and congenital defects such as collie eye anomaly, persistent hyperplastic primary vitreous, or persistent hyperplastic tunica vasculosa lentis. Hemorrhage may also arise from PIFMs or from vitreoretinal vascular membranes.[86] Labrador retrievers may be predisposed to the latter condition, which has been deemed canine ocular gliovascular syndrome in a recent article.[87] In dogs, retinal detachment has been proposed as the most common cause of hyphema.[88–90]

Key Findings

The term hyphema refers to the presence of blood in the anterior chamber, which may be accompanied by fibrin or hypopyon. Depending on the extent and duration of the hemorrhage, blood may appear as liquid admixed with aqueous humor, in the form of a clot, or as a precipitate in the dependent portion of the anterior chamber (**Fig. 14**). Other signs of uveitis may be present. Significant hyphema may prevent evaluation of intraocular structures, and long-standing hyphema may lead to corneal discoloration or endothelial decompensation and edema.

Pathogenesis

Red blood cells, inflammatory debris, or synechiae may occlude the pupil or the ICA and trabecular meshwork. Underlying causes for hyphema, such as PIFMs and neoplasms, may also obstruct the flow of aqueous.

Additional Diagnostics

A thorough physical examination allows documentation of additional injuries or hemorrhage elsewhere in the body. Owners should be queried as to potential trauma history and presence of other signs suggesting a systemic coagulation issue, such as hematuria or melena. Blood pressure measurement, laboratory tests including a complete blood count and coagulation panel, and ocular ultrasonography should be performed in all cases of unexplained hyphema (**Fig. 15**). Additional imaging, such as thoracic radiographs and abdominal ultrasonography, should also be considered.

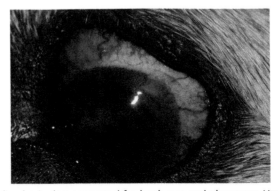

Fig. 14. This shepherd-mix dog presented for hyphema and glaucoma. Hypopyon and fibrin can also be seen in the anterior chamber. The globe is deformed dorsally and neoplasia was suspected. The owner elected not to pursue further diagnostics.

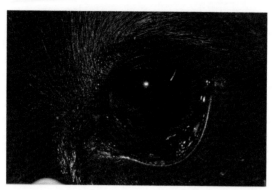

Fig. 15. Hyphema in a retriever-mix dog presenting for acute renal failure caused by lepto-spirosis. Systolic blood pressure was 230 mm Hg at the time of diagnosis. IOP was 31 mm Hg. The hyphema resorbed and the IOP normalized once systemic hypertension was controlled.

Treatment

Consensus is lacking regarding optimal treatment of hyphema in dogs or humans.[91] Management of underlying conditions, such as coagulopathies or systemic hypertension, is essential. Treatment with antiinflammatories (topical or systemic steroids or NSAIDs) is also likely warranted, although attention should be paid to the potential for NSAIDs to exacerbate bleeding. Activity restriction should be recommended to limit the possibility of further hemorrhage.

Both miotics and mydriatics have been proposed as treatments for hyphema. Miotics have been suggested to hasten resorption of hyphema by increasing iris surface area, but they may also lead to pupillary block or promote formation of posterior synechiae.[30] Mydriatics may diminish chances of synechia formation, can stabilize the blood-aqueous barrier, and can relieve ciliary spasm, but may also lead to increases in IOP and are usually contraindicated in animals that have already shown IOP increases.

As noted previously, intracameral tPA can aid in the dissolution of clotted blood and debris and may help break down synechiae of recent onset, which may be of significant benefit in normalizing IOP. However, tPA injection also may trigger recurrent hemorrhage, and iris trauma may occur in eyes with iris bombe or shallow anterior chambers when the anterior chamber is entered. Patient selection is therefore critical.

Filtering and cycloablative procedures are unlikely to be successful in pets with significant hyphema, and may lead to further deterioration.

Prognosis

Prognosis depends on the degree and duration of hemorrhage and IOP increase as well as on any underlying causes. Dogs that are treated soon after the onset of signs and in which IOP is normalized quickly may retain vision and a comfortable globe. However, prognosis should generally be considered guarded for both vision and globe retention.[88,90,92]

RETINAL DETACHMENTS

Unilateral retinal detachments in dogs frequently go unnoticed by owners, because dogs compensate well for unilateral vision loss. Animals are typically presented for evaluation when vision is lost in the fellow eye or when complications develop after the initial detachment. Rhegmatogenous retinal detachments, in which a retinal break or tear occurs followed by dissection of vitreous or fluid between the retina and retinal pigmented epithelium, have a particular association with glaucoma in both humans and dogs.[54] Rhegmatogenous retinal detachments occur in dogs with uveitis, primary glaucoma, retinal dysplasia, collie eye anomaly, persistent hyperplastic primary vitreous, lens luxations, oculoskeletal dysplasia, vitreal liquefaction or degeneration, and peripheral cystoid retinal degeneration.[93,94] They may also occur secondary to trauma or to cataract surgery.[93,94] Shih Tzus, Boston Terriers, Italian Greyhounds, and several other small breeds may be predisposed to spontaneous complete retinal tears secondary to vitreal degenerative changes; these may occur in young dogs and have been linked with activities that involve vigorous head shaking, such as playing with toys.[94,95]

Key Findings

Dogs often present with typical signs of glaucoma. Suspicion may be raised by breed. Hyphema or vitreal hemorrhage may be present, along with evidence of vitreal liquefaction (**Fig. 16**). Fundic evaluation may be prevented by corneal edema, hyphema, and other changes; ocular ultrasonography is often necessary to diagnose the retinal tear and detachment. In patients in which the fundus can be visualized, the torn retina is often seen draped or folded over the optic nerve head; the tapetum appears brighter than usual without the overlying retina, and retinal vessels are not seen in their normal position.

Pathogenesis

Photoreceptor outer segments have been documented in the anterior segment following rhegmatogenous detachments and are thought to occlude aqueous outflow pathways in some patients.[96] Long-standing retinal detachments of any kind also provide a stimulus for neovascularization and may cause PIFM formation and angle or pupil occlusion.[12,13,81,97] Intraocular hemorrhage may occur at the time of the tear or from PIFMs or previtreal membranes in more chronic cases.

Retinal reattachment surgery following rhegmatogenous detachments is becoming more common in dogs and has also been associated with development of glaucoma. Migration of silicone oil from the posterior segment into the anterior chamber following

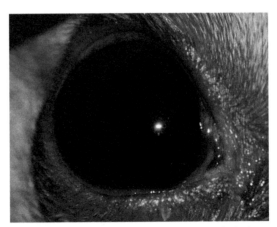

Fig. 16. This 5-year-old Chihuahua presented with hyphema and glaucoma approximately 2 years after initial diagnosis of a retinal tear and detachment in this eye. Blood has settled in the dependent portion of the anterior chamber. A Haab's stria can be seen to the right of the flash artifact.

this type of surgery occurs in up to 50% of patients and can obstruct the ICA, leading to increased IOP.[98] Inflammation and synechia or PIFM formation may also contribute. In one study, 25% of dogs developed glaucoma after retinal reattachment surgery.[98]

Additional Diagnostics

As noted earlier, ocular ultrasonography is often necessary to diagnose retinal detachments in dogs that have already developed glaucoma. Unless primary glaucoma is suspected as an inciting cause, the fellow eye should undergo pharmacologic dilation and should be examined carefully for peripheral retinal cysts, retinal breaks or tears, vitreal liquefaction or degeneration (visible as vitreal strands, opacities, or swirling motion in the vitreous), lens instability, and other conditions associated with detachment.

Treatment

Initial medical management is similar to that for other secondary glaucomas, again with attention paid to the potential undesirable effects of miotics in cases with pupillary block. Presence of uveitis or hyphema also warrants treatment with antiinflammatories. Intracameral tPA injection is a consideration if hyphema is present. Activity restriction should be recommended if hyphema is present, if pathology is noted in the other eye, or if the breed and other findings are consistent with vitreal liquefaction-related detachment.

Prompt retinal reattachment surgery has been suggested to limit photoreceptor shedding and resolve IOP increases; reattachment surgery may also preserve or restore vision.[54] Retinal reattachment surgery requires specialized equipment and training, and is offered by only a small number of veterinary ophthalmologists in North America. Prophylactic laser barrier retinopexy is more widely available and may be a consideration for the fellow eye in certain patients with focal tears, holes, or other disorders (such as colobomas in dogs with collie eye anomaly). Silicone oil in the anterior chamber following reattachment surgery must be removed.

Prognosis

Little information is available on outcomes for glaucoma secondary to retinal detachments. Dogs that receive no treatment of rhegmatogenous detachments or that are managed with medication alone seem more likely to develop intractable glaucoma than dogs that undergo retinal reattachment surgery.[99] Of dogs undergoing reattachment surgery that had not yet developed glaucoma, 90% to 99% maintained an anatomic reattachment, whereas 73% to 90% were reported to regain vision for at least some period of time following surgery.[95,98,100] Surgical outcomes are thought to be better for dogs with rhegmatogenous detachments secondary to vitreal liquefaction, and worse for dogs that have undergone prior cataract surgery or ICLE, that have sustained trauma, or that have previtreal membranes.[94,100] Success rates are likely poorer for dogs that already have increased IOP at the time of surgery. Prognosis for vision is poor to nonexistent for dogs with medically managed glaucoma secondary to retinal detachments, whereas prognosis for retention of a comfortable globe is guarded and enucleation or evisceration is often necessary. Significant hyphema is a negative prognostic indicator.[88,92,99]

PENETRATING AND BLUNT TRAUMA

Trauma to the eye may cause uveitis, retinal detachments, hyphema, lens luxations, cataract formation, infection, and other complications. Clinical findings and management for these phenomena are discussed earlier. Specific discussion of trauma-related glaucomas is therefore limited to a few special circumstances.

Angle Recession Glaucoma

Angle recession glaucoma is associated with blunt ocular trauma in humans. Angle recession is assessed by gonioscopy or ultrasound biomicroscopy and occurs in 75% of humans who have sustained blunt trauma to the eyes, a subset of whom go on to develop glaucoma.[101,102] Glaucoma occurs secondary to shearing or tearing of the ICA and trabecular meshwork, and can develop months to years after the initial trauma. Although dogs and cats should theoretically be vulnerable to the same type of injury, documentation of angle recession glaucoma in veterinary patients is limited.[81,103] Anterior chamber shunt implantation has been suggested as a viable therapy in dogs with this type of injury that fail to respond to medical management.[103]

Penetrating Trauma with Lens Damage

Penetrating trauma with lens damage is another type of ocular injury requiring special attention. This injury is common in veterinary patients, particularly in puppies, and often involves penetration of the cornea by the claw or tooth of another animal.[104] Intraocular infection is a concern with this type of injury and may show a pattern of markedly delayed onset.[81,105] Lens capsule rupture may also lead to a severe sterile uveitis, often of a granulomatous nature.[106] Eighty-five percent of canine patients with histopathologic evidence of suppurative endophthalmitis following penetrating trauma were reportedly glaucomatous.[105] Lens capsule disruption may not be obvious on initial presentation due to corneal edema, marked miosis, heavy flare, or presence of fibrin or hyphema. Attempts should be made to induce mydriasis to allow full evaluation of intraocular structures in patients with evidence of penetrating trauma, although this presents some risk if IOP is increased.

   Traditionally, management of these cases has involved immediate phacoemulsification to remove the damaged lens, along with corneal suturing or grafting as needed.[104] More recently, it has been proposed that medical management rather than immediate surgery leads to better outcomes in dogs and cats with this type of injury.[107] In the latter study, early referral to a veterinary ophthalmologist and smaller laceration size were correlated with greater likelihood of retaining vision.[107]

SPECIFIC IMMUNE-MEDIATED AND/OR PIGMENT-MEDIATED DISEASES

Several conditions characterized by pigmentary changes in the eye and known to cause secondary glaucoma have been described in dogs. Etiologies are unclear for this group of diseases, but immune dysregulation is thought to play a role in at least some of these conditions. Pigment dispersion and inflammation have been documented in canine primary glaucoma as well, which may suggest that primary glaucoma and this set of diseases share some underlying pathophysiology.[1]

Melanocytic Glaucoma/Pigmentary Glaucoma/Ocular Melanosis

This frustrating condition bears several different names, but is seen almost exclusively in Cairn Terriers, Boxers, Labrador Retrievers, and Dachshunds, with prevalence being highest in cairns.[81,108] Disease is usually bilateral (at least in cairns) and characteristic findings include deposition of pigmented cells in thickened, plaquelike lesions in the sclera, iris, ICA, and other portions of the eye (**Fig. 17**).[108,109] It is not clear whether these cells are melanocytes or melanophages (macrophages that have phagocytosed pigment granules), and underlying pathogenesis is also unclear.[110] Progression of disease is variable, but prognosis is poor for vision and globe retention in dogs that have developed glaucoma. Medical management and surgical interventions are generally

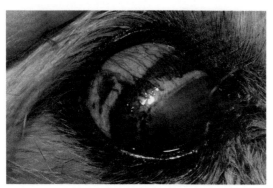

Fig. 17. A Cairn Terrier with melanocytic glaucoma. Note the prominent pigmented plaques in the sclera.

minimally effective, and enucleation or evisceration is often required to relieve discomfort. Extraocular manifestations of this condition have not been documented.

Golden Retriever Uveitis-related/Cyst-related Glaucomas

Golden retriever uveitis (GRU; also called golden pigmentary uveitis) is another frustrating condition of unknown cause, which occurs almost exclusively in middle-aged to older Golden Retrievers. The condition is thought to be inherited.[111] Both eyes are typically affected.[112] Although the term "uveitis" is used to describe the condition, the inflammatory changes seen on histopathologic evaluation of affected eyes have been unimpressive compared with the clinical findings.[113] Common clinical signs include uveal cysts, darkened irides with entropion uveae, radial deposition of pigment on the anterior lens capsule and synechiae formation, fibrinous or cobwebby debris in the anterior chamber, hyphema, and cataract formation (**Figs. 18** and **19**). Glaucoma may occur secondary to synechia formation; angle occlusion by cysts, blood, pigment, or other debris; or presence of PIFMs.[81,114] Progression and severity are highly variable. Forty-six percent of dogs with GRU in one study developed glaucoma, and all glaucomatous eyes in this study lost vision.[112] As with melanocytic glaucoma, medication and surgical interventions are often ineffective, and extraocular manifestations of disease have not been noted.

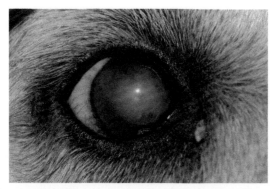

Fig. 18. Radial pigment deposition on the anterior lens capsule, pigmented debris on the corneal endothelium, corneal edema, and a cataract are present in this Golden Retriever with GRU. IOP has remained between 20–25 mm Hg in this eye.

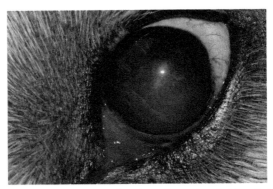

Fig. 19. Fibrinlike debris in the anterior chamber of another Golden Retriever with GRU.

Comparable cyst-related syndromes have been described in great Danes and American bulldogs; treatment and prognosis are similar.[115,116] Anterior chamber shallowing and mild IOP increases have been seen in cats with uveal cysts, and cyst-related glaucoma is also reported in humans.[117–120] Uveal cysts in dogs have typically been treated as benign findings and in many individuals they are not cause for concern.[30,121] However, documentation of cyst-related glaucomas in multiple canine breeds and in other species suggests that presence of uveal cysts in canine patients may warrant further evaluation. Ultrasound biomicroscopy and gonioscopy may be particularly appropriate ancillary tests in dogs with cysts, to assess ICA morphology and document additional cysts posterior to the iris that may be causing iris displacement and secondary angle closure.[122,123]

Uveodermatologic Syndrome/Vogt-Koyanagi-Harada–like Syndrome

Uveodermatologic syndrome (UDS) occurs most commonly in young dogs. The condition was first described in Akitas, although it has since been diagnosed in several other breeds.[30,124–127] Akitas with a particular dog leukocyte antigen haplotype are thought to be at greater risk of developing the disease, suggesting an immune-mediated pathogenesis.[128] UDS is characterized by a severe granulomatous anterior uveitis and chorioretinitis. Skin and hair-coat signs (vitiligo, poliosis, alopecia, ulceration) are variable (**Fig. 20**). In humans, neurologic signs are a component of

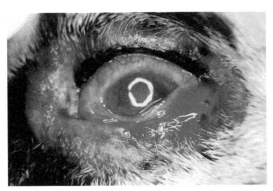

Fig. 20. Ocular and periocular changes in a great Dane with UDS and secondary glaucoma. (*Courtesy of* Stefano Pizzirani, DVM, PhD, DACVO, DECVS-I, Tufts University, North Grafton, MA.)

Vogt-Koyanagi-Harada–like syndrome; this manifestation of disease has never been definitively documented in a canine patient.[30] Pigmented cells are targeted for attack and depigmentation of the nontapetal fundus is often prominent.[81] Unilateral UDS has been reported in a Siberian Husky with heterochromia irides; in that dog the eye with a blue iris and nonpigmented retinal pigmented epithelium remained free of symptoms.[129] Ocular histopathologic changes are distinctive and in some individuals nasal planum biopsy may also be helpful in confirming a diagnosis. Treatment is often unrewarding. Topical antiinflammatories (steroids and/or NSAIDs) are used in conjunction with systemic immunomodulators, including prednisone, azathioprine, or newer agents such as cyclosporine and mycophenolate. Glaucoma occurs secondary to marked inflammatory infiltrates in the angle, and is typically poorly responsive to treatment.[130]

REFERENCES

1. Reilly CM, Morris R, Dubielzig RR. Canine goniodysgenesis-related glaucoma: a morphologic review of 100 cases looking at inflammation and pigment dispersion. Vet Ophthalmol 2005;8:253–8.
2. Mangan BG, Al-Yahya K, Chen CT, et al. Retinal pigment epithelial damage, breakdown of the blood-retinal barrier, and retinal inflammation in dogs with primary glaucoma. Vet Ophthalmol 2007;10:117–24.
3. Alyahya K, Chen CT, Mangan BG, et al. Microvessel loss, vascular damage and glutamate redistribution in the retinas of dogs with primary glaucoma. Vet Ophthalmol 2007;10:70–7.
4. Weinstein WL, Dietrich UM, Sapienza JS, et al. Identification of ocular matrix metalloproteinases present within the aqueous humor and iridocorneal drainage angle tissue of normal and glaucomatous canine eyes. Vet Ophthalmol 2007;10:108–16.
5. Fick CM, Dubielzig RR. Short posterior ciliary artery anatomy in normal and acutely glaucomatous dogs. Vet Ophthalmol 2015 [Epub ahead of print]. Available at: http://onlinelibrary.wiley.com.ezp-prod1.hul.harvard.edu/doi/10.1111/vop.12254/epdf. Accessed March 19, 2015.
6. Johnsen DAJ, Maggs DJ, Kass PH. Evaluation of risk factors for development of secondary glaucoma in dogs: 156 cases (1999-2004). J Am Vet Med Assoc 2006;229:1270–4.
7. Gelatt KN, MacKay EO. Secondary glaucomas in the dog in North America. Vet Ophthalmol 2004;7:245–59.
8. Strom AR, Hassig M, Iburg TM, et al. Epidemiology of canine glaucoma presented to University of Zurich from 1995 to 2009: part II: secondary glaucoma (217 cases). Vet Ophthalmol 2011;14:127–32.
9. Blocker T, van der Woerdt A. The feline glaucomas: 82 cases (1995-1999). Vet Ophthalmol 2001;4:81–5.
10. Wilcock B, Peiffer RL, Davidson MG. The causes of glaucoma in cats. Vet Pathol 1990;27:35–40.
11. McLellan GJ, Teixeira LBC. Feline glaucoma. Vet Clin North Am Small Anim Pract 2015, in press.
12. Zarfoss MK, Breaux CB, Whiteley HE, et al. Canine pre-iridal fibrovascular membranes: morphologic and immunohistochemical investigations. Vet Ophthalmol 2010;13:4–13.
13. Sandberg CA, Herring IP, Huckle WR, et al. Aqueous humor vascular endothelial growth factor in dogs: association with intraocular disease and the development of pre-iridal fibrovascular membrane. Vet Ophthalmol 2012;15:21–30.

14. Peiffer RL, Wilcock BP, Yin H. The pathogenesis and significance of preiridal fibrovascular membrane in domestic animals. Vet Pathol 1990;27:41–5.

15. Shazly TA, Latina MA. Neovascular glaucoma: etiology, diagnosis and prognosis. Semin Ophthalmol 2009;24:113–21.

16. Hayreh SS. Neovascular glaucoma. Prog Retin Eye Res 2007;26:470–85.

17. Simha A, Braganza A, Abraham L, et al. Anti-vascular endothelial growth factor for neovascular glaucoma. Cochrane Database Syst Rev 2013;(10):CD007920.

18. Nasisse MP, Davidson MG, English RV, et al. Treatment of glaucoma by use of transscleral neodymium: yttrium aluminum garnet laser cyclocoagulation in dogs. J Am Vet Med Assoc 1990;197:350–3.

19. O'Reilly A, Hardman C, Stanley RG. The use of transscleral cyclophotocoagulation with a diode laser for the treatment of glaucoma occurring post intracapsular extraction of displaced lenses: a retrospective study of 15 dogs (1995-2000). Vet Ophthalmol 2003;6:113–9.

20. Lutz EA, Sapienza JS. Combined diode endoscopic cyclophotocoagulation and Ex-Press shunt gonioimplantation in four cases of canine glaucoma. Vet Ophthalmol 2009;12:390–409 [abstract: 50].

21. Lutz EA, Sapienza JS. Diode endoscopic cyclophotocoagulation in pseudophakic and aphakic dogs with secondary glaucoma. Vet Ophthalmol 2009;12:390–409 [abstract: 51].

22. Lutz EA, Webb TE, Bras ID, et al. Diode endoscopic cyclophotocoagulation in dogs with primary and secondary glaucoma: 309 cases (2004-2013). Vet Ophthalmol 2013;16:E26–50 [abstract: 87].

23. Cullen CL, Corcoran K, Bartoe JT, et al. Preliminary findings from the multicenter clinical study group evaluating the Cullen canine frontal sinus valved glaucoma shunt. Vet Ophthalmol 2003;6:351–66 [abstract: 28].

24. Czepiel TM, Labelle AL, Hamor RE. Clinical experiences with a valved frontal sinus shunt for the treatment of canine glaucoma. Vet Ophthalmol 2014;17:E31–49 [abstract: 28].

25. Duke FD, Strong TD, Bentley E, et al. Canine ocular tumors following ciliary body ablation with intravitreal gentamicin. Vet Ophthalmol 2013;16:159–62.

26. Naranjo C, Dubielzig RR. Histopathological study of the causes for failure of intrascleral prostheses in dogs and cats. Vet Ophthalmol 2014;17:343–50.

27. Wiggans KT, Vernau W, Lappin MR, et al. Diagnostic utility of aqueocentesis and aqueous humor analysis in dogs and cats with anterior uveitis. Vet Ophthalmol 2014;17:212–20.

28. Pate DO, Gilger BC, Suter SE, et al. Diagnosis of intraocular lymphosarcoma in a dog by use of a polymerase chain reaction assay for antigen receptor rearrangement. J Am Vet Med Assoc 2011;238:625–30.

29. Linn-Pearl RN, Powell RM, Newman HA, et al. Validity of aqueocentesis as a component of anterior uveitis investigation in dogs and cats. Vet Ophthalmol 2014 [Epub ahead of print]. Available at: http://onlinelibrary.wiley.com.ezp-prod1.hul.harvard.edu/doi/10.1111/vop.12245/epdf. Accessed March 19, 2015.

30. Hendrix DVH. Diseases and surgery of the canine anterior uvea. In: Gelatt KN, Gilger BC, Kern TJ, editors. Veterinary ophthalmology. 5th edition. Ames (IA): Wiley-Blackwell; 2014. p. 1146–98.

31. Gelatt KN, MacKay EO. The ocular hypertensive effects of topical 0.1% dexamethasone in beagles with inherited glaucoma. J Ocul Pharmacol Ther 1998;14:57–66.

32. Krohne SG, Gionfriddo J, Morrison E. Inhibition of pilocarpine-induced aqueous humor flare, hypotony, and miosis by topical administration of anti-inflammatory and anesthetic drugs to dogs. Am J Vet Res 1998;59:482–8.

33. Millichamp NJ, Dziezyc J, Olsen JW. Effect of flurbiprofen on facility of aqueous outflow in the eyes of dogs. Am J Vet Res 1991;52:1448–51.
34. Pirie CG, Maranda LS, Pizzirani S. Effect of topical 0.03% flurbiprofen and 0.005% latanoprost, alone and in combination, on normal canine eyes. Vet Ophthalmol 2011;14:71–9.
35. Pirie CG, Maggio F, Maranda L, et al. Combined effect of topical prednisolone and latanoprost on normal canine eyes. A controlled study. Vet Ophthalmol 2006;9:414–25 [abstract: 11].
36. Gilmour MA, Lehenbauer TW. Effect of dexamethasone sodium phosphate 0.1% on intraocular pressure in normal dogs treated with latanoprost 0.005%. Vet Ophthalmol 2009;12:390–409 [abstract: 22].
37. Acheampong AA, Shackleton M, Tang-Liu DD, et al. Distribution of cyclosporin A in ocular tissues after topical administration to albino rabbits and beagle dogs. Curr Eye Res 1999;18:91–103.
38. Fujita E, Teramura Y, Shiraga T, et al. Pharmacokinetics and tissue distribution of tacrolimus (FK506) after a single or repeated ocular instillation in rabbits. J Ocul Pharmacol Ther 2008;24:309–19.
39. Sallam A, Sheth HG, Habot-Wilner Z, et al. Outcome of raised intraocular pressure in uveitic eyes with and without a corticosteroid-induced hypertensive response. Am J Ophthalmol 2009;148:207–13.
40. Kovalcuka L, Birgele E, Bandere D, et al. Comparison of the effects of topical and systemic atropine sulfate on intraocular pressure and pupil diameter in the normal canine eye. Vet Ophthalmol 2015;18:43–9.
41. Hacker DV, Farver TB. Effects of tropicamide on intraocular pressure in normal dogs. J Am Anim Hosp Assoc 1988;24:211–415.
42. Taylor NR, Zele AJ, Vingrys AH, et al. Variation in intraocular pressure following application of tropicamide in three different dog breeds. Vet Ophthalmol 2007; 10:8–11.
43. Grozdanic SD, Kecova H, Harper MM, et al. Functional and structural changes in a canine model of hereditary primary angle-closure glaucoma. Invest Ophthalmol Vis Sci 2010;51:255–63.
44. Mori M, Araie M, Sakurai M, et al. Effects of pilocarpine and tropicamide on blood-aqueous barrier permeability in man. Invest Ophthalmol Vis Sci 1992;33:416–23.
45. Horsley MB, Chen TC. The use of prostaglandin analogues in the uveitic patient. Semin Ophthalmol 2011;26:285–9.
46. Markomichelakis NN, Kostakou A, Halkiadakis I, et al. Efficacy and safety of latanoprost in eyes with uveitic glaucoma. Graefes Arch Clin Exp Ophthalmol 2009;247:775–80.
47. Chang JH, McCluskey P, Missotten T, et al. Use of ocular hypotensive prostaglandin analogues in patients with uveitis: does their use increase anterior uveitis and cystoid macular oedema? Br J Ophthalmol 2008;92:916–21.
48. Johnstone McLean NS, Ward DA, Hendrix DVH. The effect of a single dose of topical 0.005% latanoprost and 2% dorzolamide/0.5% timolol combination on the blood-aqueous barrier in dogs: a pilot study. Vet Ophthalmol 2008;11: 158–61.
49. Crasta M, Clode AB, McMullen RJ, et al. Effect of three treatment protocols on acute ocular hypertension after phacoemulsification and aspiration of cataracts in dogs. Vet Ophthalmol 2010;13:14–9.
50. Heinz C, Koch JM, Zurek-Imhoff B, et al. Prevalence of uveitic secondary glaucoma and success of nonsurgical treatment in adults and children in a tertiary referral center. Ocul Immunol Inflamm 2009;17:243–8.

51. Lerner LE, Patil AJ, Kenney MC, et al. Use of intraocular human recombinant tissue plasminogen activator as an adjunct treatment of posterior synechiae in patients with uveitis. Retin Cases Brief Rep 2012;6:290–3.

52. Skolnick CA, Fiscella RG, Tessler HH, et al. Tissue plasminogen activator to treat impending pupillary block glaucoma in patients with acute fibrinous HLA-B27 positive iridocyclitis. Am J Ophthalmol 2000;129:363–6.

53. Gerding PA, Essex-Sorlie D, Vausane S, et al. Use of tissue plasminogen activator for intraocular fibrinolysis in dogs. Am J Vet Res 1992;53:894–6.

54. Plummer CE, Regnier A, Gelatt KN. The canine glaucomas. In: Gelatt KN, Gilger BC, Kern TJ, editors. Veterinary ophthalmology. 5th edition. Ames (IA): Wiley-Blackwell; 2014. p. 1050–145.

55. Klein HE, Krohne SG, Moore GE, et al. Postoperative complications and visual outcomes of phacoemulsification in 103 dogs (179 eyes): 2006-2008. Vet Ophthalmol 2011;14:114–20.

56. Biros DJ, Gelatt KN, Brooks DE, et al. Development of glaucoma after cataract surgery in dogs: 220 cases (1987-1998). J Am Vet Med Assoc 2000;216(11):1780–6.

57. Sigle KJ, Nasisse MP. Long-term complications after phacoemulsification for cataract removal in dogs: 172 cases (1995-2002). J Am Vet Med Assoc 2006; 228:74–9.

58. Fischer C. Lens induced uveitis in dogs. J Am Anim Hosp Assoc 1972;8:39–48.

59. Leasure J, Gelatt KN, MacKay EO. The relationship of cataract maturity to intraocular pressure in dogs. Vet Ophthalmol 2001;4:273–6.

60. Van der Woerdt A, Nasisse MP, Davidson MG. Lens-induced uveitis in dogs: 151 cases (1985-1990). J Am Vet Med Assoc 1992;201:921–6.

61. Wilkie DA, Gemensky-Metzler AJ, Colitz CMH, et al. Canine cataracts, diabetes mellitus, and spontaneous lens capsule rupture: a retrospective study of 18 dogs. Vet Ophthalmol 2006;9:328–34.

62. Allgoewer I, Heinrich CL, Renwick PW, et al. Spontaneous posterior lens rupture associated with rapidly progressive cataracts in nondiabetic dogs. Vet Ophthalmol 2008;11:413–29 [abstract: 88].

63. Miller PE, Stanz KM, Dubielzig RR, et al. Mechanisms of acute intraocular pressure increases after phacoemulsification lens extraction in dogs. Am J Vet Res 1997;58:1159–64.

64. Smith PJ, Brooks DE, Lazarus JA, et al. Ocular hypertension following cataract surgery in dogs: 139 cases (1992-1993). J Am Vet Med Assoc 1996;209:105–11.

65. Crumley W, Gionfriddo JR, Radecki SV. Relationship of the iridocorneal angle, as measured using ultrasound biomicroscopy, with post-operative increases in intraocular pressure post-phacoemulsification in dogs. Vet Ophthalmol 2009;12:22–7.

66. Moeller E, Blocker T, Esson D, et al. Postoperative glaucoma in the Labrador Retriever: incidence, risk factors, and visual outcome following phacoemulsification. Vet Ophthalmol 2011;14:385–94.

67. Myrna KE, Pot S, Bentley E, et al. Toxic anterior segment syndrome and are we missing it? Vet Ophthalmol 2009;12:138.

68. Scott EM, Esson DW, Fritz KJ, et al. Major breed distribution of canine patients enucleated or eviscerated due to glaucoma following routine cataract surgery as well as common histopathologic findings within enucleated globes. Vet Ophthalmol 2013;16:64–72.

69. Lannek EB, Miller PE. Development of glaucoma after phacoemulsification for removal of cataracts in dogs: 22 cases (1987-1997). J Am Vet Med Assoc 2001;218:70–6.

70. Strubbe T. Uveitis and pupillary block glaucoma in an aphakic dog. Vet Ophthalmol 2002;5:3–7.
71. Curtis R, Barnett KC, Lewis SJ. Clinical and pathological observations concerning the aetiology of primary lens luxation in the dog. Vet Rec 1983;112:238–46.
72. Farias FH, Johnson GS, Taylor JF, et al. An ADAMTS17 splice donor site mutation in dogs with primary lens luxation. Invest Ophthalmol Vis Sci 2010;51: 4716–21.
73. Gould D, Pettitt L, McLaughlin B, et al. ADAMTS17 mutation associated with primary lens luxation is widespread among breeds. Vet Ophthalmol 2011;14: 378–84.
74. Luo L, Li M, Zhong Y, et al. Evaluation of secondary glaucoma associated with subluxated lens misdiagnosed as acute primary angle-closure glaucoma. J Glaucoma 2013;22:307–10.
75. Alario AF, Pizzirani S, Pirie CG. Histopathologic evaluation of the anterior segment of eyes enucleated due to glaucoma secondary to primary lens displacement in 13 canine globes. Vet Ophthalmol 2013;16:34–41.
76. Stuhr CM, Shilke HK, Forte C. Intracapsular lensectomy and sulcus intraocular lens fixation in dogs with primary lens luxation or subluxation. Vet Ophthalmol 2009;12:357–60.
77. Lutz EA, Wilkie DA, Gemensky-Metzler AJ. Combined lensectomy and diode laser endoscopic cyclophotocoagulation as prophylactic therapy in non-glaucomatous canine eyes with primary lens instability. Vet Ophthalmol 2013; 16:E1–21 [abstract: 81].
78. Montgomery KW, Labelle AL, Gemensky-Metzler AJ. Trans-corneal reduction of anterior lens luxation in dogs with lens instability: a retrospective study of 19 dogs (2010-2013). Vet Ophthalmol 2014;17:275–9.
79. Binder DR, Herring IP, Gerhard T. Outcomes of nonsurgical management and efficacy of demecarium bromide treatment for primary lens instability in dogs. J Am Vet Med Assoc 2007;231:89–93.
80. Glover TL, Davidson MG, Nasisse MP, et al. The intracapsular extraction of displaced lenses in dogs: a retrospective study of 57 cases (1984-1990). J Am Anim Hosp Assoc 1995;31:77–81.
81. Dubielzig RR, Ketring KL, McLellan GJ, et al. Veterinary ocular pathology: a comparative review. Edinburgh (United Kingdom): Saunders Elsevier; 2010.
82. Labelle AL, Labelle P. Canine ocular neoplasia: a review. Vet Ophthalmol 2013; 16:3–14.
83. Radcliffe NM, Finger PT. Eye cancer related glaucoma: current concepts. Surv Ophthalmol 2009;54:47–73.
84. Wilcock B, Peiffer RL. Morphology and behavior of primary ocular melanomas in 91 dogs. Vet Pathol 1986;23:418–24.
85. Dubielzig RR, Steinberg H, Garvin H, et al. Iridociliary epithelial tumors in 100 dogs and 17 cats: a morphological study. Vet Ophthalmol 1998;1:223–31.
86. Zeiss CJ, Dubielzig RR. A morphologic study of intravitreal membranes associated with intraocular hemorrhage in the dog. Vet Ophthalmol 2004;7:239–43.
87. Treadwell A, Naranjo C, Blocker T, et al. Clinical and histological characteristics of canine ocular gliovascular syndrome. Vet Ophthalmol 2014 [Epub ahead of print]. Available at: http://onlinelibrary.wiley.com.ezp-prod1.hul.harvard.edu/doi/10.1111/vop.12209/epdf. Accessed March 19, 2015.
88. Bliss CD, Sila JH, Morreale RJ, et al. Concurrent findings in canine and feline patients presenting for hyphema at a private referral clinic in Michigan from 2004 to 2008. Vet Ophthalmol 2009;12:390–409 [abstract: 77].

89. Book BP, van der Woerdt A, Wilkie DA. Ultrasonographic abnormalities in eyes with traumatic hyphema obscuring intraocular structures: 33 cases (1991–2002). J Vet Emerg Crit Care 2008;18:383–7.

90. Paul TA, Ward DA. Clinical features, outcomes, and etiologies of hyphema in dogs: a retrospective study (1999-2002). Vet Ophthalmol 2003;6:351–66 [abstract: 44].

91. Gharaibeh A, Savage HI, Scherer RW, et al. Medical interventions for traumatic hyphema. Cochrane Database Syst Rev 2013;(12):CD005431.

92. Nelms SR, Nasisse MP, Davidson MG, et al. Hyphema associated with retinal disease in dogs: 17 cases (1986-1991). J Am Vet Med Assoc 1993;202:1289–92.

93. Hendrix DV, Nasisse MP, Cowen P, et al. Clinical signs, concurrent diseases, and risk factors associated with retinal detachment in dogs. Prog Vet Comp Ophthalmol 1993;3:87–91.

94. Vainisi SJ, Wolfer JC, Hoffman AR. Surgery of the canine posterior segment. In: Gelatt KN, Gilger BC, Kern TJ, editors. Veterinary ophthalmology. 5th edition. Ames (IA): Wiley-Blackwell; 2014. p. 1393–431.

95. Vainisi SJ, Wolfer JC. Canine retinal surgery. Vet Ophthalmol 2004;7:291–306.

96. Smith PJ, Mames RN, Samuelson DA, et al. Photoreceptor outer segments in aqueous humor of a dog with rhegmatogenous retinal detachment and glaucoma. J Am Vet Med Assoc 1997;211:1254–6.

97. Narfstrom K, Peterson-Jones SJ. Diseases of the canine ocular fundus. In: Gelatt KN, Gilger BC, Kern TJ, editors. Veterinary ophthalmology. 5th edition. Ames (IA): Wiley-Blackwell; 2014. p. 1303–92.

98. Spatola RA, Nadelstein B, Leber AC, et al. Preoperative findings and visual outcome associated with retinal reattachment surgery in dogs: 217 cases (275 eyes). Vet Ophthalmol 2015 [Epub ahead of print]. Available at: http://onlinelibrary.wiley.com.ezp-prod1.hul.harvard.edu/doi/10.1111/vop.12246/epdf. Accessed March 19, 2015.

99. Grahn BH, Barnes LD, Breaux CB, et al. Chronic retinal detachment and giant retinal tears in 34 dogs: outcome comparison of no treatment, topical medical therapy, and retinal reattachment after vitrectomy. Can Vet J 2007;48:1031–9.

100. Steele KA, Sisler S, Gerding PA. Outcome of retinal reattachment surgery in dogs: a retrospective study of 145 cases. Vet Ophthalmol 2012;15:35–40.

101. Ng DS, Ching RH, Chan CW. Angle-recession glaucoma: long-term clinical outcomes over a 10-year period in traumatic microhyphema. Int Ophthalmol 2014 [Epub ahead of print]. Available at: http://download.springer.com.ezp-prod1.hul.harvard.edu/static/pdf/582/art%253A10.1007%252Fs10792-014-0027-5.pdf?auth66=1426818123_cb54db0676e1fa2d660928827b613b0d&ext=.pdf. Accessed March 19, 2015.

102. Girkin CA, McGwin G, Long C, et al. Glaucoma after ocular contusion: a cohort study of the United States Eye Injury Registry. J Glaucoma 2005;14:470–3.

103. Lew M, Lew S, Brzeski W. Short-term results of Ahmed glaucoma valve implantation in the surgical treatment of angle-recession glaucoma in dog. Pol J Vet Sci 2008;11:377–83.

104. Spiess BM, Ruehli MB, Bolliger J. Eye injuries in the dog caused by cat claws. Schweiz Arch Tierheilkd 1996;138:429–33 [in German].

105. Bell CM, Pot SA, Dubielzig RR. Septic implantation syndrome in dogs and cats: a distinct pattern of endophthalmitis with lenticular abscess. Vet Ophthalmol 2013;60:180–5.

106. Wilcock BP, Peiffer RL. The pathology of lens-induced uveitis in dogs. Vet Pathol 1987;24:549–53.

107. Paulsen ME, Kass PH. Traumatic corneal laceration with associated lens capsule disruption: a retrospective study of 77 clinical cases from 1999 to 2009. Vet Ophthalmol 2012;15:355–68.
108. Van de Sandt RR, Boeve MH, Stades FC, et al. Abnormal ocular pigment deposition and glaucoma in the dog. Vet Ophthalmol 2003;6:273–8.
109. Petersen-Jones SM, Forcier J, Mentzer AL. Ocular melanosis in the Cairn Terrier: clinical description and mode of inheritance. Vet Ophthalmol 2007;10:63–9.
110. Petersen-Jones SM, Mentzer AL, Dubielzig RR, et al. Ocular melanosis in the Cairn Terrier: histopathological description of the condition, and immunohistological and ultrastructural characterization of the characteristic pigment-laden cells. Vet Ophthalmol 2008;11:260–8.
111. Townsend WM, Mankey A, Gerlach JA. Association between dog leukocyte antigen haplotype and Golden Retriever pigmentary uveitis. Vet Ophthalmol 2009; 12:390–409 [abstract: 66].
112. Sapienza JS, Simo FJ, Prades-Sapienza A. Golden Retriever uveitis: 75 cases (1994-1999). Vet Ophthalmol 2000;3:241–6.
113. Esson D, Armour M, Mundy P, et al. The histopathological and immunohistochemical characteristics of pigmentary and cystic glaucoma in the Golden Retriever. Vet Ophthalmol 2009;12:361–8.
114. Deehr A, Dubielzig RR. A histopathological study of iridociliary cysts and glaucoma in Golden Retrievers. Vet Ophthalmol 1998;1:153–8.
115. Spiess BM, Bolliger JO, Guscetti F, et al. Multiple ciliary body cysts and secondary glaucoma in the Great Dane: a report of nine cases. Vet Ophthalmol 1998;1:41–5.
116. Pumphrey SA, Pizzirani S, Pirie CG, et al. Glaucoma associated with uveal cysts and goniodysgenesis in American Bulldogs: a case series. Vet Ophthalmol 2013;16:377–85.
117. Gemensky-Metzler AJ, Wilkie DA, Cook CS. The use of semiconductor diode laser for deflation and coagulation of anterior uveal cysts in dogs, cats and horses: a report of 20 cases. Vet Ophthalmol 2004;7:360–8.
118. Azuara-Blanco A, Spaeth GL, Araujo SV, et al. Plateau iris syndrome associated with multiple ciliary body cysts: 3 cases. Arch Ophthalmol 1996;114:666–8.
119. Vela A, Rieser JC, Campbell DG. The heredity and treatment of angle-closure glaucoma secondary to iris and ciliary body cysts. Ophthalmology 1984;91: 332–7.
120. Lois N, Shields CL, Shields JA, et al. Primary cysts of the iris pigment epithelium. Clinical features and natural course in 234 patients. Ophthalmology 1998;105: 1879–85.
121. Corcoran KA, Koch SA. Uveal cysts in dogs: 28 cases (1989-1991). J Am Vet Med Assoc 1993;203:545–6.
122. Dada T, Gadia R, Sharma A, et al. Ultrasound biomicroscopy in glaucoma. Surv Ophthalmol 2011;56:433–50.
123. Taylor LN, Townsend WM, Heng HG, et al. Comparison of ultrasound biomicroscopy and standard ocular ultrasonography for detection of canine uveal cysts. Am J Vet Res 2015;76:540–6.
124. Herrera HD, Duchene AG. Uveodermatologic syndrome (Vogt-Koyanagi-Harada-like syndrome) with generalized depigmentation in a Dachshund. Vet Ophthalmol 1998;1:47–51.
125. Kang MH, Lim CY, Park HM. Uveodermatologic syndrome with concurrent keratoconjunctivitis sicca in a miniature poodle dog. Can Vet J 2014;55:585–8.
126. Blackwood SE, Barrie KP, Plummer CE, et al. Uveodermatologic syndrome in a rat terrier. J Am Anim Hosp Assoc 2011;47:56–63.

127. Laus JL, Sousa MG, Cabral VP, et al. Uveodermatologic syndrome in a Brazilian Fila dog. Vet Ophthalmol 2004;7:193–6.
128. Angles JM, Famula TR, Pedersen NC. Uveodermatologic (VKH-like) syndrome in American Akita dogs is associated with an increased frequency of DQA1*00201. Tissue Antigens 2005;66:656–65.
129. Sigle KJ, McLellan GJ, Haynes JS, et al. Unilateral uveitis in a dog with uveodermatologic syndrome. J Am Vet Med Assoc 2006;228:543–8.
130. Lindley DM, Boosinger TR, Cox NR. Ocular histopathology of Vogt-Koyanagi-Harada-like syndrome in an Akita dog. Vet Pathol 1990;27:294–6.

Index

Note: Page numbers of article titles are in **boldface** type.

A

Adrenergic agonists
  α_2-
    in primary glaucoma management, 1239–1240
  in feline glaucoma management, 1326–1327
Adrenergic antagonists
  β-
    in primary glaucoma management, 1240–1243
Adrenoceptor(s)
  drugs acting on
    in primary glaucoma management, 1239–1243
Age
  as factor in canine glaucoma, 1128–1130
AH. *See* Aqueous humor (AH)
Anterior chamber shunt procedures
  in feline glaucoma management, 1328
Anterior segment
  glaucoma-induced changes in, 1214–1223
    concurrent lesions *vs.* insights on pathogenesis, 1219–1223
    goniodysgenesis, 1214–1217, 1223
    histopathologic diagnosis and challenges related to, 1217–1219
Anterior-segment optical coherence tomography (AS-OCT)
  in ICA evaluation, 1203
Applanation tonometry
  in IOP evaluation, 1196–1197
Apraclonidine
  in primary glaucoma management, 1239–1240
Aqueous flare and cell
  mild
    as early to midstage sign of primary angle-closure glaucoma, 1193
Aqueous humor (AH)
  in cats, 1307
  described, 1101–1102
Aqueous outflow
  pathways of, 1104
Aqueous production, 1102–1104
AS-OCT. *See* Anterior-segment optical coherence tomography (AS-OCT)
Autoimmune system
  canine glaucoma related to, 1145–1148

Vet Clin Small Anim 45 (2015) 1365–1377
http://dx.doi.org/10.1016/S0195-5616(15)00130-8
0195-5616/15/$ – see front matter © 2015 Elsevier Inc. All rights reserved.

vetsmall.theclinics.com

United States Postal Service

Statement of Ownership, Management, and Circulation
(All Periodicals Publications Except Requester Publications)

1. Publication Title
Veterinary Clinics of North America: Small Animal Practice

2. Publication Number
0 0 3 – 1 5 0

3. Filing Date
9/18/15

4. Issue Frequency
Jan, Mar, May, Jul, Sep, Nov

5. Number of Issues Published Annually
6

6. Annual Subscription Price
$310.00

7. Complete Mailing Address of Known Office of Publication (Not printer) (Street, city, county, state, and ZIP+4®)
Elsevier Inc.
360 Park Avenue South
New York, NY 10010-1710

Contact Person
Stephen R. Bushing

Telephone (Include area code)
215-239-3688

8. Complete Mailing Address of Headquarters or General Business Office of Publisher (Not printer)
Elsevier Inc., 360 Park Avenue South, New York, NY 10010-1710

9. Full Names and Complete Mailing Addresses of Publisher, Editor, and Managing Editor (Do not leave blank)

Publisher (Name and complete mailing address)
Linda Belfus, Elsevier Inc., 1600 John F. Kennedy Blvd., Suite 1800, Philadelphia, PA 19103

Editor (Name and complete mailing address)
Patrick Manley, Elsevier Inc., 1600 John F. Kennedy Blvd., Suite 1800, Philadelphia, PA 19103-2899

Managing Editor (Name and complete mailing address)
Adrianne Brigido, Elsevier Inc., 1600 John F. Kennedy Blvd., Suite 1800, Philadelphia, PA 19103-2899

10. Owner (Do not leave blank. If the publication is owned by a corporation, give the name and address of the corporation immediately followed by the names and addresses of all stockholders owning or holding 1 percent or more of the total amount of stock. If not owned by a corporation, give the names and addresses of the individual owners. If owned by a partnership or other unincorporated firm, give its name and address as well as those of each individual owner. If the publication is published by a nonprofit organization, give its name and address.)

Full Name	Complete Mailing Address
Wholly owned subsidiary of	1600 John F. Kennedy Blvd., Ste. 1800
Reed/Elsevier, US holdings	Philadelphia, PA 19103-2899

11. Known Bondholders, Mortgagees, and Other Security Holders Owning or Holding 1 Percent or More of Total Amount of Bonds, Mortgages, or Other Securities. If none, check box ☐ None

Full Name	Complete Mailing Address
N/A	

12. Tax Status (For completion by nonprofit organizations authorized to mail at nonprofit rates) (Check one)
The purpose, function, and nonprofit status of this organization and the exempt status for federal income tax purposes:
☐ Has Not Changed During Preceding 12 Months
☐ Has Changed During Preceding 12 Months (Publisher must submit explanation of change with this statement)

13. Publication Title
Veterinary Clinics of North America: Small Animal Practice

14. Issue Date for Circulation Data Below
September 2015

15. Extent and Nature of Circulation			Average No. Copies Each Issue During Preceding 12 Months	No. Copies of Single Issue Published Nearest to Filing Date
a. Total Number of Copies (Net press run)			1421	1180
b. Legitimate Paid and/Or Requested Distribution (By Mail and Outside the Mail)	(1)	Mailed Outside-County Paid/Requested Mail Subscriptions stated on PS Form 3541. (Include paid distribution above nominal rate, advertiser's proof copies and exchange copies)	770	649
	(2)	Mailed In-County Paid/Requested Mail Subscriptions stated on PS Form 3541. (Include paid distribution above nominal rate, advertiser's proof copies and exchange copies)		
	(3)	Paid Distribution Outside the Mails Including Sales Through Dealers And Carriers, Street Vendors, Counter Sales, and Other Paid Distribution Outside USPS®	236	262
	(4)	Paid Distribution by Other Classes of Mail Through the USPS (e.g. First-Class Mail®)		
c. Total Paid and or Requested Circulation (Sum of 15b (1), (2), (3), and (4))		▲	1006	911
d. Free or Nominal Rate Distribution (By Mail and Outside the Mail)	(1)	Free or Nominal Rate Outside-County Copies included on PS Form 3541	97	89
	(2)	Free or Nominal Rate In-County Copies included on PS Form 3541		
	(3)	Free or Nominal Rate Copies mailed at Other classes Through the USPS (e.g. First-Class Mail®)		
	(4)	Free or Nominal Rate Distribution Outside the Mail (Carriers or Other means)		
e. Total Nonrequested Distribution (Sum of 15d (1), (2), (3) and (4))			97	89
f. Total Distribution (Sum of 15c and 15e)		▲	1103	1000
g. Copies not Distributed (See instructions to publishers #4 (page #3))		▲	318	180
h. Total (Sum of 15f and g)		▲	1421	1180
i. Percent Paid and/or Requested Circulation (15c divided by 15f times 100)		▲	91.21%	91.10%

* If you are claiming electronic copies go to line 16 on page 3. If you are not claiming Electronic copies, skip to line 17 on page 3

16. Electronic Copy Circulation	Average No. Copies Each Issue During Preceding 12 Months	No. Copies of Single Issue Published Nearest to Filing Date
a. Paid Electronic Copies		
b. Total paid Print Copies (Line 15c) + **Paid Electronic copies** (Line 16a)		
c. Total Print Distribution (Line 15f) + **Paid Electronic Copies** (Line 16a)		
d. Percent Paid (Both Print & Electronic copies) (16b divided by 16c Ⅹ 100)		

I certify that 50% of all my distributed copies (electronic and print) are paid above a nominal price

17. Publication of Statement of Ownership
If the publication is a general publication, publication of this statement is required. Will be printed in the **November 2015** issue of this publication.

18. Signature and Title of Editor, Publisher, Business Manager, or Owner
Stephen R. Bushing
Stephen R. Bushing – Inventory Distribution Coordinator

Date
September 18, 2015

I certify that all information furnished on this form is true and complete. I understand that anyone who furnishes false or misleading information on this form or who omits material or information requested on the form may be subject to criminal sanctions (including fines and imprisonment) and/or civil sanctions (including civil penalties).

PS Form 3526, July 2014 (Page 3 of 3)

PS Form 3526, July 2014 (Page 1 of 3 (Instructions Page 3)) PSN 7530-01-000-9931 PRIVACY NOTICE: See our Privacy policy in www.usps.com

Moving?

Make sure your subscription moves with you!

To notify us of your new address, find your **Clinics Account Number** (located on your mailing label above your name), and contact customer service at:

Email: journalscustomerservice-usa@elsevier.com

800-654-2452 (subscribers in the U.S. & Canada)
314-447-8871 (subscribers outside of the U.S. & Canada)

Fax number: 314-447-8029

Elsevier Health Sciences Division
Subscription Customer Service
3251 Riverport Lane
Maryland Heights, MO 63043

*To ensure uninterrupted delivery of your subscription, please notify us at least 4 weeks in advance of move.